T0360397

OPERATIVE CHYMIST

THE WELLCOME INSTITUTE SERIES IN THE HISTORY OF MEDICINE

Forthcoming Titles

Social Medicine and Medical Sociology in the Twentieth Century
Edited by Dorothy Porter

Ashes to Ashes: The History of Smoking and Health
Edited by Stephen Lock

Out of Otherness: Characters and Narrators
in the Dutch Venereal Disease Debates 1850–1990
Annet Mooij

Academic enquiries regarding the series should be addressed
to the editors W. F. Bynum, V. Nutton and Roy Porter at
the Wellcome Institute for the History of Medicine,
183 Euston Road, London NW1 2BE, UK.

OPERATIVE CHYMIST

Anthony Morson

Amsterdam – Atlanta, GA 1997

First published in 1997

by Editions Rodopi B. V., Amsterdam – Atlanta, GA 1997.

© 1997 Anthony Morson

Design and Typesetting by Christine Buckley,

the Wellcome Trust.

Printed and bound in The Netherlands by Editions Rodopi B. V.,
Amsterdam – Atlanta, GA 1997.

British Library Cataloguing in Publication Data
A catalogue record for this book is available from the British Library

ISBN 90-420-0366-9 (Paper)
ISBN 90-420-0376-6 (Bound)

Anthony Morson

Operative Chymist – Amsterdam – Atlanta, GA:
Rodopi. – ill.

(Clio Medica 45 / ISSN 0045-7183;
The Wellcome Institute Series in the History of Medicine)

Front cover:
Thomas N. R. Morson (1799–1874)

© Editions Rodopi B. V., Amsterdam – Atlanta, GA 1997

Printed in The Netherlands

I dedicate this book to Margaret, Jane, Peter and Angela;
and my grandchildren

Contents

Acknowledgements

In 1972, Professor G.R. Paterson of Toronto University approached me for some details of T. N. R. Morson's production of alkaloids. Later, he suggested that Morson's achievements were 'worthy of attention'. It was not until 1981 that I got in touch with Leslie Matthews, doyen of pharmaceutical historians, to discuss a possible project. He wrote later that 'Morson's story is well worth telling in detail'. These two men were responsible for sowing the seeds.

When I decided to retire in 1985, I began a study of some sources, particularly the papers I had been given and collected over a period of thirty years. I discovered I had a major project on my hands if justice was to be done to one whose eminence I had not realised.

So many debts of gratitude for encouragement, help and advice are owed that I hope the majority will understand why only a few can be mentioned here. More than forty librarians, curators and others have helped me to find records, sources of information and made useful suggestions for investigation.

I am indebted especially to the librarians of the Societies to which Morson belonged: The Royal Society of Medicine, successor to the Medico-Chirurgical Society, The Linnean Society and the Royal Pharmaceutical Society, whose staff provided me with sight of archival material and helped in numerous other ways.

I am grateful to the Royal Pharmaceutical Society for giving me access to the minutes of their Council for the period until Morson's death.

The staff at the libraries of the Royal Society, the London Guildhall, the Society of Apothecaries and the British Library provided valuable assistance. I am grateful to the staff of the Wellcome Library whose unstinting help was much appreciated.

I wish to thank colleagues in Merck & Co. Inc., for their help and encouragement. I am indebted to the Merck, Sharp & Dohme Development Laboratories at Hoddesdon for the use of their library.

The guidance I have received from Dr J. G. L. Burnby, editor of the *Pharmaceutical Historian* and from Professor W. F. Bynum, Professor of the History of Medicine at the Wellcome Institute has been vital. Nita encouraged me from the outset, guiding me to sources, discussing many aspects of my work and commenting on the drafts of my text. Bill stimulated a rather more than mature student to search for the context of Morson's scientific life, directing me to many important sources and suggesting improvements to my text.

While any mistakes are mine, this project would not have been completed without Nita's and Bill's contributions. I thank them both very much.

Preface

The first book on pharmaceutical history that I read was Bell and Redwood's *Progress of Pharmacy*, a title that Morson had used years previously for his first address to the newly-formed Pharmaceutical Society in 1841. As I learnt a little more about the history of the Society, I became aware of the contrast between Bell's history written in 1842 and Redwood's account of events after that date. Bell's broader and informed approach was different from Redwood's description, stressing legislative aspects, of the years following the Society's incorporation.

Morson was quickly forgotten by the Society to which he had contributed so much and his achievements were ignored by pharmaceutical historians, with few notable exceptions, even to the extent that his name did not appear in the official centenary history of the Society.

This provided a spur to discover more about an eminent scientist whose obituaries pointed out that he had a circle of famous scientific friends. Letters from some of these indicated that he played a part in the professionalisation of pharmacy and the creation of the fine chemical industry which had been overlooked. As the first manufacturer in Britain of the new alkaloids and for twenty years the foremost manufacturer of opiate alkaloids, he was the founder of the British alkaloid industry.

There has, rightly, been much written about Jacob Bell whose skills and courage in the face of chronic illness attract attention. His letters to Morson, however, show that he was dependent upon support from at least one person. The condition of the Pharmaceutical Society at his death, revealed by the minutes of the Council, left his successors with very serious problems.

These matters, and Morson's life as the proprietor of an important business, together with his activities in several learned societies, all occurred against a background of change. The assertiveness of the middle class, religious prejudice in education and the appearance of virtually self-educated men wishing to contribute to the management of their scientific societies – all this was happening while the medical professions debated questions of power and privilege and attempted to reconcile themselves to scientific method. Research in recent years has changed our perception of medical history during the nineteenth century. An attempt has been made to relate to this a life which was central to a culture which developed science into a part of everyday life.

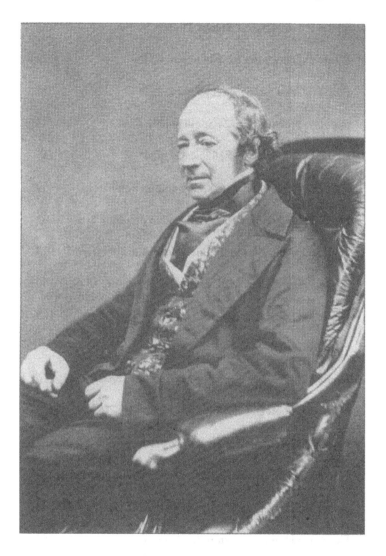

Thomas N. R. Morson
(1799-1874)

List of Illustrations

1

Early Life

It seems improbable that an only son, whose parents, only sister and apprentice master all died before he was nineteen, and whose father had emigrated from country to city in the social and economic turmoil at the turn of the eighteenth century and gone bankrupt, would have an outstanding career in a science-based industry in London. Thomas Newborn Robert Morson overcame these handicaps to become an eminent scientist, a successful pharmacist-entrepreneur and a driving force in making British pharmacy a respected profession.

Morson's family had been stonemasons in Wilbarston, a village six miles west of Corby in Northamptonshire, for generations and were prosperous. They ran a successful business, owned small amounts of land and property; they joined in the social life of their village.[1] Two eighteenth-century Morsons saw service in the militia, one serving in Europe. They seem to have had good constitutions for there is less early death, especially among the women and children, than would be expected at a time when the lack of medicine and hygiene caused many deaths.

All the Morsons' wealth was bound up in their business, part of which involved ownership of building land, because Morsons were, in today's parlance, house-builders, in addition to their work in repairing churches and carving headstones. In 1741 when Thomas Mauson the elder (T. N. R. Morson's great-grandfather) died he left his wife Elizabeth 'my dwelling house and ye house yt joynes to it with ye barn and ye yard'. Another provision was that, on his wife's death, his married daughter Mary inherited a plot at the east end of the barn, measuring eighteen feet by sixteen, large enough on which to build a house. The two elder sons inherited the business which

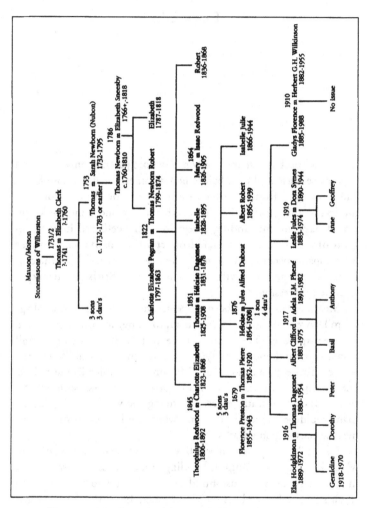

Figure 1: Genealogical Table compiled by Anthony Morson.

had mortgaged some land, and £37 was owed from 'the money the land is sold for'. So provision was made for the continuation of the business and housing all members of the family.

The name Thomas had been given for several generations. Morson's grandfather, Thomas, married Sarah Newborn in 1753. She came from Stoke Dry, a hamlet about seven miles away across the valley of Eye Brook in the rich rolling sheep-farming country of Rutland. It is a hamlet on the west side of the ridge at the top of which runs the Rockingham to Uppingham road. It was called 'Dry' because it is well above the marshes which the Eye Brook made, and flooded in winter. Stoke is from the Saxon word stoc, meaning wood. Years ago the brook was dammed so there is now a lake inhabited by many kinds of waders. The stream has always been the parish and county boundary. The area of the parish was only 1000 acres and its population towards the end of the eighteenth century was only 60 people or so – greatly exceeded by the cattle and especially by the sheep. Stoke Dry church was originally a twelfth-century building and looks west across the river towards Holyoake, a large house held by the Hospitallers at the beginning of the thirteenth century.

To reach his future wife's farmhouse, Thomas walked or rode from Wilbarston along the east-west ridge above the River Welland, which he crossed at Rockingham. In summer, it was possible to save some distance and walk across the marshes of Eye Brook near Holyoake; then up the steep hill to the farm.

Coming from different parishes, Thomas and Sarah had to apply for a licence[2] for their marriage; unlike their parents and grandparents, they were both able to sign their names in the register.

Sarah's mother, who died in 1776, had been the tenant of a farm at Stoke Dry. Although she was illiterate, she made wealth enough to decide to make a Will bequeathing everything to her daughter. She hoped that her landlord, the great landowner the Earl of Exeter, would permit Sarah to continue the tenancy. This was allowed and Sarah Morson ran the farm until her death in 1795.

We do not know if her husband Thomas left her any money when he died, which was in 1783 or earlier for she remarried in 1784. Her second husband, Richard Wade[3] was a farmer and horse breeder and may too have left her some money. At all events, Sarah left nearly £600 to which may be added the value of the farm stock and the contents of the house. Since her mother had left only £159, Sarah certainly exploited the good farmland of Rutland, famed then for its sheep and wool. Perhaps her coffin was lined with wool, a

Rutland custom in those days, presumably as a sign of affluence and of gratitude for its source. Her Will makes reference to her investments as well as the farm stock and furniture. Sarah Morson had had the help of two friends in managing her affairs; one was Thomas Bryan who was an important local figure and the other Benjamin Peach, again from a local family of graziers and successful enough to live in a large house, Hallyoak Lodge, a mile or so from Stoke Dry, and, incidentally, still standing. These two were pillars of the little community. There are many Bryan gravestones in the churchyard. The church silver includes a cup inscribed 'Conyers Peach, Churchwarden 1708, Stoke Dry'.

Sarah's Will[4] made in 1793 directed that all her assets should be liquidated, added to her other funds and placed in trust for her grandchildren. The resulting capital was to be under the control of her trustees, Bryan and Peach. The income was left to her daughter-in-law because her son, who was born about 1760 and christened Thomas Newborn Morson, was a bankrupt. Only if he discharged his debts could he have up to £300 for a business and then only if his wife approved. There can be no doubt of Sarah's opinion of her son's business acumen, nor of the regard she held for her very young daughter-in-law. The distaff side were in control!

Thomas in his twenties had decided to leave the country and moved to London. He was married on 14 December 1786 to Elizabeth Sneesby, who was a minor, at St Clement Danes Church in the Strand. There is no record of what he did for a living, although there is one indication because a Thomas Mauson (the alternative spelling frequently used in the eighteenth century) of Tokenhouse Yard, City, was a 'merchant and insurer'; he had not discharged his debts by 1801.[5]

There were two children of this marriage, the first being Elizabeth (of whose baptism no trace has been found) and Thomas Newborn Robert, born on 8 November 1799 when the family were living at Stratford-le-Bow, in Essex then, but now very much part of East London.

Instead of depending solely on her husband's earnings, if any, Elizabeth from 1795 onwards could rely upon the income from her mother-in-law's trust fund. In addition, she had the use of all the farmhouse furniture and other contents. With four mouths to feed, she was confident that they would have sufficient. If money was needed, then Bryan and Peach could be approached for some of the capital. The Will was drawn up in such a way that the monies would be looked after, no matter what happened to either Elizabeth or her husband. It was not necessary for them to make Wills and, in view of what was to happen, this proved fortunate.

As soon as he was old enough, young Morson attended a school at Stoke Newington where he must have received a good grounding judging from his literacy and later interests. Stoke Newington[6] was then a village only 3¹/₂ miles from Cornhill on what was originally the Roman Ermine Street to the North. There were only 300 houses in 1811 when Morson was in the middle of his schooling. It was known as a place where Dissenters lived. William Allen, the famous Quaker, subsidised a school there in 1820 near his own house. The population was about 2000 making it a substantial place. It was quite rural, the farms and market gardens growing food for London's expanding population. The numerous schools provided good education, some including science in their curricula, or as they termed it 'Natural and Experimental Philosophy', which included chemistry and geology, magnetism and natural history. It was while Morson was at school in 1810 that his father died and was buried at St Mary's, Lambeth.

When he was fourteen he was apprenticed to a surgeon-apothecary, Charles Dunn at 65 Fleet Market in the City of London. Like so many of his profession at that time, Dunn had been an Army Surgeon before he settled in the City in 1784,[7] so he did not serve in the Army during the Napoleonic Wars. Like their Naval colleagues, they combined surgery and pharmacy and, on entering civilian life, were the educators of many eighteenth- and early nineteenth-century apprentices. The records[8] show that Dunn had received a premium of 100 guineas[9] in 1802 for an apprentice but his fee was reduced to 60 guineas in 1807 when Thomas Gale was apprenticed to him. Like Morson, Gale went on to found his own business and was an important colleague in the Pharmaceutical Society. Inland Revenue apprenticeship records were not kept after 1810 but such sums were being paid around 1825 when Morson's father-in-law left money for a nephew's apprenticeship. We can safely assume that a similar sum was paid for Morson's apprenticeship.

The Book of English Trades in 1824, one of a series of books on careers published by Richard Phillips in London, held the opinion that applicants for apprenticeships in surgeon-apothecaries' shops should at least be 'good scholars'. We can assume that Dunn was satisfied that Morson was such. He needed to know 'as much Latin as to be able to read the best writers in the various sciences connected with medicine: botany, materia medica, chemistry, anatomy and the outlines of medicine'.

In the Army, Dunn would have stitched wounds and performed amputations as well as minor surgery; he dealt with fractures and dislocations. He may well have been called upon to do this in civilian life as well as routine extraction of teeth and the lancing of boils. Thus Morson knew what such surgery was like at an early age. St Bartholomew's Hospital up the hill at Smithfield was the place for more serious surgical attention. Nonetheless, it was a wide experience when added to the preparation of medicines and tending the shop; time also had to be made for study. The hours of work were long – 12 hours a day with only Sunday free. As in the nature of any business there would have been times during the day when few customers called and, if stocks of medicines allowed, apprentices could use a little time for study. Otherwise books were read upstairs after or before shop hours.

Dunn taught Morson the basic techniques for preparing the medicines of those days and their uses; he would also have shown him something of the purchasing of the roots, barks and other ingredients as well as the routines of the shop. Dunn had a good reputation, if we base our comment on the inspections[10] carried out by the 'censors' from the Royal College of Physicians, whose premises were in Warwick Lane, not five minutes' walk away and also close to Apothecaries' Hall in Blackfriars Lane.

To get some idea of the censors' expectations it is necessary to look at the comments on such famous pharmacies as those of Bell, Corbyn and also Allen at Plough Court. While the latter two were described as very good, Bell's premises in 1805 had 'not much to commend', though it had been 'very good' in 1800. The censors' standards were as much a variable as the condition of a shop; the attitude seems also to have been affected by the presence or otherwise of medicines bought from Apothecaries' Hall, because the presence of these was recorded with approval.

Sometimes the censors encountered a 'surly and unmannerly' reception[11] from both masters and assistants whose attitude provoked them into writing a warning for subsequent visits in the hope that they would not 'meet with the same insolence'. The most extreme action was meted out to a Mr Nichols in Tottenham Court Road; in 1803 he had two of his products 'thrown into the street after due admonitions'!

Inspections of 65 Fleet Market are recorded for 1808, 1809 and 1810. In the first year it was 'a very good shop' with the scales and weights in good order, but Dunn was criticised for not having a pharmacopoeia, only *Lewis' Dispensatory*. He was described as 'moderate' on 23 June 1809, but the following year he was rated only 'tolerable'.

65 Fleet Market was in a terrace[12] of typical Georgian shops of four storeys at the top end of the Market on the west side; it was between George Alley and Eagle and Child Alley. The premises were quite modest with a door on the right-hand side, the rest of the frontage being a window, the whole being only about fourteen feet wide. For many years, they were assessed at £3 10s. 0d.[13] for land tax, another indication of the small size.

The view from the top floor looked towards St Paul's and so you could see the spires of the City churches. On a fine evening it must have been an unforgettable sight – some compensation for the days when fog, made worse by the mist rising from the Thames flowing putrid with sewage, and smoke from innumerable chimneys, obscured the views. The atmosphere cannot have been improved by the habit of throwing most waste, especially that of the market stalls, into the street where it waited to be swept down towards the river to form large piles at the water's edge.

Dunn not only ran the surgeon-apothecary's shop, he was also the proprietor of a patent medicine warehouse at 35 West Smithfield,[14] a short distance up the hill to the east from Fleet Market. With Morson's search for knowledge, it seems likely that he was allowed to see what the running of the warehouse involved. It is equally likely that the making of some of the medicines was carried out at the Fleet Market shop – an early experience in manufacture for a keen and energetic young man.

The apprenticeship must have been for five years. There are no records of what was agreed but a review of Morson's life in the *Chemist and Druggist* of 14 May 1870, four years before his death, provides the clues. It states that Morson went to Paris 'after the expiration of his apprenticeship'. If he was apprenticed on his fourteenth birthday, a five-year term would have expired in 1818, the date he went to Paris.

Morson was 'placed in charge' of the shop by Dunn. This may have been necessitated by Dunn's health. Such a move was not unusual as there were complaints at this time about young boys giving advice, and about their dispensing of medicines. Such criticism did not extend to druggists' wives who were assumed to have learnt sufficient of the craft by helping their husbands.

In June 1815, Dunn died, having been in Fleet Market for 31 years. So, before he was sixteen Morson had lost first his father and then his master, two men who could be expected to provide guidance in his early years. He was now dependent upon his own character and judgement only.

The interview with Morson published in the *Chemist and Druggist* records that 'the business, stock-in-trade, goodwill and apprentice were transferred all together to' Henry Morley, a young man whose interest was mainly in surgery. He was born in 1791 and had been educated at a Mr Chandler's in Canterbury before going to Guy's Hospital where he registered on 30 November 1813 as a surgeon's pupil for one year.[15] He was granted his certificate on 24 January 1815, whereupon he sat the examination for his M.R.C.S. which was granted on 3 March 1815, giving his address as 65 Fleet Market. He was therefore only just qualified to take on an apprentice when he purchased Dunn's business a few months before the latter's death. Not only did he afford to purchase the business, but two years later he paid 200 guineas for the Freedom of the Society of Apothecaries; it was a redemption as his master was not an apothecary.[16]

This was shortly after the enactment in 1815 of the Apothecaries Bill, which exempted chemists and druggists from the supervision of the Society of Apothecaries. The Act secured their existing rights by a clause providing that nothing in the Act 'shall extend to prejudice, or in any way affect the trade and business of a chemist and druggist, in the buying, preparing, compounding, dispensing and vending of drugs, medicines and medicinable compounds, wholesale or retail'. Everyone in business could therefore continue in the same way as before the passing of the bill.[17]

One of the main purposes of the Act was to improve medical education. Sir Zachary Cope described the results in his Gideon De Laune lecture on 16 November 1955.[18] New powers to organise medical, as distinct from surgical, education outside London where the College of Physicians retained its privileged position, were given to the Society of Apothecaries. The educational requirements, which included apprenticeship and the study of chemistry, were quickly established as was the appointment of examiners. Between 1815 and 1858 when the Medical Act was passed, the Society exerted a powerful influence on medical training and practice throughout England. There can be little doubt that the authorities were pleased that the Society responded so decisively in pursuing this aim of the Act. The curriculum was improved and the standards of training raised. The numbers of candidates passing the Society's examination increased dramatically. The training also went a long way to keeping pace with the rapid increases in medical knowledge. The establishment of provincial medical schools was a direct result of the Society's policies and, in turn, stimulated the London schools to raise their standards. The Society cooperated with the University of London to arrange its medical course. The Medical Act of 1858 created the General Medical Council which became responsible for medical education.

The 1815 Act also provided an opportunity, for it was passed at a time when demand for medicines was growing due to an increase in the population and of incomes. Both Morson and Morley grasped this opportunity.

Throughout the country these changes were evident. An example is Sheffield, where the number of chemists quintupled between 1800 and 1840 while the population doubled.[19] While chemists became better off, the ordinary practitioner found his income falling. 'The practice of medicine was, for the large majority, their main source of income.'[20] Physicians' charges were such that only the comfortably off could afford them. Their charges were $1/2$ guinea for a visit to the surgery, 1 guinea for a visit in town and 4 guineas out of town. Medicines were charged for as well.[21]

Growing demand was facilitated by a change in the law. The public had a wider choice depending on their location and their means. Nor must it be assumed that they distinguished between any of those dispensing medicines, whether physician, apothecary or druggist, on the basis of their skill. It was later snobbishness, combined with jealousy created by the changes in income, that created strains between these groups. The public were being better served. Thus, at the time when Morson entered his career his occupation was a respected one and increasingly used. The occupation of druggist, was well regarded and perceived as a good career. Roy Porter[22] has pointed out that 'a scrupulous man such as Corbyn could easily have chosen to practise medicine as an apothecary but preferred the manufacture of drugs because it interested him and he realised that the drugs trade was a far more lucrative business'.

While money was to be made from all kinds of medicine and nostrums, intense competition led to cheating. Even the Society of Apothecaries was accused in 1818 of selling 'at an exorbitant rate preparations and drugs made by servants who are not esteemed for their chemical knowledge'. They were said to have purchased spurious cinchona bark, perhaps because they were hoodwinked by a dishonest trader or due to incompetence. The editor of the *Monthly Gazette of Health*[23] who wrote these criticisms was also running a rival establishment that he called the Medical Hall at 171 Piccadilly, London. Maybe he was just knocking the opposition.

More serious was the sale of completely useless medicines given the label of a recognised preparation: quackery or fraud in serious cases. This was motivated by no more than the desire for a quick profit. Some chemists ignored the need to raise standards. As Irvine Loudon[24] has written: 'In the final years of the eighteenth century and the early years of the nineteenth, there was an unparalleled outburst against the evils of quackery' and it was the surgeon-apothecaries who led the attack. Morson cannot have missed being influenced by this and confirmation is provided by a cutting, dated 1740, found in his diary. It is a short poem on 'A Character of a Quack':

> Till by long travels he acquires the Knack
> To make the sweepings of a drugster's shop
> Into some unknown universal slop, and
> Thus by base means to live, does worse pursue
> And culls the Poor of life and money too.

While Morson was learning his trade and now serving a recently qualified man, he must have realised that the job could be done with greater skill and so greater knowledge was necessary. For him, chemistry was the key to progress. He may also have been shamed a little by the censors who inspected the shop in July 1816 calling it 'not a bad, but a dirty shop'. In addition they rated Syr. Papav. 'very bad', another medicine as 'deficient' and only three as 'good'. The only mitigating factor could have been the difficulties which may have arisen after Dunn's death and before Morley had settled in, although his greater interest in surgery may also have been a cause. His lack of interest in pharmacy probably provided an opportunity for Morson to exploit. The 1815 Act required Morson to attend some chemical lectures; he also arranged to join the City Philosophical Society in order to learn about the wider aspects of science and especially of chemistry.

It is recorded[25] that surgery was uncongenial to Morson and that he preferred chemistry and scientific pharmacy. He persuaded Morley that he should study chemistry and was given permission to attend additional lectures at Guy's and the Royal Institution, where he attended Brande's lectures, an important influence on him and others as well as an opportunity to meet fellow scientists. A renowned teacher at the former was Dr William Wollaston who had been one of the censors visiting Dunn's shop and with whom Morson had also a brief contact in the mid-1820s. Morson was fortunate that several learned men were responding to the increasing demand for lectures. It was William Babington[26] who persuaded

William Allen to join him at Guy's in February 1802 and they were joined by Alexander Marcet, whose wife Jane wrote *Conversations on Chemistry*, which had delighted Faraday as an apprentice. These lectures[27] covered general and applied science including references to industrial processes, thus widening the scope of Morson's scientific education beyond the needs of a purely medical one. Morson attended their lectures from 1815; the chemical lectures being in the morning, he would have had to stay late in Morley's shop to make up the time. Apprentices like Morson had the same training as other medical men and this included anatomy and clinical lectures and, later, ward rounds. Attendance at chemical lectures was made easier by Morson discontinuing his attendance at demonstrations of dissections. They had been one of the factors persuading him that he did not wish to be a surgeon.

For some years dissections had been filling the public mind with dread. Unlike Paris, London hospitals were confined to using the bodies of executed criminals. Grave robbing was the result; the infamous Borough Boys delivering bodies surreptitiously for four guineas or, when demand and supply did not match so well, their charge rose to twenty guineas. The effrontery of using the professional man's measure gives us an insight into the circumstances of the trade. However, we must not blame only the grave robbers for this repulsive activity. The conditions of dissecting rooms were awful, and usually provoked disgust.

The circumstances are described vividly by Edward Osler, who as a student at Guy's wrote on 14 June 1816 to his friend James Cornish who had recently qualified and was in practice in Falmouth:[28]

> I entered the dissecting room where the body of an old man was stretched on a shutter in the court, the brains taken out and the scalp hanging about his ears, while his straggling white locks were matted together by his blood. A hungry wolf was snarling at it and straining as far as his leash allowed. A tub of human flesh was standing near it, some pieces of which I gave the eagles* who devoured it with avidity. On entering the room the stink was most abominable. About twenty chaps were at work, carving limbs and bodies in all stages of putrefaction and of all colours; black, green, yellow, blue, white. The pupils carved them apparently with as much pleasure as they would carve their dinner. One ..., was striking with his scalpel at the maggots as they issued from their retreats.
>
> * These were probably buzzards.

The list of men, some to become very famous, whose reaction was similar and some, like Morson, who were helped by such reaction to divert their interest to other sciences, is a long one, Charles Darwin being the best known. The remarks written by Rousseau sum up their feeling: 'What an awful place an anatomy lecture theatre is; with its stinking bodies, bloated flesh of lurid colours, blood, sickening intestines, frightful skeletons and pestilential stenches. Upon my word, it is not there that I shall look for my entertainment.'[29]

In the same year that Morson had this experience, Michael Faraday gave a series of lectures at the City Philosophical Society. It is clear that these were not only more congenial to him, he was listening to a subject which fascinated him and to a master in the art of presentation. Faraday gave seven lectures,[30] the first one on 17 January on 'The General Properties of Matter'; another was on chemical affinity and he finished by describing the properties of oxygen, chlorine, iodine, fluorine, hydrogen, and nitrogen. This was when Faraday immersed himself entirely in chemical research and lectures. He did not begin until 1831 on the research for the discoveries which would make him world famous – electricity.

Both Morson and Faraday belonged to the City Philosophical Society. Unfortunately it did not last long and none of its proceedings has survived. There can be no doubt, however, that Faraday's lectures and the contact with him in this Society were the circumstances for these two men to become lifelong friends. Faraday's influence 'assisted and improved his early efforts in chemical science'.[31]

Having found the idea of surgery uncongenial, his experience at Morley's shop and the influence of Faraday and other students led Morson to select the scientific field to which he was best fitted – chemistry.

In the early months of 1818 Morson's mother and sister died. No record of their burial has been found nor the cause of their deaths. Perhaps they died in the epidemic of typhus which, according to Thomas Bateman[32] in the *Reports on diseases in London*, was at its height in 1818, only declining in April 1819, Morson was now without relatives and so was truly alone in the world. A result of this misfortune was that he was now sole beneficiary of his grandmother's Will; and would inherit the capital and all the so-called chattels when he reached his majority. One wonders if the trustees visited him in London. He was still a minor and they may have consulted him, his master and others about the way the money should be spent. It is clear from his notes that Morson did not

travel to Stoke Dry.[33] It is probable that he had the advice of his
close and valued friend, Thomas Lott, who was studying to become
a lawyer and who acted for him in later years. His scientific friends,
especially Faraday, must have been asked for their advice. The
decision was crucial to his whole career.

How this decision was taken can be surmised from the roles of
those who were probably involved. At the meetings of the City
Philosophical Society, Morson met two men among several who
were influential in London scientific circles. The pharmacist
Richard Phillips, at the time of Faraday's lectures, had left his
pharmacy at 29 The Poultry, City of London, and was working at
Apothecaries' Hall besides lecturing in chemistry at the London
Hospital. It is not unlikely that he met Morley who took an interest
in the production of medicines at Apothecaries' Hall, later
becoming one of its proprietors. Phillips was one of two older men
in the City Philosophical Society, both being aged 38 in 1816,
whereas the others were ten years or more younger. The second was
Richard Horsman Solly with whom Morson became a close friend
when he went to live in Bloomsbury. Solly was already an F.R.S. by
1816. His reputation as a scientist and his considerable wealth,
inherited from his father and uncle, placed him in an influential
position. Being very widely known he was able to introduce to one
another people he knew had similar interests. His record of
proposals for membership of such societies as the Linnean, Royal
Institution and Society of Arts is a very long one and includes
people of title as well as of humbler circumstances like almost all the
members of the City Philosophical Society.

This Society included in its aims that of mutual help. Without
relations Morson was dependent for advice upon his meeting men
in London's scientific circle. Faraday had recently returned from
visiting Paris with Humphry Davy. It is certain that the situation
regarding chemistry there would have been the subject of
conversation, just as the lack of facilities for learning chemistry in
England was regretted. Morson must have impressed his colleagues
for them to offer advice, which came from not only Faraday but
also men like Solly and Phillips with whom Faraday had a close
personal and scientific liaison.

Morson seems to have been shrewd enough to cultivate men of
influence and talent, a trait referred to in obituaries of him, the one
in the Linnean Society's proceedings referring to him 'surrounding
himself with men of talent and high position'. He did this from an
early age and his later success ensured that it continued.

There is no record of a formal agreement between Morley and Morson. At the time of the 1815 Act, the period of apprenticeship was reduced from the seven years of the Elizabethan Act; four or five years became usual. Morson was still a minor and had not passed any official examination; it is likely that he made an agreement with Morley, especially if his original apprenticeship had been for five years. He went to Paris in September 1818 two months before the expiry of the full term. The agreement may have included the arrangement for Morson 'to succeed to the shop'. It is equally possible that some such arrangement could have been made earlier; by Morson's mother and Charles Dunn, who probably wanted to retire from the business at 65 Fleet Market. In this context, the absence of a reference to the disposal of his business in Dunn's Will[34] may be significant.

If there was no agreement involving the apprentice and the shop either with Morson or with Morley before Dunn died, a deal allowing Morley to pursue his main interest as surgeon and accoucheur while disposing of the chemist and druggist side of the business to Morson may have been promised. In this way Morson would have a business on his return from Paris and by that time he would have reached the age of 21. This seems the most likely, suiting Morley both professionally and financially; and suiting Morson by providing him with some security in his profession. We must not overlook that Solly was a barrister. His assistance in such a situation could only have benefited Morson.

Whatever the exact circumstances, Morson was launched into a career as a scientific chemist.

We are lucky that Morson decided to write a diary[35] starting with his journey from London on Saturday, 5 September 1818. Perhaps keeping the diary was a reflection of his loneliness. He was not quite nineteen, orphaned and leaving for a foreign country having travelled very little in his own and he could not speak French. But he had a few introductions and found it easy to make friends, both casual and otherwise. His personality must have been an attractive one – a fact mentioned years later when he was described as having 'pleasing manners'.

He left London at 7.30 a.m. and enjoyed the journey, noting a castle on top of Shooters' Hill and the crops of hops in the Kentish fields. On reaching Canterbury at 4.30 p.m. he went 'directly to Mrs Morleys' in St Paul's Street. He made a particular point of making a second visit to her to 'take his leave'. He also called on Mr Chandler. The conclusion that these were his master's mother and teacher is inescapable. He delivered a letter for his friend Lott to a Miss March at the Deanery; Lott practised in the Ecclesiastical Courts.

The next morning he attended divine service in the French Protestant Chapel beneath the Cathedral. He was critical of the condition of the Black Prince's armour for it was 'in a very decayed state'. He was taken round the hospital, opposite St Augustine's Monastery, by a Mr Cullen and noted that it was very comfortable and clean; then a visit to the prison – he does not seem to have wanted to miss anything.

On the Monday, having risen at 4 a.m. and breakfasted with a friend in Dover, he boarded the *Princess Augusta* which sailed at 11.30 a.m. but he was 'in a calm for three hours: very sick all the time' before reaching Calais at 6.30 p.m. In spite of the journey, he had 'a good appetite for dinner'. There must be many of us who have had the same experience!

Soon after Waterloo, which was preceded by so many years of wars, the French countryside and small towns presented a run-down aspect and the people were poorly clad. Morson found the streets of Calais 'filthy' and the 'bread is bad', though he enjoyed the coffee and eggs after an early morning walk to see the town and the ramparts, from which he saw the Dover cliffs.

Having paid two francs (less than two shillings) to get back his passport, he started in a diligence for Boulogne. They arrived in Samer, 'which is a pretty town for France, the villages in general being the most miserable that can be conceived'. He had the impression that the women did 'all the work which the men do in England and vice versa'. The village girls ran after the diligence presenting the passengers with baskets of flowers filled with fruit and fixed to a long pole; 'it is done with inexpressible grace'. The beggars left their huts and asked for sous, saying 'How do you do, Sir', 'How do you do, Mr Bull – Mr Goddam* etc.' – 'there being no Poor Laws is the cause of this'. They went through the forest of Crécy 'so famed in English history'. He compared a vineyard near Abbeville to a plantation of raspberries.

Eventually they reached Paris at half past eight. He 'directed a conductor' to show him Meurice's Hotel 'but that being engaged, took up residence at the Hotel des Indes' in the Rue Traversière, St

---

* This was the favourite swear-word of Wellington's soldiers during their campaigns across France, so much so that the French made it their nickname.

Honoré; Rue Traversière ran towards the Seine at the Place Mazas and the Quai de la Rapée. So after a long day which had started at half past five, he had 'some soup and retired to sleep'.

Morson's powers of observation (much later in his life he was described as having a remarkably keen eye) and his ability to express himself are clear from his diary and these very qualities would serve him well in his study of chemistry.

Although several people must have influenced his decision not to use his inheritance merely to buy Morley's shop and stay where he was, we must admire the character of a man who, nevertheless, decided to study and prepare himself well for his chosen career in chemistry.

Notes

1. Northamptonshire Record Office; Parish records folio 8; Morson Wills, 1740–1795.

2. Marriage Licence bond, 12 November 1753. Thomas Morson of Wilbarston, mason, was supported by William Burditt, grazier of Pipwell. Both signed. Morson was first spelt Mawson but was altered to the former spelling. Sarah's name is spelt Newbourn.

3. Personal Archive, T. N. R. Morson's Genealogical Notes. Most are irrelevant but there is an added note stating that his grandmother remarried to become Mrs Wade. Without this it would not have been possible to trace his ancestors. The fact that his notes were compiled in 1870 is indicative of Morson's busy life and a lack of speculation about his forebears. Not until he had retired from all activity, except some in his business, did he spend time searching for his grandparents. His notes do not refer to his mother and he is vague about the date of his father's death, writing that it was about 1808. The actual date was 1810.

4. Peterborough, Wills Office; Folio 18, Will of Sarah Wade, née Morson, née Newborn.

5. P. R. O. *Minute Books of Orders in Bankruptcy, 1800–1809*. No reference in electoral or Guild Records can be found to T. N. Morson, who would have needed to have been in a Guild, but the records are far from complete.

6. Whitehead, J., *The Growth of Stoke Newington*, London: Camden History Society, 1985.

7. Guildhall Library Ms. 11316 Land Tax Assessments, Precinct of St Andrew, Market Side.

8. I am grateful for a letter, including these details, from Dr J. G. L. Burnby, F.R.Pharm.S., 7 July 1988.

9. References to money will always be in our earlier (pre-1971) coinage i.e. 20 shillings in a pound and 12 pence in a shilling. A guinea, £1 1s. 0d. was in use especially for professional fees.

10. Royal College of Physicians' Library; Ms. 6151, Visitation of Apothecaries' Shops.

11. Dopson, Laurence, 'The State of London Chemists' Shops in the eighteenth and early nineteenth century' *Chemist and Druggist,* Vol. 163, 25 June 1955, 718.

12. Guildhall Library; Print Room. John Tallis' *London Street Views, 1838–40,* part 18, Page 72; London: Nattali and Maurice, 1969.

13. *Op. cit.,* note 7 above. Assessments dated 1784–1815. In the years 1784–7, the assessment was £2-8-0; 1789–95, £3-15-0 and 1787–1815, £3-10-0.

14. *Holden's Trade Directory,* 1799–1802.

15. Guy's Hospital Medical School, Register of Pupils and Dressers, 1755–1823, 19.

16. Guildhall Library; Society of Apothecaries Records Ms. 8200, Vol. 10, Court Book, October 1806–August 1817.

17. Savage, A. W., 'Historical Notes of Chemists & Druggists', *Chemist and Druggist,* 15 September 1869, 679.

18. 'The influence of the Society of Apothecaries upon Medical Education', *BMJ* Ser. No. 4957, 7 January 1956, 1–6.

19. Bud, Robert and Roberts, Gerrylyn K., *Science v. Practice, Chemistry in Victorian Britain,* Manchester: Manchester University Press, 1984, 18.

20. Loudon, I. S. L., 'A doctor's cash book: the economy of General Practice in the 1830's' *Medical History,* 27 (1983) 267.

21. Matthews, L. G. 'Pharmacy & Medicine in nineteenth century England', *Pharmaceutical Journal,* Vol. 209, 28 December 1972, 595.

22. Porter, Roy and Porter, Dorothy, 'The rise of the English Drugs Industry: the role of Thomas Corbyn', *Medical History,* 33 (1989) 294

23. *Monthly Gazette of Health,* Vol. III, No. 26, Feburary 1818, 105.

24. Bynum, W. F. and Porter, R. (eds), *Medical Fringe and Medical Orthodoxy,* London: Croom Helm, 1987, 108.

25. *Chemist and Druggist,* Obituary of T. N. R. Morson, 14 March 1874; 96.

26. William Allen (1770–1843) F.R.S. Joined Bevan, 1792 at Plough Court, which was to become the premises of Allen & Hanbury. 1st President, Pharmaceutical Society of Great Britain. Dr Alexander Marcet, M.D. (1770–1822) Physician & Lecturer. Dr William Babington, M.D. (1756–1833) Physician & Lecturer.

27. Inkster, I. and Morell, J. (eds), *Metropolis and Province, Science in British Culture, 1780–1850*, London: Hutchinson, 1983, 135.

28. Wilkinson, Anne, *Lions in the Way*, London: Macmillan, 1957. Edward was an uncle of Sir William Osler, Bart., M.D., F.R.C.P., F.R.S. (1849–1919) whose father emigrated from Falmouth to Canada. He had a memorable career in Canada, the U.S.A. and in England.

29. Walker, Margot, *Sir James Edward Smith, 1759-1828*, London: The Linnean Society of London, 1988, III, 7. The quotation used by Smith is from the seventh promenade of Rousseau.

30. Bence Jones, H. C., *Life & Letters of Faraday*, London: Longmans, 1870, (9)1:13.

31. *Annual Register*, 1874; Obituary of T.N.R. Morson.

32. Bateman, Thomas, M.D., F.L.S., *Report on the diseases of London 1804–1816*, London, 1819.

33. *Op. cit.,* note 3 above.

34. Will of Charles Dunn dated June 1815, Public Record Office, Register of Wills, PROB11/1569.

35. Personal Archive, T. N. R. Morson's Diary, 1818–20.

2

Paris 1818

The morning after his arrival on 8 September 1818 at the Hôtel des Indes, Morson called on a Dr Tupper,[1] but had to call again on the 11th and the 13th before finding him at home. Tupper had 'promised to obtain information respecting a situation for me'. He went to the house again on the 15th only to learn that there had been no progress. Morson seemed determined to make contact straightaway and from Dr Tupper's response and Morson's choice of words, it appears that a prior introduction, if not a meeting in London, had been arranged.

Which of his London friends had suggested that Dr Tupper would be able to assist Morson to find a position in Paris which would satisfy his ambitions, is not known. Solly was so widely known that he would have had little difficulty in selecting a suitable person even if he did not already know one. He may have known Tupper through their positions in London's scientific life. Tupper may have met Morley at Guy's, where they were students but at different times, or as is more likely at the Society of Apothecaries. What is certain is that Tupper knew Phillips since they were both members of the Asksian Society. They were also members of the British Mineralogical Society before these two societies amalgamated in 1806. It is likely that Phillips provided the link to Tupper and that the two most senior members of the City Philosophical Society, Phillips and Solly, gave their young friend the help he needed.

In the days following their meeting on 15 September, Morson visited a number of apothecaries' shops, but nothing particular occurred. It was after this that they put an advertisement into the *Gazette d'Affiches*.

The first response was from a Frenchman who proposed that Morson should 'enter his house and dispense British medicines'. One must assume that the large colony of English in post-Waterloo Paris provided a good market. Morson declined the offer because he did not want 'to be so much my own master'; this is explained by the fact that he was in Paris to complete his education and he had no intention of starting a business there.

On Saturday 19 September he went to Dr Tupper who sent him to M. Planche in the Rue de Mont Blanc. Morson could not make Planche understand and proposed a meeting for the following day when he took Dr Tupper with him. The result was an arrangement for Morson to 'enter his establishment on 10th October and receive my board and lodging and 15 francs² per month'. Other offers were turned down – wisely since Louis Antoine Planche³ was to provide more than can have been expected at the time of the interview, even if Morson had not felt instinctively that this arrangement was 'right'. Planche was a noted *pharmacien* or apothecary – in the true meaning, as always used on the Continent, restricted to those who prepared and sold medicines. It is only in England that it came to mean a medical practitioner.

The role that Dr Tupper played was vital to the success of Morson's visit to Paris. Morson's whole career would be affected by what he learnt and the colleagues, both French and English, that he met and worked with. Tupper's selection of Planche may have had something to do with their scientific interests and also with the demand of English doctors in Paris for English medicines which Planche dispensed. It was also a measure of the regard in which he held both men.

On 21 September, Morson was offered a job by a *pharmacien* named Renard in the Rue Vivienne. He merely records the fact. It was the day after he had accepted the arrangement with Planche.

On 27 October, Morson records that he visited Dr Tupper and 'communicated my wish to visit Italy or Germany'. As Morson was a minor, it is possible that Dr Tupper played a role beyond that of adviser. His approval may have had to be sought, especially if expense was involved, on behalf of the Trustees of the Morson Will.

Morson wondered if he should use some of the interval before he started work in learning French. He was offered lessons at three francs each – half a crown in his money, but at one lesson a day, a month's money from M. Planche would be spent in a week. He did pay threepence to have his fortune told; it is a pity that he did not confide the result to his diary.

In the three weeks between the interview and starting work, Morson saw as much of Paris as possible. Not a day passed without a visit to one of the museums or galleries, a trip to Fontainebleau, the Palais Royale or another of the sights. He went several times to the theatre, ballet and opera – this last he found the 'most beautiful amusement in Paris'. His interest in the theatre, opera particularly, is an indication of his early cultural pursuits. At this time it was popular but the cost of seats confined the clientele to the better-off. Although the Opera House was smaller than Covent Garden, he thought the music and performance much better; an indication that the theatre and opera had been one of his recreations. This interest lasted all his life. His collection of playbills and theatre programmes was of great interest many years later to his great-grandchildren when they visited his house, by then occupied solely by his daughter.

The Palais Royale intrigued him; he thought it beautiful with its immense square filled with trees and full of flowers, chairs being placed so that one could sit and enjoy the scene, watching the people visiting the little shops and stopping at the coffee houses – 'superb, beyond description in fact; it is impossible to compare them with anything in London'. His favourite was the Café de la Paix where he went for breakfast on Sundays.

On another afternoon he visited the Tuileries and dined at the Hôtel; 'the dinners are very grand, generally consisting of 15 or 16 dishes'. After dinner he went to the Théâtre Français, commenting that the house was large but very plain and that 'No women are permitted to sit in the pit at any of the theatres.'

The Gallery of the Luxembourg with 'a most splendid collection of pictures by modern artists' was enjoyed following a visit to Notre Dame where he climbed to the top of the tower to see the view over Paris. The day was completed with a visit to the Opéra Comique which put on a performance of the P*etit Chaperon Rouge.*

He did not neglect his technical interests. He visited the Ecole des Mines and the Conservatoire des Arts, where patentees had to deposit models of their inventions which were put on display at the expiration of the patent. He was particularly interested by the model of a chemical laboratory.

The comments in his diary reveal an appreciation of art, architecture and music which does credit to an 18 year-old. They are not, however, confined to these. He observed everyday life as well. After a visit to St Cloud on a festival day, he comments that:

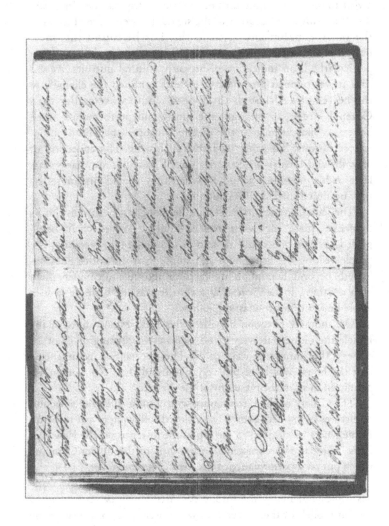

Figure 2: Diary entry for 10 October 1818.

a great concourse of people were there from all parts. It has a great
resemblance to our fairs but the exhibitions are much inferior. One
feature, however, differs considerably viz. that although a most
immense number of persons are there, there is nothing in the shape
of a riot or pilfering.

The *cabinets d'aisence* were used by women without their being
considered 'as particular or in any way indecent'. Use of them cost a
penny.

It is hardly surprising that after ten days of sight-seeing, he
spent most of the next day in the hotel. He was off again, however,
the following morning to the Jardin des Plantes where he found
'every plant you can name'. He went on to the Natural History
Museum. Another morning, after breakfasting in the Palais Royale,
he went to the Rue Vivienne where he read the English papers and
joined a subscription library.

Several of these visits were made in the company of casual
acquaintances as well as of English friends. One such was with a
Mrs Goddard. They visited St Sulpice together, where they saw a
statue which had been hidden during the time the Allies were in
Paris 'lest they should take it away'. On a second visit to Mrs.
Goddard he found her 'very dull on account of her niece, Miss
Larkin being very ill'. His diary notes that he suggested she should
send for an English doctor!

After spending the day with Dr Tupper's son, he dined with
them on the evening of 9 October at their house in the Rue de la
Paix, 'the cleanest street in Paris'. The next day he started work at
M. Planche's at '1 o'clock and was soon preparing Pil.Cal P. L. and
much English medicine'.

At first, he was unhappy, commenting that M. & Mme Planche
with their three sons and a daughter lived 'in a miserable way'. He
felt better when he had the use of a 'good laboratory'. He attended
lectures on chemistry, anatomy and some clinical subjects,
continuing the studies that he had begun at Guy's. He described a
visit to the Hospital of Charity. He was appalled by the state of the
dissecting room, calling it 'a stable'. However, the bodies were
'tolerably fresh with up to twenty in the room at a time'. They cost
eight francs, coming legally from other Parisian hospitals. London
would have to wait a few years before a change in the law in 1828
stopped the illicit trade that had been thriving there.

In the company of one of M. Planche's sons, Morson toured the
wards seeing a great many cases of ulceration of the legs, a few of

fistula in ano and a badly fractured leg. The wards were not well ventilated, but the patients clearly had every attention from the Sisters of Charity. It is interesting that Reece had visited the same hospital and also in that year. In his *Monthly Gazette of Health*[4] he wrote that the hospital had 350 beds, with further wards for another 250 being built. 'The Government pays all the staff and pupils attend free; a medical education at the first school in the known world may be obtained gratuitously.' The wards were lofty and airy but with less space between beds than in London, whose hospitals did not use screens or curtains.

Medical and surgical cases were in separate wards - again different from London. The salary of a surgeon was '£100 a year whereas in London they were paid six guineas an hour'. Reece does not say whether this fee covered services in addition to the surgeon's own; Reece's views on such matters may not be wholly reliable, for his Gazette contains several statements which seem to owe more to bias than accuracy.

Morson's French was clearly improving quickly for he attended lectures, without a comment that he could not understand. At the College of France on 25 November he went to a lecture on 'Osteology, the spine and the ribs', in a very large lecture theatre which was dirty. Soon after he accompanied a Mr Bresmontier to the College of Passy, Rue St Jacques, to hear Thénard[5] on the subject of specific heat. Thénard was then at the height of his powers as a forceful and dramatic lecturer. So popular was he that some 600 people packed themselves into a 400-seat theatre, some sitting on the window-sill and others on their friends' knees. The theatre was 'even more filthy than the others without any plaster on the roof'. Thénard was dressed in a blue coat and pantaloons, was of middle stature with hair erect 'like the caricatures of the French'. He spoke without notes for an hour and a half in a clear and distinct voice. Morson was in a good position to judge a lecturer after listening to that artist among lecturers – Michael Faraday. Morson went into the laboratory afterwards and wanted to speak to Berzelius[6] who had accompanied Thénard but 'there was no opportunity'. The latter, with Gay-Lussac, worked out in 1811 the analytical methods for determining the amounts of carbon, hydrogen, oxygen and nitrogen in vegetable and animal substances. This paved the way for progress in organic chemistry, a subject of vital interest to Morson.

By the date of his 19th birthday he was finding life more congenial. He celebrated with a visit to the waxworks in the Boulevard du Temple: 'very fine and very indelicate' was his comment. He no longer complained that he had not heard from his friends in London, particularly Thomas Lott, the young lawyer whose friendship and advice he valued throughout his life.

Morson's skill at chemistry and in the preparation of medicines soon impressed Planche, who put him in charge of the laboratory, the word then meaning the place where the manufacturing operations were carried out. The great advantage of this move for Morson was that Planche had to make sure that his new assistant was learning all the new processes necessary to produce the substances recently discovered in Paris and, also, to keep abreast of all the new discoveries and developments, otherwise Planche would have lost trade. Besides he was himself contributing to the discussions in the learned societies and, for instance, to the discovery, in cooperation with Henry[7] and Caventou,[8] of Gentianine, announced in 1821.

Planche was a founder of the *Bulletin de Pharmacie* and had published papers in the journal – an activity he continued until his death in 1840.

His papers ranged from purely chemical to pharmaceutical ones and to reporting his investigations into mineral waters, including that from Cheltenham. Pharmacists at this time looked upon mineral waters as being close to medicines. Planche invented machinery for his mineral water factory; the enterprise being one of the earliest in a long line of French mineral water producers.

A man so well known in the scientific world in Paris introduced Morson to his colleagues at many meetings. Discoveries of new alkaloids were being made quite frequently – eleven were announced in Morson's time in Paris, apart from process improvements and changes in formulations. The most important discoveries were strychnine in 1818, emetine and cinchonine in 1819, quinine in 1820 and caffeine in 1821. Work on morphine had already been published but process improvements continued as well as clinical work. Morson must have operated all these processes, not just because Planche's dispensary needed them but because of the speed with which he announced their availability from his premises when he returned to London.

All these discoveries were the result of the encouragement given to pharmacy and chemistry by the Academy of Sciences. To be in the mecca of phytochemical science and to know the principal contributors to this great achievement was a stimulating experience; similar to attending university and doing postgraduate work concurrently, while your colleagues, lecturers and professors make frequent discoveries.

The most important discovery was Pelletier's[9] and Caventou's of quinine. Morson saw the process being operated by Henry whose responsibility it was to supply the Paris hospitals. Morson knew Pelletier, whose firm became the largest manufacturer of this alkaloid. In those days, professors were allowed to be entrepreneurs as well. In view of contacts with Pelletier later, it is likely that this factory was also visited.

The habit of French scientists to encourage younger men meant that attendance at different scientific meetings brought Morson into contact with all the great men of this extraordinary time. In addition to those already referred to, there was Robinet[10] who, some twelve years later, sponsored Morson's membership of the Société de Chimie Médicale, an honour valued as highly as his later membership of the Linnean and the Pharmaceutical Societies. At the time he was admitted in 1832, Robinet was secretary, and the great toxicologist, Orfila[11] was President.

Taking account of all that happened during his nearly three years in Paris, it is not surprising that Morson held French science in such high esteem. He could not have obtained this depth of knowledge and skill in Britain for there were no facilities, the timing made it an extraordinary experience and he made full use of his opportunity.

The superiority of medical education in France had been commented upon by Alexander Marcet in an introductory lecture given at Guy's on 17 January 1818. His comments were used by the editor of the *London Medical Repository*[12] to review the subject, especially the point about clinical lectures and the attitude of lecturers to students. Clinical lectures had long been used at Edinburgh, Paris and other European medical schools but only at Guy's in England; even then it was not until 1817 that they had been restarted after a lapse of more than 25 years. This neglect of good training applied at least as much to pharmacy and even more to medical chemistry.

In contrast to the encouragement given by French professors and lecturers was the 'distant manner which the medical officers assume towards their pupils' in England. This attitude resulted in inferior teaching for a very long time. It took another twenty years for the education of pharmacists to be placed on a logical basis. And this was achieved against furious opposition by the established institutions of physicians and surgeons which had few positive ideas of their own. Indeed medical education was to be a subject of

26

discussion for a long time; the corporate influence of the Royal Colleges prevented any legislation and this allowed them to run the medical schools as they saw fit.

Morson's attitude to these matters was much influenced by his Parisian experience. He saw the branches of the medical profession as interdependent; the interminable quarrelling of the English ones he viewed as irrelevant, preventing progress towards a well-educated, scientific and expert profession.

France was 'distinguished by rigorous hospital medicine and an institutionalised commitment to research'.[13] English attitudes were severely practical and tended to avoid the pursuit of knowledge for its own sake. The results seem to have been a torrent of discovery and progress in the one and very few outstanding men struggling to make progress amid *laissez-faire* attitudes in the other.

Morson was experiencing in Paris the results of state sponsorship and patronage of science. This applied to Germany as well. In Britain, the situation was quite different. Individuals were left to initiate and support their own activities. A wide range of specialised societies flourished. Morson never wanted state sponsorship for the Pharmaceutical Society and his work there always aimed at professionalisation by means of high standards in education and performance. 'If differences of function, location and social class are made, the variegated structure of institutionalised British Science at the accession of William IV seems almost tailor-made to satisfy the needs and aims of professionals, devotees and amateurs alike.'[14]

Planche's reputation could hardly have been greater. He was a Chevalier of the Legion of Honour, awarded in recognition of his services to the Royal Academy of Medicine and his achievements in chemistry and pharmacy. To be working so closely with such a well-respected pharmacist of great reputation was good fortune indeed for Morson; and some credit for this must go to Dr Tupper, who no doubt had contacts among his French colleagues. There may be some connection in the fact that Planche's pharmacy was preparing 'much English medicine'.

Planche was born in 1776. His mother was widowed when young and so Louis Antoine was left to fend for himself at an early age. He decided to go into pharmacy when he was sixteen and soon proved a good pupil, accurate and careful. In 1793, he joined up as a soldier with a battalion of Parisian volunteers; France at that time feeling threatened on all military fronts. It was not long before he was employed in a military hospital. He was able to study at the Ecole de Mars and had the good fortune to be taught there by Fouquier[15] with

27

whom he became friendly. He returned to France very ill after a period of service in Spain, and, still convalescent, left the Army. He returned to his studies, qualifying at the College of Pharmacy in 1798.

These last years of the 18th century saw the beginning of French successes in chemistry. When F. W. A. Sertürner,[16] who gave the world one of its most beneficial, even indispensable substances – morphine in 1816 – was eventually given due recognition with the award of the Prix Montyon in 1831, the citation stated that it was 'for having recognised the alkaline nature of morphine and for having opened up pathways that led to great medical discoveries'. It was some of these pathways that Planche trod.

He soon reached the first rank of chemists, his research being described as delicate and varied and carried out with precision. His health, however, was not of the best and prevented him from undertaking lengthy investigations while running his dispensary. His first paper was published in the *Annales de Chimie* in 1802 on the 'Decomposition of Lead Acetate by Zinc'. He published papers throughout his life, even leaving one which was presented after his death. His work on the etherification of alcohol was taken up by others, even twenty years later when the German chemist Mitscherlich quantified the use of sulphuric acid for this purpose. According to Félix Boudet,[17] this was but one of a number of instances of his instigating work followed up by others.

It was medical chemistry which was Planche's main interest. He was the first to discover the therapeutic importance of lupuline, a substance extracted from hops, and then used as a sedative. It was one of the first products which Morson offered for sale.

Among Planche's varied work was the translation of Brande's *Manual of Chemistry*. In the review in the *Journal de Pharmacie* in January 1821, this was described as an elegant and faithful translation. 'The work has the appearance of having been written in French. One translates best when one has deserved to be translated oneself.' It is surprising, therefore, that less than three years earlier he and Morson could not understand one another at their first meeting. Perhaps there was a mutual improvement during Morson's sojourn. One can also wonder if the book was one of those that Morson had in Paris and he may have been involved in the translation.

Boudet, whose father and uncle were pharmacists and knew Planche well, makes particular mention in his eulogy[18] of the confidence that physicians placed in Planche. A contributory factor in this was the scrupulous care he brought to the preparation of medicines. This was of great importance at a time when adulteration and quackery were rife. Ascertaining the source and purity of materials used as well as skill in their preparation as medicines was not universal. Reliability was important for the patient. Earning the confidence of prescribing physicians was essential to business. These same qualities were passed on to Morson whose reputation with doctors was one of the reasons for his early success.

Planche died in 1840, having achieved the highest reputation in pharmacy at a time when France had many outstanding men in this field.

Working with such a man in the forefront of his profession provided Morson with an opportunity, of which he took full advantage, to meet the most eminent and successful scientists in that golden age for French phytochemistry. The lists of the famous who were entertained at his house in London, published in his obituaries, are long ones. Naturally, it was his attendance at scientific meetings and listening to the lectures on new processes, ideas and especially discoveries that brought him into contact with the great men of the day.

Apart from the Société de Pharmacie and the other institutions of similar interest, many were members of the Société de Chimie Médicale. When he was established in London, he was invited to be a member, thus recognising his growing European reputation as a scientist. The Society published the *Journal of Medical Chemistry, Pharmacy and Toxicology,* so there was a wide scope for discussion of phytochemistry, chemical production, preparation of medicines, their uses and effects. They also interested themselves in the growing of opium and other similar sources of what were then called 'principles'.

Robinet made important contributions to the analysis of opium, first publishing his researches in 1825. It was Guibourt[19] who published, with the aid of an impressive list of his fellow countrymen, the *Journal de Chimie Médicale.* He was the author of the *Natural History of Simple Drugs* in 1820. With Henry, senior, he wrote a textbook on pharmacy in 1828. He had organised the temporary hospitals in Paris in 1814–15, when such large numbers of injured soldiers were too much for the established ones. It was Henry's son, Ossian[20] who ran the Central Pharmacy for Paris hospitals. Only a year older than Morson, he was an expert in mineral analysis. Production of quinine became one of his most important tasks when demand for it increased so rapidly in the middle of the decade. His demonstration of the process resulted in Morson using it on his return to London. There can be no doubt that this and the processes for morphine, strychnine, emetine, and of lupuline previously mentioned, were all operated by Morson for the benefit of Planche's business and the acquisition of the necessary experience.

It was to be expected that if a new process was announced, there would be attempts to improve it or even to disprove some aspect of another's work. These scientists were nothing if not competitive. Robiquet,[21] who taught at the Ecole de Pharmacie, is famous for his improvements to opiate alkaloid processes. His greatest single achievement is the discovery of narcotine, the stimulant which is the second-largest alkaloidal constituent of opium, being about 5% of it. He published this work in 1821 just at the time that Morson was starting manufacture in London. Robiquet operated a chemical factory, it then being permissible to hold an academic appointment without restricting business activity. An English visitor, besides Morson, to this factory was Joseph Ince. He was there with his father, who was so appalled at the untidiness of the premises that he remarked upon it there and then; fortunately in English which Robiquet did not understand.

Some of Robiquet's work was followed up by Pélouze[22] who was described as 'a young chemist of well-recognised merit'. Pélouze was a professor when only 23 and rose to be President of the French Mint in 1848. The correspondence between him and Morson was assisted on one occasion by a young Russian, Nicolai Witt,[23] who had been staying in London in 1840 in order to study pharmaceutical developments in England. He went on to Paris and, when returning to St Petersburg, was asked by Pélouze to despatch a parcel of books and samples from Le Havre.

Pélouze was born in 1807 and in the 1830s became a friend of Liebig[24] with whom he worked in Germany and in 1836 they discovered aenanthique acid. He wrote, with Frémy, a textbook of chemistry which ran to six volumes. Numerous works of his appeared in the prestigious journals, the *Annales de Physique et Chimie* and the *Comptes Rendus de l'Académie des Sciences*.

The activity of French chemists was matched by progress in physiology. No one made a greater contribution in this field than Magendie[25] who published his work on the effect of prussic acid on chest illnesses while Morson was in Paris. This was followed by his *Formulaire*, which provided physicians with the opportunity to prescribe medicine of precise dosage and of which the effects were to a great extent predictable because there had been experiments on animals and, in some cases, clinical trials. Magendie succeeded the famous Laennec[26] as Professor of Medicine at the Collège de France. In 1832 he went to live in Sunderland to avoid the cholera epidemic in Paris. He must have felt relieved at escaping the disease for it caused the death of his colleague Noel Henry, even though he chose to stay in the very town where the cholera epidemic had started in England in 1831, spreading to Newcastle and other north-eastern towns, reaching Scotland in 1832 almost at the same time that the first outbreak was reported in London.

Some of these scientists were collaborators in the *Journal de Pharmacie* which Planche helped to start in 1809. It later incorporated the *Bulletin of the Société de Pharmacie*. Félix Boudet was one of the most distinguished of these. He was the great-nephew of a pharmacist who served in Napoleon's army in Austria, Prussia and Egypt and whose biography he wrote. With such experience it is not surprising that his advice was sought when Jacob Bell and Morson were working on the *Pharmaceutical Journal* in 1841. Bell wrote to Morson in Paris in August that year to remind him to visit Boudet, so that 'you can tell me what he says'. The recently formed Council of the Pharmaceutical Society in London had just authorised a scientific correspondence with Boudet, whom they appointed an Honorary Member.

The wide range of interests represented by these men broadened Morson's horizons. His experience of chemistry, pharmacy, medicine and physiology meant that he was now more than qualified to start his own business. Evidently he was keen to do so if we judge by the speed with which he commenced production. There was a flurry of activity at 65 Fleet Market in the middle of 1821.

Notes

1. Tupper occurs several times at this period in Munk's Roll; the family was 'an ancient Saxon' one and settled in Guernsey in the mid-sixteenth century. Morson knew at least one other member of the family in the middle of the nineteenth century. From the dates of both qualifications and the locations, it can only have been Dr Martin Tupper (1779–1844), whom Morson met in Paris. Tupper was trained at Guy's, being apprenticed to Richard Stocker in 1796. He joined the Society of Apothecaries in 1811. He developed a large practice from 1816 in New Burlington Street. He had extensive scientific connections through his membership of various societies. He became a member of the Medico-Chirurgical Society in 1819. He became a F.R.S. in 1835. Tupper was 39 when Morson went to Paris.
2. There were 24 French francs to the pound sterling.
3. Planche, Louis Antoine, born and died in Paris (1776–1840); see

Fritz Ferchl, *Bio and Bibliographikon; Biographie General,* Paris, 1855; and Boudet's Eulogie in *Journal de Pharmacie,* Vol. 27, 1841.

4. *Monthly Gazette of Health,* Vol. III, 1818, 981.
5. Thénard, Louis Jacques (1777–1857). Taught by Vauquelin and attracted the attention of Gay-Lussac with whom he discovered hydrogen peroxide in 1818. He held three chairs of chemistry.
6. Berzelius, John Jacob (1779–1848), world-renowned chemist; inventor of Berzelian Theory of Salts. Was in Paris August 1818–June 1819.
7. Henry, Noel Etienne (1762–1832), Director of the Central Pharmacy for Paris Hospitals; discovered Gentianine with Planche and Caventou.
8. Caventou, Joseph Bienaimé (1795–1877), Professor of Chemistry and Toxicology at the Ecole de Pharmacie; discoverer of many alkaloids, especially quinine with Pelletier.
9. Pelletier, Joseph (1788–1842), Professor, Ecole de Pharmacie; Professor of Natural History, Ecole Supérieure de Pharmacie, 1815. Discoverer of more than a dozen alkaloids, sometimes with others.
10. Robinet, Etienne (1796–1869). Parisian pharmacist. Many contributions to *Journaux de Pharmacie, de Chimie Médicale, et d'Agriculture pratique.*
11. Orfila, Matthieu Joseph Bonaventure (1787–1853). Father of experimental toxicology. *Traité de Toxicologie* published 1814. Lectured on medical chemistry for 29 years.
12. *London Medical Repository,* 9, 1818, Editorial.
13. Petersen, M. Jeanne; *The Medical Profession in Victorian London,* Berkeley: University of California Press, 1978.
14. Morell, J.B., 'Individualism and the structure of British Science in 1830', *Historical Studies in the Physical Sciences,* 2 (1971), 192.
15. Fouquier, Pierre-Cloy (1776–1850). Studied medicine in Paris. An expert on febrifuges.
16. Sertürner, Friedrich Wilhelm Adam (1783–1843). First publication on morphine, 1805; republication attracted attention in 1817.
17. Boudet, Félix Henri (1806–1878), Professor, Ecole de Pharmacie; Editor *Journal de Pharmacie.* Publications include: *De l'action de l'acide hyponitrique sur les huiles, et des products qui en résultent,* Paris, 1822; *Essai Critique et Expérimental sur le Sang,* Paris, 1833.
18. *Journal de Pharmacie,* Vol. 27, 1841,175. Éloge de Louis-Antoine Planche, prononcé le 3 Fevrier 1841 par M. Félix Boudet.
19. Guibourt, Nicolas Jean Baptiste Gaston (1790–1867). Professor of Medicine, Ecole de Pharmacie 1832–65; Head of the Central Pharmacy for Public Hospitals; author of several books and learned

articles in the *Journal de Chimie Médicale* ;Paris 1818. Professor of Materia Medica, Ecole de Pharmacie,1832–65.

20. Henry, Ossian Etienne (1798–1873); son of Noel. Professor Ecole de Pharmacie. Discoverer of quinidine with Delondre, 1833. Director of Central Pharmacy for Paris Hospitals.

21. Robiquet, Pierre Jean (1780–1840). Editor, *Manual of Analysis of Water*, 1825. Treatise with Guibourt on theoretical and practical pharmacy, 1828. Owner of a chemical factory. Director, Ecole Supérieure de Pharmacie, Paris. Member of the Academy of Science. Discoverer of asparagine, 1805; of cantharidine and narcotine, 1817; of codeine, 1832; &c. &c.

22. Pélouze, Théophile Jules (1807–1867). Studied with Gay-Lussac,. Professor of Chemistry, Lille 1830. Worked with Liebig in Giessen, 1836; Assayer, 1833, then in 1848 President of the French Mint. Published learned papers throughout his life.

23. Personal archive; letter Nicolai Witt, St Petersburg to T. N. R. Morson, 29 September 1840.

24. Liebig, Justus von (1803–1874); Professor of Chemistry, Giessen. His greatest contribution was to organic chemistry.

25. Magendie, Francois (1783–1855); French physiologist. Professor at the College of France. Studied the effects of many medicines on animals. Joint discoverer of strychnine and brucine. His *Formulaire* ran to nine editions.

26. Laennec, Théophile-Réné-Hyacinthe (1781–1855). Physician at the Hospital de la Charité. Father of chest medicine. Professor at the Collège de France, 1822.

3

19 Southampton Row

The urgency which was necessary in starting to make alkaloids in a
small room at the back of the shop[1] where Morson put his sign over
the entrance, was dictated by the need to earn. After the expense of
being in Paris for nearly three years and following the cost of
whatever arrangement had been made over the well-established
business in Fleet Market, there was the purchase of essential
equipment and an initial stock of raw materials. There can have
been little left of his inheritance.

The first requirement was to advertise his presence. This was
done in two ways: a list was prepared for circulation among his
circle of medical and trade acquaintances; and a technical paper on
quinine sulphate was published in the *London Medical Repository*.

Morson's 'Price List of New Chemical Preparations',[2] issued in
1821, lists eight alkaloids and their salts. This little piece of paper,
only three inches square, includes quinine sulphate, strychnine and
'morphia' free of narcotine, the first time that these substances were
made in Britain, as well as 'opium deprived of narcotine'.

Starting with quinine sulphate was, no doubt, due to his
realising that there was a large demand for a medicine effective
against 'fevers' and, the market being so competitive, it was
important to be first. The French were already manufacturing in
quantity and had announced in the previous autumn that it was
effective. They had the confidence to send a large quantity to
Barcelona, together with clinical results obtained in Paris. It would
be exported to England and obtain a distinct advantage if
substantial quantities arrived before his production was on sale.
Besides, other chemists would soon be offering it for sale.

Morson's paper on the process was published in the *London*

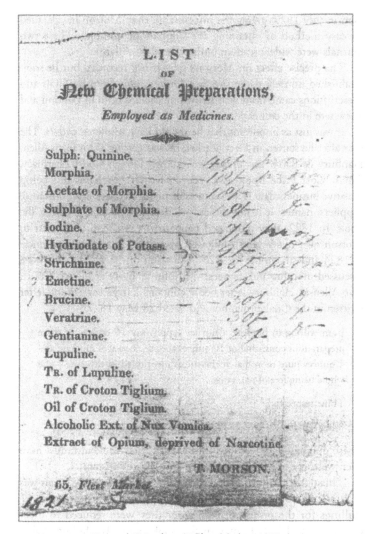

Figure 4: Price list, 65 Fleet Market, 1821.

Medical Repository in the latter half of 1821[3]. The effect was as great as he could have hoped, for there followed, two issues later, a report on its medical use, quoting French experience, with a footnote by the editor referring to the earlier paper and giving Morson's name and address with the comment that he was 'a zealous and scientific young chemist who has paid considerable attention to the preparation of this substance'[4]. It was sufficiently noteworthy for the editor of the *Philadelphia Medical & Physical Journal* to report the item in July 1822, giving the information that 'Morson has detailed an easy method of obtaining the sulphate of quinine'. These two journals were widely read on both sides of the Atlantic.

The precise effect on Morson's sales is not recorded but he soon established himself as the supplier. Orders came from hospitals and prescriptions came from well-known physicians both in London and elsewhere in the country.

It was just as important that he should have wholesale orders. The year after he started in Fleet Market, he was getting them from Allen, Hanbury & Barry,[5] the already well-known Plough Court Pharmacy. Their 'Cost Price Book' is a record of their purchases but being sensitive business data it uses some shorthand to conceal, for instance, suppliers' names. It is not difficult to detect these after studying the book. In 1822, they purchased peppercorns (an item of interest to Morson over many years), followed by acetate of morphine solution in 1824 and strychnine in 1826. As a result of the earliest orders, he discussed morphia and its sales with John T. Barry at Plough Court. The Allen & Hanbury letter book[6] contains Barry's confirming letter written in the Quaker manner and dated 28 May 1827:

> I am willing to bespeak a further supply, say 16 ounces of these preparations consisting of 10 ounces acetate, 2 ounces sulphate and 4 ounces pure morphia, at the prices mentioned in thy note – the whole being free of narcotine.
>
> Thine respectfully
>
> John T Barry.

These purchases are recorded in the Cost Price Book and must have been welcome to Morson for the quantities are substantial.

This trade continued for a long time and in the early stages was at high prices: 45 shillings per ounce for the acetate and 51 shillings for the pure morphia. Later they were reduced to meet competition. The last entry in the book shows 10 shillings being paid in 1842, when MacFarlan in Edinburgh was the main competitor for opiate alkaloids.

During the 1830s the book records his supplying eight alkaloids: veratrine, delphine (also purchased from Robiquet and Pelletier), aconitine, quinine, cinchonine, emetine, gentianine and strychnine, which were regularly supplied until 1837.

These business dealings between the two firms were conducted, as their size and the habit of the time dictated, on a very personal basis. Daniel Bell Hanbury, who kept his firm's books and dealt with 'the business side', rarely needing to join assistants on the counter, used to visit 19 Southampton Row. He recorded some visits in his diaries; the entries are brief: 'went up to T. Morson in the afternoon' (17 September 1832). Their purpose was to settle the account but it is certain that they discussed the state of trade and of their profession while Daniel Bell was the recipient of the Morsons' famous hospitality. 1832 was the year of a cholera epidemic so discussion will have turned on their own precautions as well as the increased business it created. By November the epidemic was dying down but Allen & Hanburys had earlier had so many customers for cholera remedies and bowel complaints that 'we can scarcely serve them'.

The purchase book shows frequent trade continuing until the book's end in 1844 but it continued for many later years with alkaloids, inorganic salts, chloroform and creosote when Morson introduced these substances.

Within a year of returning to London, Morson was running two businesses: a retail side, dealing with prescriptions, 'patent' medicines and pharmacopoeia items over his counter, and household items like soaps and scents; and a manufacturing operation supplying other firms in bulk.

For a man of only 22 it was remarkable that he did all those things which established him in business over such a short period. Premises, customers and scientific reputation were making progress within months of his return from Paris. Additionally he made the contacts so important in running a business. He realised membership of one of the London Guilds was essential, so he joined the Makers of Playing Cards[7] in February 1824 and was still paying quarterage in 1851. His membership cost him £2 6s. 8d. in redemption, not having a father or other close relative who had been accepted. He was helped by friends, for example by Charles Dinneford, who was also a chemist and had an extensive business in London. He was later, like Morson, to be one of the founders of the Pharmaceutical Society. He died in 1846 aged 57.

For Morson, the most important of the coffee houses where business was conducted was Garraway's whose auction rooms were built in 1820, though they had been in business since 1657 as a coffee house. Importers of bark, opium, scammony and the whole range of roots, spices and other raw materials for manufacture, plied their trade here. Commercially it was essential to keep in touch with a market whose prices fluctuated appreciably, where information, even gossip, was important, both having an effect on the costs which most affected his profit because they were the largest items of his purchases.

The trade was affected to a great degree by the purchases made by the Quaker firms who had such a large proportion of the business in medicines. Barred from Oxford and Cambridge, Quakers had to go to Edinburgh or, for instance, Leiden University to become medically qualified, so many established themselves in pharmacy in the eighteenth century and did a great deal of business with one another. Their own rules resulted in intermarriage, so the ties of belief and family created a common interest when it came to business.

Firms like Bell, Corbyn and Allen & Hanbury were very important in the trade, so a little combination by others was to be an expected defence. However, Morson never conducted himself in a way that excluded him from close contact with groups to which he had no formal ties. It is greatly to his credit that he established and maintained friendships and contacts with all the business and professional groups in his spheres of interest.

As he had been in Paris, Morson was accepted by colleagues and physicians as well as business acquaintances and customers. So business soon increased and he became known in London, as both a chemist and an entrepreneur. After little more than a year he felt sufficiently established to think of getting married.

His wedding took place in November 1822. His bride, Charlotte Elizabeth Pegram was the only child of Joseph and Ann, who were married in 1778. Ann was four years older than her husband. It is noteworthy that the couple waited nineteen years for a child, by which time Ann was 46. Joseph came from a very humble home, but became a successful mahogany merchant – and what better time than the late eighteenth century to be in that trade. He had premises in Savoy Hill and a house in St Giles High Street – the heart of the furniture business for a very long time.

Charlotte was born on 20 November 1797 and baptised at the Pegrams' parish church, St Clement Danes, on 4 February 1798, so she was almost exactly two years older than her husband. A little portrait, dated 1821, as well as photographs taken many years later, depict a kindly face with expressive eyes; it is not unkind to describe her as plain.

The couple were married at St Pancras Church and set up home at 65 Fleet Market, which continued to be Morley's home as well. He was married, with a son born in 1822. Charlotte must have found the change from St Giles High Street considerable. Her new home was small and there were many stairs. The odours of her husband's chemical activities, as well as those from stored drugs, were added to the stenches of the Thames and the smoky London atmosphere; rather different from the smell of fresh sawn timber and the better air of St Giles.

The Morsons' first child was a girl, named after her mother. Arriving in the height of summer, she was baptised at Christ Church, Greyfriars on 21 August 1823. The happiness this brought was diluted by her grandmother's death, aged 72, the month before.

In less than a year the house in Fleet Market had changed from being the living quarters of two bachelors to housing six people in addition to the shop, surgery, chemical and pharmaceutical production. Much of the space was used by Morson for his raw materials, process work and the shop with its work benches, mortars, scales, boxes and bottles. His hours were very long; customers in those days called for medicines whenever the need arose, night or day. Even Sundays were not exempt. There can have been only short periods when it was quiet and these were perhaps broken by Morley being summoned to deliver a baby, for his surgeon-accoucheur's practice was growing.

The success of these two young men brought problems. Quite apart from the shortage of space, the Fleet Market was no longer the area for the sort of practices they wanted theirs to become.

When it was first built[8] in 1737 the Market was handsome, well built and even provided parking space for carts bringing supplies, whether of meat, vegetables and fruit from the country or any of the other wide range of goods for the stalls. It had attracted good custom for many years, surrounded as it was by handsome properties.

In the 1820s that had changed. The influence of the wharves on the river and their constant expansion, especially in the post-Waterloo era, was not good, introducing people and activities more connected with the free and easy ways of seamen and others away from home than the more respectable trades for which the Market had been known. Eventually spurious parsons 'married' couples for a fee and prostitution was far from unknown.* All this was quite alien to the aspirations of two capable and ambitious young men.

They had an example in front of them. The Royal College of Physicians who had been at Warwick Lane Castle, just on the other side of the Fleet Market, for 146 years had moved in 1820 to Pall Mall, one of the reasons being the deterioration of the surrounding

---

* There is a detailed description in *London Scenes*, a small guidebook of 1863 published by Collingridge.

area. The Market lasted until 1829 when it was cleared to make way for Farringdon Road running down to Blackfriars Bridge. It was transferred to the west side and thus immediately behind No. 65, which disappeared in this redevelopment. Farringdon Market was opened in 1829.

This was not the only change that impressed itself on anyone returning to London after some years away. London was changing quickly, reflecting the greater wealth and importance of the greatest city in the world, the hub of its international commerce and the centre of a huge Empire. Blackfriars Bridge was the western boundary of the warehouses on the river, which was a forest of the masts of sailing ships, many of which had to wait weeks for unloading because of the congestion, causing boredom among the crews. Further west had become fashionable and the area for recreation as well. Opera at the Haymarket and the Lyceum were favourite entertainments; there was the Royal Academy, more popular than before; a walk in Hyde Park on a Sunday or a visit to Kew Gardens; the new Vauxhall Gardens were open three nights a week, admission being 3s. 6d.

Improvement in London was needed. Edward Osler, soon after his arrival in London, wrote: 'As people travelled to these places, they notice the new buildings going up all over town.' The names of Nash and Burton have only to be mentioned to remind us of the extraordinary activity at this time and of the wonderful results in fine houses, public buildings and, not least, of layout. The elegance of the Nash creations round Regent's Park and Portland Place, some 125 feet wide, are there for us to feel the excitement of Regency times. Southwark Bridge was completed in 1829, the spaces between Russell Square and Euston Road were filled up in Georgian times and the King's Library was opened in 1823; these areas being amongst those that the Morsons knew and where they hoped to find a house and business premises.

Morley decided to move to Hatton Garden to pursue his interest in gynaecology. He made good progress in his practice and in his profession, eventually being held in such esteem by his colleagues that he became Master of the Society of Apothecaries in 1870. He remained in practice until 1875 and died two years later at the great age of 84.

He was a lifelong supporter of Apothecaries' Hall, paying to be a proprietor so that he could buy his medicines at a discount and receive a dividend, all in return for a fee of £294 in 1846 when he transferred from second-to first-class proprietorship. There were then about 100 first- class proprietors. The annual fee rose to £448 in 1856 but fell to £413 in 1860.[9]

The two men kept in touch for many years, meeting at the Royal Society of Arts, Morley's membership of which Morson sponsored on 9 March 1825.

At the time that discussions about leaving Fleet Market were taking place, Charlotte's father died. Since his wife's death he had moved from Tottenham Court Road, as St Giles High Street had become, to live at 115 Long Acre. He was 69 and was buried next to his wife at St Clement Danes Church in the Strand on 12 January 1824.

Joseph Pegram had a generous nature. He had provided his daughter with a dowry of £1,000, the capital being held for his grandchildren. Generating an income of about £30 a year, this was a helpful addition to the family budget. Pegram's Will[10] directed that Charlotte should have a legacy of £500. He left an annuity to his brother, a labourer in Kent and directed that his nephew should be educated at his expense and have £50 for buying an apprenticeship. His spinster sister, maid and executors were each to receive £20, the executors being in businesses associated with his own: upholstery, piano and cabinet making. The remaining capital was to provide an income for Charlotte and then go to her children after their mother's death. Fortunately, the Trustee accounts and share transfers have been preserved[11] and show that each of Charlotte's children received £1,274 7s. 4d. as 3% consols in 1864, just after her death. This means that Pegram's estate was worth £8,000 so Charlotte's income from 1824 onwards was £240 a year.

It is interesting that both the Newborn and Pegram Wills stipulated that the female beneficiaries retained control over their inheritance and, for instance, that their money could not be used to pay the debts of husbands; somewhat contrary to the impression often given that women at that time were not given such control.

Although they were now financially secure, neither partner had living parents or other near relatives. Morson had lost his in his teens and now Charlotte too was alone. While this was not uncommon, the circumstances can only have strengthened the bond between them.

Of immediate importance was the legacy of £500 so they could straightaway search for a new home. The business and its reputation 'had so much increased that more extensive premises were necessary for carrying out his operations'.[12]

They found premises in Bloomsbury, at 19 Southampton Row.

Those chosen met all their requirements. They were located in a good residential district, which included the houses of eminent medical men, judges and lawyers, and academics connected with the British Museum and University College. Such a move would be seen as a step up into a better world, in both style of living and reputation, both business and scientific. Bloomsbury was far healthier than being by the river and would suit better the growing family.

In the spring of 1824, they took over the buildings occupied since 1816 by a John Baster and paid £60 a year to the Bedford Estate[13] for a full repairing lease. For insurance purposes the premises were valued at £1,000.

Their immediate neighbours included a confectioner and a baker, so the operations of the pharmacy and chemical production were not alone in making their presence known even if the chemical smells were less pleasant, however brief the discharge!

The furnishing of a home was probably the least of their problems. After all, they had both inherited furniture and other household needs like cutlery. With her contacts in her father's business, Charlotte was in a position to find good furniture and furnishings. Even so, the expense of this and that of fitting out a shop and laboratory meant some careful calculations, albeit with a 'cash injection' of £500.

It was calculated in 1804 that a 'London Druggist' could set up in business for between £500 and £2,000.[14] When he was in a similar business situation to Morson, John Bell had the help of £400 from his father in 1798 to prepare and stock his shop in Oxford Street. Even with the transfer of furnishings and equipment from Fleet Market, the initial expense at Southampton Row ran into hundreds of pounds.

Fortunately Charlotte's income could comfortably meet the domestic expenses so vagaries of business income were not a worry. At this period, prices were falling, wages rising slowly and 1825 was a boom year in the trade cycle. One lady estimated that 'for a gentleman, his lady, three children and a maid-servant a total income of £250 would be adequate'.[15]

An income like Charlotte's was that of a successful shopkeeper, and this before the addition of the business profit. In fact, the Morsons were not to know hard times for the rest of their lives. Not that their lives had been affected by shortage of money: one has only to recall Morson's interests in opera and other cultural pursuits to appreciate that his Newborn inheritance had enabled him to live a life which was not deprived in any way, while Charlotte's home had

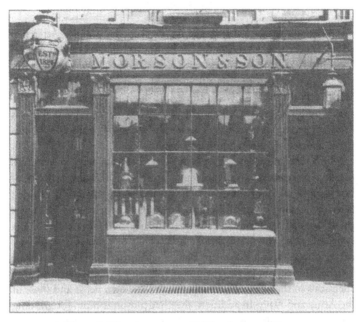

Figure 4: The pharmacy at 124 Southampton Row.

been a comfortable one.

All the Morsons' children, except the eldest, were born at 19 Southampton Row: Thomas junior in 1825, followed by Isabel (1826) and Mary (1828) – somewhat later came Robert (1836). They were baptised at St George the Martyr which was only a couple of minutes' walk along the street. It is probable that the Morsons thought that they had completed their family with four children because in about 1835 enamel miniatures were made of them. They are charming, if a little naive. A small painting of Robert was added to complete the group which is still in its original frame.

The family home was on the three upper floors of the house which faced west and was entered by its own door on the right of the large shop window. In 1841, Thomas junior was away at the time of the census; at 15, he had been sent to Paris to study and work in the Pharmacie Béral. The rest of the family was at home together with a nurse and two servants, one of whom was the daughter of the nurse. Two assistants lived in, together with a third who was described as a 'foreigner of independent means' staying temporarily. There was some accommodation in the roof which may well have been the servants' bedrooms.

Although the house frontage was18 feet, the premises stretched some 77 feet to the rear, or east. The house itself was about 30 feet long and behind it was a yard with a small room, beyond which was the laboratory; this had a half-basement. It measured 18 feet by 16 feet. Beyond this again was a small area open to the sky with a two-storey building 27 feet long and 14 feet wide – one suspects this was used for storage for it had access from a gap between two houses three doors away down Southampton Row.

This yard must have been kept pretty busy for the raw materials needed were bulky vegetable products, barrels and carboys of liquids and sacks of inorganic chemicals; and in addition coal for furnaces, drying ovens and domestic needs. His operation was not a small one. His laboratory occupied nearly 300 square feet. This compares with the 1,500 square feet which Apothecaries' Hall had fitted out as a laboratory at Blackfriars in 1786. This was their 'principal workshop' for the manufacture of medicines and fine chemicals so that they could supply both their own needs and those of the Army and Navy. In addition, they had a mortar room for grinding vegetable materials. This was an activity that Morson carried out for himself and occasionally for customers' materials; there is a record of Allen & Hanbury's purchasing this service. With a total production area of over 1,000 square feet, Morson's facilities, while not needing the space necessary at Apothecaries' Hall, confirm that he was running a large-scale operation by the standards of the 1820s.

In the 1850s an extension was built at the rear. This was about20 feet square. While greatly increasing the space available, the premises still really consisted of five buildings with three stairways to reach the different levels, apart from the staircase to the four storeys in the domestic part. The situation was accepted for 75 years, so the frustrations cannot have been so bad.

About a year after moving to Southampton Row, Morson produced his first catalogue.[16] It is obviously the result of careful thought. He went to an engraver for his frontispiece which was used by the firm until the 1950s. W. J. White operated from Brownlow Street, Holborn, describing himself as an engraver and print-seller. The tiny engraving has superb detail. The catalogue gives notice, after an interesting foreword, of the new medicines with 'their doses as far as they are at present known'; it lists a wide range of the usual preparations; includes some articles which we would term toiletries and offers a list of chemicals for those interested in carrying out some chemical experiments at home. All in the same volume, he

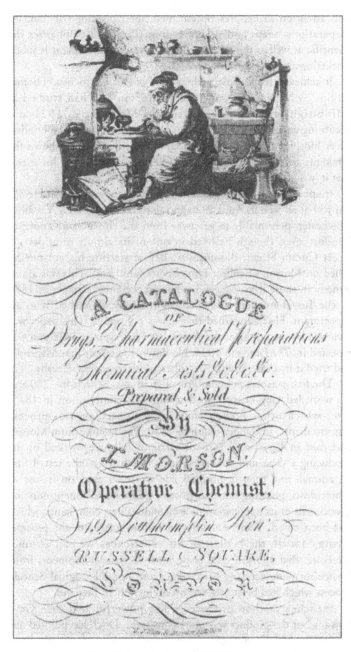

Figure 5: Frontispiece of 1825 Catalogue.

calls attention to his prescription medicines; his range of standard preparations, soaps and perfumes from Paris and emphasises the scientific as well as the purely medical. By any standards, it is subtle marketing and promotion!

It achieved its purpose with at least one of his friends. Thomas Filkin,[17] who was the same age as Morson and had studied at Edinburgh graduating as Doctor of Medicine in 1821 and becoming an LRCP in 1824, when he was physician to the London Fever Hospital, wrote in 1826 to say that he had already shown the catalogue to some of his medical colleagues and assured his friend that it 'would be shown to more'.

It appears that Filkin was suffering from a severe cough. He did not feel at all well in April 1826 and decided to visit a Dr Vassall in Chichester, presumably to get away from the climate and smoke of London, even though he lived in one of its almost rural parts – Great Coram Street, Bloomsbury. Before starting his journey he called on Morson to collect some hydrocyanic acid. This was a new remedy in those days; Magendie, having presented a paper in 1818 to the Royal Academy of Sciences in Paris, described it as an expectorant. He had warned that it was poisonous. This paper was reviewed by the editor of the *Journal de Pharmacie* in 1822 and was repeated in *The Lancet* in 1824. No doubt the report that Magendie had tried it in a case of phthisis (tuberculosis) was very relevant.

The first person to obtain 'Prussic Acid' was Scheele in 1780 and his work led Gay-Lussac[18] to determine its composition in 1815, after which other French chemists proposed various process improvements. In the period up to 1820, Vauquelin, whom Morson had met in Paris, and Morson's friend Pélouze worked on it, producing a clear and colourless acid, which Magendie tested first on animals and then in hospital. He wrote an essay on its use in tuberculosis, pointing out that it was a palliative treatment only; he gave details of its application to less serious chest complaints, which had been cured. Planche developed improvements in the process, giving Morson the benefit of his experience. We can assume, therefore, that Morson used these most recent developments from France in manufacturing his product and not the original Scheele process which had been used almost exclusively in England.

Planche's method produced a less powerful acid than Gay-Lussac's but the product was more consistent. Lesch has pointed out that some of Magendie's cases came from physicians in Britain, Italy and the United States as well as France – a reflection of his reputation as well as widespread interest in a new medicine. Even so,

Magendie complained in his 1820 paper of the 'prejudice of some physicians against the sciences which at this moment declaims against the utility of physiological experiments and the rational and restrictive application of chemistry to medicine'.[19]

There had in any case been much criticism of the lack of uniformity of strength – an occurrence not confined to hydrocyanic and one to be discussed in future years. In fact variable quality was a problem until the latter part of the nineteenth century, when better chemical techniques and proper standards became established. Magendie criticised the variation in strength when publishing his suggestion that the acid should be diluted with $8^1/_2$ times its weight of distilled water when made by Gay-Lussac's process. The criticism was echoed by Gully, the translator of Magendie's *Formulaire*, who reported a review by Everitt, the Professor of Chemistry at the Medico-Botanical Society. Hanbury's had sold acid yielding 5.8%, Apothecaries' Hall 2.1–2.6% and 'several other sources' only 1.4%, when he had asked for Scheele's strength.

In the *Philadelphia Medical and Physical Journal* in 1824, Dr Milton Antony of Augusta, Georgia described his clinical work although the editor had pointed out the previous year that American experience had not been so good and it was 'rarely prescribed in this city'. Dr Antony makes an interesting comment which is relevant to much more recent times than his. After paying tribute to the chemists for introducing new substances, he goes on to write: 'that a substance is no sooner discovered to possess some virtues than it is seized with avidity and is expected to accomplish nearly all things'. He also criticises the tendency to stop using a medicine because it has been disappointing after a 'few desultory trials'. He was afraid that this would occur with hydrocyanic acid so he described his cases with precise details about treatment and the preparation of the medicine.

In England, Dr John Elliotson, whose acid was made by Vauquelin's method, published a book in 1820, as also did Dr Granville, both men well-known London physicians. The latter gives details of consumption which had 'increased in the five years since he had drawn attention to its use'. Apothecaries' Hall had sold eight or nine quarts in 1819 and his supplier, Garden of Oxford Street, had sold forty pints. A dose was about 16 drops a day, so a very large number of doses was being prescribed. Granville was critical of the Apothecaries' Hall product, believing it less pure than Garden's. This led to some correspondence in the medical press between him and W. T. Brande.[20] At this time Brande was the leading chemist in London and for many years was the link between chemists and medical men, providing the basis for the latter to take an interest in a science without which they could never make progress.

Brande published a reviewer's criticism of Granville's book. The exchange between these two men was typical of the time – prolix and acerbic.

Morson's interest in hydrocyanic acid continued throughout his life. It was regularly manufactured; the firm's price lists included it until the 1950s when it was being made in batches of scores of gallons.

Salts of the acid were used by Lord Lister at one period because of the belief that they had antiseptic properties. Large quantities were supplied for impregnating surgical dressings in the early years of this century, especially for the Army in the 1914–18 War.

After he had been in Chichester for some days, Filkin wrote[21] that he had used all the medicine without poisoning himself 'increasing the dose by one drop daily'. We can assume that Morson had made improved Scheele's acid, and that it was a 1% solution.

> Yesterday I took 6 minims, 3 times – no peculiar effects. Are you sure your acid is good? Has it not been too long made, or too much exposed in the light? Be that as it may, I want some more.

He was soon better in every respect without definitely attributing the improvement to the acid. He intended increasing the dose until some 'sensible effects are produced'.

A week later Filkin said he did not have time to write sooner. He was busy translating Riessessen's work on the lungs* which he expected 'a gentleman to take to town' but his friend forgot; 'they say he is in love and is consequently much to be pitied and certainly to be excused'! Morson got the job of sending the translation to the Medico-Chirurgical Society, of which he was a member and was described as 'Surgeon'. Perhaps this was a device by his friends to allow him to attend meetings for it is certain that he was not in practice.

The dose of hydrocyanic was increased to ten minims three times per day. It alleviated the cough; 'two or three days I omitted it and the cough increased'.

Filkin's side became very painful at the weekend and so Dr Vassall applied fourteen leeches. Filkin then reported that he had 'less expectoration, pulse 86 and natural'. In a footnote he said he

---

* Published in the Saltzburger Zeitung Medizin und Chirurg.

went out riding all day on the 17th and planned to return to London on 28 April. Meantime Morson was keeping an eye on his affairs in London; 'your appointments are in good order and Mr. Nunn had found a kindly servant to wait on you'.

The improvement in his health was not sustained for this talented young doctor died in April 1828 and was buried in Bloomsbury Cemetery.

Here surely is a case of a courageous man, pioneering the use of new medicines of so recently known purity and strength.

Thomas Filkin asks Morson in his letter of 10 April 1826, for all the chit-chat of London: 'How is *The Lancet,* and Dr Johnson?' – a reference to attacks by the latter on The Lancet which is referred to as 'an infamous abomination'. Dr. Johnson was editor of the *Medico-Chirurgical Review.* The two friends were enjoying watching some medical politics. That they were close friends is indicated by the familiar form of address: 'My dear Morson' and an enquiry after 'my little favourite' – a reference to Isabel, or Biddy as she was called. She was then aged two and had not been well when Filkin left London.

Perhaps as interesting as this history of the use of hydrocyanic acid is another of Filkin's letters on the subject of intestinal worms – that bane of nineteenth century and early-twentieth century life. The fact that the letter has survived is a reminder that harbouring these parasites was a frequent and uncomfortable occurrence for people of all ages and was not to be virtually eliminated until kitchen hygiene reached a higher level in the early twentieth century.

It is best to quote the letter in full while reminding ourselves that, even with Morson's income, the bathroom and lavatory arrangements were minimal and crude; no central heating, and cold and hot water carried upstairs; drainage very simple. In spite of Filkin's elegant prose and sense of humour, the discomfort of the procedure cannot be hidden.

> I lay in bed last night and thought of you and your friends the Oxyures Vermiculares, or as you would term them, the ascarides; and my advice would be that you should first of all clear out the whole alimentary canal by a good brisk cathartic which would be necessary to do in the first place before the latter part of the remedy would have its full effect – as these mischievous little gentry like many larger ones are not content with a single habitation viz: the rectum or large intestine, but they also have what may be termed a country house or a shooting box at the end of the small intestine

49

which you cannot touch by the means I am going to recommend. Consequently they must be compelled to take up their headquarters near the tail before you can reach them with a lavement. The brisk purgative would effect this. Then when the intestines are fully emptied of their contents by the said purgative dose I would recommend you to fill them as completely as you can by the same end from which their former contents were evacuated. The lavement should be composed of an infusion of some of the Bitters recommended as vermifuges, as tanacetum vulgare, the seeds or leaves, or of the seeds of the Artemisia santolina. To this add two or three ounces of olive oil and inject at least a pint into the gut so as to distend it pretty fully and retain it as long as possible. Half an ounce of Ol.Terebinthino would be no bad addition to the above enema .As I am aware you will be in the city tomorrow when I go out, I send you this information tonight that it may afford you subject of meditation during your perambulations. And if you approve of it you can put it in force Dimanche.

Ever truly yours,

Thos. Filkin

This was an unenviable start to a Sunday! No mention here of Ching's Worm Lozenges[22] or any other 'patent' remedy, in which Filkin can have had no faith. Nor did he agree with Dr William Howison, of Edinburgh, whose remedy in 1823 was to cover the middle finger with candle grease and waggle it about in the rectum so as to pull the worms out in a ball.

It was often the case that more than one person in a family or household was infected, including the children. It is an unpleasant thought that a whole household might need to undergo Thomas Filkin's procedure. Even children had to get used to such treatments in an age when bleeding, purging and vomiting were prescribed along with medicines whose precise dosage and benefits were not known.

Morson's clientele extended ever more widely during the twenty years following his return to London. The records of his technical liaisons show how he made his reputation with physicians, but his contacts also extended to firms all over the country.

There is a record[23] of his supplying the Highgate Pharmacy between 1820 and 1842 with 'Tinct. Morph.Mur.' or tincture of morphine hydrochloride. It is referred to as a Proprietary Medicine, which cannot have been literally true, but is nonetheless a flattering recognition of Morson's reputation. Scheele's Hydrocyanic acid is mentioned in the same context. A little further afield was Isaiah Deck in Cambridge. A page from his ledger of 1846 records a payment of £3.0s.0d.[24] Deck was an important pharmacist, and was an original member of the Pharmaceutical Society and of the Cavendish Society, forerunner of the Royal Society of Chemistry.

There is mention in *The Forceps*[25] of an incident in 1844 illustrating the neglect of chemistry in England in contrast to Morson's quite different approach and the resulting reputation that he had earned. A celebrated physician called at a fashionable West End chemist about eighteen months after the new chemical nomenclature had been introduced. He asked for two ounces of bicarbonate of soda, only to be told they had none, but that they 'would send to Southampton Row for it'. Seeing a bottle labelled 'Sodae carb' on the shelf behind the chemist, the doctor replied that he would 'procure it for himself'. *The Forceps* classed Morson among 'the scientific men of the country' because of his reputation and his obtaining the patronage of the leading physicians.

In London were also some of Morson's most valued customers, one of whose letters he carefully preserved. The Bishop of London had a note[26] sent from Fulham Palace on 13 January 1842 asking that 'Mr. Morson send to London House [the Bishop's other official residence which was in St James's Square] between 11 and 2 o'clock tomorrow, the ointment mentioned by Mr. Gaskoin and tell the person who brings it to ask for payment.' One wonders if all such customers paid cash on delivery!

John S. Gaskoin, though not formally qualified, was a member of the Medico-Chirurgical Society; he specialised in skin diseases and practised in Clarges Street on the other side of Piccadilly from St. James's Square.

Morson's widening scientific circle extended to the continent of Europe as well as London. He had met a young Russian, Nicolai Witt,[27] who stayed in London and visited Paris before returning to his native St Petersburg. Witt sent a letter in 1840 via a Mr. Lehmann of Hamburg and it was accompanied by a book and samples of Siberian minerals 'for your collection'. These included a 'small quantity of Platin, or Iridium (which may contain some percents of Osmium) and of Titanate of Iron', which Witt suggested was Nigrin. The samples came from the Siberian 'platin sand'; more were promised. This interest of Morson's in mineralogy explains the presence in his laboratory of a cabinet with hundreds of samples, some of which were sent in later years by friends from as far away as Australia.

Witt's letter contains confirmation of Morson's friendship with Pélouze, who had arranged for Witt to despatch from Le Havre, where he called on his journey to St Petersburg, a letter and a packet of books. He mentions a recent visit to Paris by Morson. In thanking his host for his hospitality, Witt asks to be remembered to 'your friends, Bennett, Solly, Giles and White'.[28] He finishes his letter with a request for a few grains of white crystallised Aconitin, about which Poggendorf[29] had reported that it was used for facial twitches in an ointment and detailed Morson's method of extraction.

Two years before, in 1838, Heinrich Rose had written[30] that it was 'not necessary for me to re-introduce my friend Poggendorf as you met him during your short stay in Berlin. He is currently making a scientific trip to England with my friend Professor Weber from Göttingen.'

Although Morson knew Solly from his earlier days in Fleet Market, he met Bennett soon after his move to Bloomsbury. John Joseph Bennett became Keeper of Botany at the British Museum, having been Brown's assistant, and looked after the famous herbarium of Joseph Banks. Living at the Museum, he was only a little further away from 19 Southampton Row than Richard Horsman Solly whose house, 48 Great Ormond Street, was the other side of Queen Square. We can date their more intimate friendship from the entry in the archives of the Library of the British Museum as well as Morson's move to Southampton Row.

Solly proposed Morson as a reader on 12 June 1827[31] and this was approved by 'Mr. Ellis', later to become Sir Henry Ellis. The readership was renewable every six months, so 25 February 1828 sees another entry. In his turn Morson proposed some of his friends including Thomas Lott in 1838. The proposal was approved by J. E. Gray, another senior British Museum official who joined the circle of Morson's friends. Gray was the son of Samuel Frederick Gray, whose *Supplement* to the *Pharmacopoeia* and his book on operative chemistry was very well-known. John Edward trained as a surgeon-apothecary but, like Morson, preferred science. He became a world-famous zoologist.

Thus Morson, while well established in business and chemical science in the 1830s, also achieved the respect and friendship of eminent men. His life ,however, extended to many social activities. He held musical evenings at 19 Southampton Row to which his widening circle of friends was invited. Nicolai Witt in his letter asks if the family had enjoyed the Russian music. One of these friends was the artist William James Muller,[32] who often spent his winter Sunday evenings with the Morsons after lunching with Solly in Great Ormond Street. In summer the two men visited the house at Hornsey Rise that Morson purchased in 1834.[33] It was on high ground sloping to the south with views over the whole of northern London. 'Hornsey Expeditions' were a part of family life and nearly always included friends.

It was on one of these visits in 1842 or 1843, that Muller wandered down the garden and into the chemical factory at the end of the garden that Morson had built to house his much-increased output, particularly of creosote and alkaloids. Muller was 'impressed by the artistic possibilities'[34] and made a sketch from which he subsequently painted a watercolour. He called it 'Laboratory' and presented it o Morson.

Solly's cousin, N. N. Solly, wrote a biography[35] of Muller in 1875 and recalls the circumstances of their friendship. He also mentions Morson as 'a man of the most unassuming pleasing manners as well as of great intelligence'. Morson, Solly and Muller remained close friends until Muller's early death in 1845. His brother, having nursed Muller for several months, wrote to Morson to advise him of the death and to request that R. H. Solly be told. The picture was photographed by the daguerrotype process by the photographer Antoine Claudet;[36] the daguerrotype was used to produce an engraving which was published in the *Pharmaceutical Journal*.[37]

All of this was a far cry from the humble beginnings in the Fleet Market. The operative chymist with an enviable reputation had made his name in about a dozen years. He was financially well-off; supported by his wife who was an excellent hostess; and with a wide circle of friends. His interests extended to the arts so his social life was full and varied.

This was the foundation on which he would build to make a contribution to the creation of the profession of pharmacy. However, we must first recall his technical achievements.

Notes

1. *Pharmaceutical Journal*, 4 (1874),726.
2. Personal archive; Price List, T. Morson, 1821.
3. *London Medical Repository*, Vol. XVI (1821) 447–9.
4. *Ibid.*, Vol. XVIII, (1822),. 270.
5. Pharmaceutical Society archives, Ms. 2006, Allen, Hanbury & Barry Cost Price Book, 1822–44.
6. Glaxo Pharmaceuticals Ltd Archives; Plough Court letter book

1820–26; Letter No. 35, John T. Barry to T. N. R. Morson,
28 5mo. 1827.

7. City of London Record Office; records of Livery Companies,
   CF1/1503.
8. Jackson, Peter, *George Scharff's London: Sketches and
   Watercolours of a Changing City, 1820–50*, London: Murray, 1987.
9. Guildhall Library, Ms. 5963, Society of Apothecaries' Records,
   Vol. 5.
10. Personal archive; Will of Joseph Pegram, 1823.
11. Personal archive, Stock & Cash Accounts; Trustees of
    Joseph Pegram's Will, 1864.
12. Morson Company publication, 1924.
13. Bedford Estate Archives; rental agreement and plan of premises.
14. Stander, S. S., 'A history of the Pharmaceutical Industry with
    particular reference to Allen & Hanbury, 1775–1843', M.Sc (Econ)
    thesis, University of London, 1965; a quotation from Montefiore.
15. Burnett, John, *A History of the Cost of Living*, London:
    Penguin, 1969.
16. Personal archive; Morson's Catalogue, 1825.
17. Filkin, Thomas, MD(Edinburgh), cf. *Munk's Roll*, 1824, vol. 3,
    Royal College of Physicians. He qualified in Edinburgh, 1821 with a
    thesis entitled: '*Quaedam de Diabete Mellito.*'
18. Gay-Lussac's research on prussic acid was published in September
    1815. Davy's comment on this piece of research was that it was very
    elaborate and ingenious (cf. Crosland, Maurice, *Gay-Lussac,
    1778–1856, scientist and bourgeois*, Cambridge University Press,
    Cambridge: 1978, 129). Davy's work had stimulated Gay-Lussac
    and Thénard to work together. This was an example of Gay-
    Lussac's ability to apply chemical techniques to practical
    problems. The other strand of this great man's achievement
    was the development of volumetric analysis. Morson used these
    techniques immediately and they were well understood by Andrew
    Ure when he met Gay-Lussac in Paris in 1816.
19. Lesch, J. E., 'The Origins of Experimental Physiology and
    Pharmacology in France, 1790–1820. Bichat and Magendie',
    Ph.D. Thesis, Princeton University, 1977, 400–425.
20. Brande, William Thomas (1788–1866); the son of an apothecary,
    Brande was apprenticed to his brother, a Licentiate of the Society
    of Apothecaries, whose Master William Thomas became in 1851.
    He was an F.R.S. in 1809 and was Secretary 1816–26; Vice-
    President 1836–7. He was Professor of Chemistry at the Society of
    Apothecaries in 1812 and of Materia Medica in 1813, posts he

held for almost fifty years. He was responsible for the Laboratory and published a booklet in 1823 on the facilities for chemical and pharmaceutical production. He was a founder member of the Chemical Society in 1841 and its President in 1847–8. As Professor of Chemistry, following Humphry Davy, at the Royal Institution, he was a popular lecturer from 1815 to 1848. Morson attended these lectures as an apprentice from 1815 to 1818. Brande was one of his proposers for membership of the Royal Institution. Their contacts continued for many years, Brande being a guest at Morson's 1848 Reception. Brande lectured on theoretical and practical chemistry in the R. I. Laboratory for about thirty years. These were the first lectures in London in which an extended view of chemistry was attempted and included the technical, mineralogical, geological and medical applications – a stimulating experience for the young men fortunate enough to be present. Brande was among the first to demonstrate the link between chemistry and medicine. In this context, he formed a friendship with Andrew Ure. At the Royal Institution, on 3 April 1852, after his last lecture: he commented 'I listened to Davy; I acquired the patronage of Sir Joseph Banks; was singled out by Wollaston as his successor in the Secretaryship of the Royal Society.'

21. Personal archive letters, Thomas Filkin to T. N. R. Morson, April 1826.

22. *Gazette of Health*, 1820,51. See also Wootton's *Chronicles of Pharmacy*, 1910, Vol. II,166 and Jackson, W.A., 'Ching's Worm Lozenges', *Pharmaceutical Journal*, 209(1972),614. John Ching patented his 'Medicine for destroying worms' on 11 July 1796. Two types of lozenge, yellow and brown, were made; the morning lozenge (brown) contained jalap in addition to 'panacea mercuric alba', (calomel), which was the basis of the night (yellow) lozenge with the addition only of sugar and saffron as colouring matter. The lozenges were made by rolling out the mixture of ingredients to an exact thickness and then cutting out the lozenges with an oval tinplate cutter. Ching's lozenges were sold until the 1860s; in their early days they were very popular, allowing Ching to move from Cornwall to the City of London. After his death, his widow Rebecca amended the formula and continued their sale from premises in Lambeth.

23. *Pharmaceutical Journal*, 185, 4th series 131 (1960), 208.

24. Personal archive; letter, Reginald Deck to W. Ballantyne, 5 March 1948.

25. *The Forceps*, No. 2 (1844), 13.

26. Personal archive; letter, Bishop of London to T. N. R. Morson 13 January 1842.

27. Personal archive; letter, Nicolai Witt, St Petersburg to T. N. R. Morson, 29 September 1840.

28. Bennett, John Joseph (1801–1876), M.R.C.S. 1825, F.L.S. 1828, F.R.S. 1841, Secy Linnean 1828–52. Richard Horsman Solly (1778–1858) M.A. Cantab. 1803, F.R.S. 1807, F.L.S. 1826. Giles not traced. Alfred White, F.L.S., chemist and founder of A. White & Son, chemical manufacturers and traders, who were absorbed by Burgoyne, Burbidge of Goswell Road, Clerkenwell.

29. *Poggendorf's Annalen*, XLII (1837),175–6.

30. Personal archive; letter, Heinrich Rose to T. N. R. Morson 28 May 1838. Rose was born 1795, died 1864 in Berlin. Studied pharmacy but after working in Stockholm with Berzelius in 1819, taught chemistry; became Professor of Chemistry, Berlin University, 1823; foreign member, Royal Society, 1842 (*Proc. Roy. Soc.* 14, 1865). The reputation of the Rose pharmacy extended throughout Europe. Even at this early date in Morson's career he was well known in such circles. The date of Morson's visit to Berlin must have been around 1835, taking account of Rose's remark about their meeting and also Poggendorf's publication of his Aconitine process. Their scientific and social contacts lasted until very late in Rose's life. Rose published over 200 research papers and achieved an unrivalled position in research into inorganic chemistry and analysis.

31. British Museum Archives; Admissions Register.

32. Muller, W. J. (1812–45). Exhibited at Royal Academy 1836–45; was living at 22 Charlotte Street, Bloomsbury at this time. Cyril G. E. Burt, *Life & Work of W. J. Muller*, London: F. Lewis, 1948.

33. Shackell Edwards archives; Contract, 24 July 1834, for purchase of two parcels of land.There were further purchases in 1842 and 1844; in all a little more than an acre.

34. *Chemist and Druggist*, Vol. 92, 15 February 1908, 25.

35. Solly, N. N., *A Memoir of the Life of W. J. Muller*, London, 1874,96.

36. Claudet, Antoine François Jean, (1798–1867). See *Photographic Journal*, Vol. 107, December 1967, 405–9.

37. *Pharmaceutical Journal*, 6, (1846–47), 252.

4

Quinine

The discovery that the bark of the cinchona tree could be used to treat all kinds of fevers was made by the Spaniards in South America, but only some hundred years after their conquests had started. Like all such substances from places far away from Europe, romantic legends sprang up and quinine gave rise to one of the best. The story about the Countess of Chinchon being cured of a fever led to Linnaeus adopting cinchona instead of quina quina as the generic name. Three hundred years passed before this story was proved untrue[1] – the Countesses (there had been two) never having suffered from fever!

The bark reached Europe in the seventeenth century. The fact that it was called Jesuit's powder is possibly a reflection of the importance that Jesuits had in medicine. It is probable that the Spaniards were the first to benefit but there are references to the Italians being so. Both countries had a great need for a cure for malaria and if the one started using it the other would have followed quickly.

The symptoms of fever, aching limbs, high temperature, sweating, are familiar to us all. Three hundred years ago, they occurred quite frequently and no distinction was made between malarial and other kinds of fevers – in other words people were concerned with symptoms because they had no knowledge of causes.

By the beginning of the eighteenth century bark had become widely used but only among those of middle income since it was expensive. The arguments about the efficacy of their medicine frequently arose because the material itself may have been spurious or the preparation made from good bark was faulty. Because of the foul taste and texture of the medicine (and in those times they were used to strong flavours and had strong stomachs) it was often swallowed down with sweet wine. A glass of port left a better after-taste than that of a very bitter cold soup made from the ground-up bark of a strange tree! This habit was fortunate for the alkaloid is soluble in alcohol and it would have made quinine available for absorption in the stomach. It is more likely that bark was effective when administered this way than placing reliance on stomach acids to do the extraction of the alkaloid. Even so, the result of taking bark was often a fit of vomiting because it was not only unpleasant but very indigestible.

By the time of the start of the nineteenth century, bark was one of the two most important vegetable medicines, the other being opium which has a much longer history. For some years at the beginning of the century attempts had been made to find what it was that the vegetable contained. Progress in chemistry made this possible. The work of men like Scheele, Thénard, Gay-Lussac and Berzelius laid the foundations for others to develop the extraction techniques necessary for finding the 'active principle'.

Chemical education in Paris received much attention following Napoleon's changes in education and thus in the attitude to science and medicine. It is not surprising that the most important discoveries were made there when everyone had such belief in these two sciences – something that has been taken for granted in the twentieth century.

It was Gomez, in Lisbon in 1810, who was the first to isolate crystals of cinchonine, Duncan in Edinburgh being the first to translate his article – and within a year of its publication. Work was also carried out in other countries, even Russia. It was the French, however, who were to succeed and in such spectacular fashion.

Morson had been in Paris using the new extraction techniques for a little over eighteen months when Pelletier and Caventou announced in September 1820 that they had prepared quinine – albeit in a non-crystallisable form, but they then converted some to quinine sulphate, obtaining white crystals, thus demonstrating its purity.

It was almost immediately used clinically by Dr Chomel (who was reported in the Philadelphia Journal of August 1821 to have been supplied with a 'large quantity') at the Hospital de la Charité after Magendie had been given some to test and 'this ingenious experimentalist soon proved them [the chinchonine alkoloids] to be innocent'. Magendie then included it in the first edition of his Formulaire.

The success of Pelletier's and Caventou's work followed that of Sertürner and Robiquet, with the extraction of two opiate alkaloids,

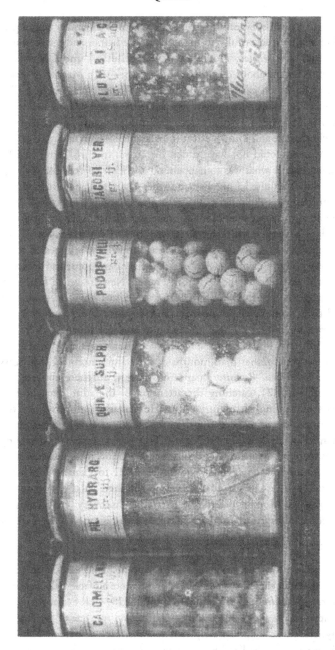

Figure 6: Phials of pills, including quinine sulphate in a miniature dispensary.

and their own isolation of strychnine. The new chemical techniques were applied successfully to many plant medicines and resulted in a spate of discoveries. However, it was Pelletier's and Caventou's announcement about quinine and their work with Magendie which caused so much excitement throughout Europe and America. The demand for quinine created a new industry – alkaloid manufacture. Also it was the start of modern pharmacy – pure ingredients of precise dosage and known effect in palatable formulation.

Morson could not have timed his arrival in Paris better had he known exactly what was to happen. So 'the high degree of knowledge and skill'[2], acquired from Planche who so ungrudgingly helped and stimulated, was exploited on his return to London. It is probable that he had already operated Henry's process in Planche's laboratory.

His price list was the first way he called attention to his presence. Confining it to alkaloids was shrewd, for it appealed to all those who were paying attention to the new developments in science and the discoveries reported from France. News travelled fast, even in those days, otherwise Duncan would not have been able to publish Gomez's paper in his *Edinburgh Medical and Physical Journal* in January 1812, nor would medical journals there, in London and Philadelphia have been publishing news from Paris written weeks rather than months of their announcement. Morson's *London Medical Repository* paper on quinine sulphate appeared in December 1821, catching the attention of the editor* as the first news of its English manufacture. He was also impressed by the important details concerning the preparation of an alkaloid and the chemical analysis of cinchona bark. This was necessary for detecting false material. Morson had also drawn attention to the discovery of cinchonine in a letter of 12 November 1821 to Planche which the latter ensured, as an editor, was published in the *Journal de Pharmacie*. Morson points out that the discovery 'enables us to detect adulterations used in commerce'. It is one of the earliest

---

* The editor was James Copeland (1791–1870), who had studied in Paris and in Germany after qualifying in 1815 and becoming F.R.C.P. in 1837. Apart from his clinical and editorial work, he wrote his famous *Dictionary of Practical Medicine* between 1832 and 1858 – an extraordinarily comprehensive and learned textbook. Copeland was one of the English physicians who made an early visit to Paris. He understood Morson's achievement very well and having spent some time in West Africa realised the clinical implications of quinine. He had supported Dr Martin Tupper's application for membership of the Medico-Chirurgical Society in 1819.

references to attempts to introduce some technical quality control of the materials used in pharmacy. As an example of the need for this, Morson mentions that he had found a formula for preparing extract of 'quinine' which had been used extensively in various places in England and the Continent: 'Take 200 parts of chestnut bark and 25 of yellow resin and mix.'

By the end of 1820, Double, who was Pelletier's brother-in-law, had published his successes in using quinine sulphate on his patients in Paris. The news reached America, being published in the *Philadelphia Medical & Physical Journal*, in early 1821. They followed this in July 1822 with a note drawing attention to French successes and a specific reference to Morson's work. The French were very confident, so much so that the Académie Royale de Médecine sent no less than 2,000 ounces of quinine sulphate to help in the yellow fever epidemic in Barcelona. This was a huge quantity in those times.

Copeland states that he used Morson's sulphate of quinine 'with complete success' in a case when the 'irritability of the stomach' precluded the use of bark. Along with his comment that the mode of preparation of bark detracts so little from the activity of the substance, we have some confirmation of the great stride forward that had been made. Patients and physicians alike welcomed the new medicine.

There were exceptions and a few influential people were among them. Correspondence published in the *London Medical Repository* immediately after Pelletier's discovery, between Richard Battley[3] and the College of Physicians, is very revealing of the attitudes of those who were so imbued with the existing ideas and practices that new techniques were misunderstood, even resented.

Battley was a successful chemist and druggist with an established practice relying substantially on prescription business. He decided to make an extraction of bark, which he said was soluble, and presented it with a few other medicines to the College of Physicians. Dr Paris gave a lecture three months later on the 'Preparation of Medicine' criticising Battley's product, saying that his experiments with it, and similar ones carried out by Michael Faraday at the Royal Institution, showed that two-thirds of the medicine consisted of a substance insoluble in water and spirits of wine.

Battley took great offence, partly no doubt because he was told he was wrong, but also because samples of his products had been frequently displayed at lectures at the Royal College in order to impress his name and products on the students. Instead of agreeing to the proposal to perform his experiment in Faraday's presence, there was a great deal of artificial difficulty about dates and the nature of the experiment, especially when Faraday said it was 'an affair of not more than five minutes'.

More words than sense were generated in this incident which went on for six months. While it is easy to have some sympathy with a man who is defending his reputation, he was exhibiting an ignorance of the new techniques. Most of all, he had put himself in an impossible position, tactically with the Royal College and technically in disagreeing with Faraday, whose reputation was already high.

Battley made other technical errors in his chemical analysis. He expressed the opinion that there was muriatic acid in hemlock, henbane, nightshade and garden lettuce; also in opium. The editor of the *Pharmaceutical Journal* wrote: 'This would be remarkable and is not believed.'[4]

This incident and many others exemplifying the same unscientific attitude is part of the justification for the poor opinion in which English pharmacy was held by other countries. Even in America, the English 'neglect of scientific and analytical pharmacy' was a matter for comment in the *Philadelphia Medical & Physical Journal* in 1822.[5]

Another paper, important for establishing quinine sulphate and, consequently for Morson's business, was that of Dr John Elliotson. In July 1823 his clinical paper,[6] including two cases of Dr Roots', was published. Both men were eminent physicians working at St Thomas'. As in Paris, there were very few cases that did not respond to this treatment. One comment of Elliotson's is of interest in relation to Morson's claim that his medicine had 'elegance as a pharmaceutical preparation'. Elliotson wrote:

> The patient has only to take a pill and is spared the annoyance of
> swallowing any of the mass of inert powder which so disgusts him,
> or so oppresses his stomach and deranges his system at large, that
> bark cannot be borne in efficient quantity, or at all.

For this wholly new medicine, Morson was charging, in 1821, forty shillings an ounce, although competition almost immediately started to lower the price. Elliotson, however, was so pleased with his clinical results that he wrote that the 'article we [St Thomas'] have at present is very beautiful' and he went on to point out that 'it cannot be afforded at a lower price than three guineas an ounce'. It seems that he did not realise that his retail chemist had added fifty per cent and rounded the sum up to guineas to make it sound better!

One response to Morson's paper was a contribution from the naval surgeon to whom he had supplied some quinine sulphate. Dr. D. J. H. Dickson,[7] in Clifton, published a paper in the *Edinburgh Medical and Surgical Journal* in 1823 and this was reviewed in the *Medico-Chirurgical Journal* in 1824. Both men were members of the Medico-Chirurgical Society. With Morson being described as 'surgeon' in 1827, one must assume that it was his medical friends, including Filkin, who arranged his membership and ensured that he met many influential surgeons and physicians, among them Elliotson, Roots and Dickson, along with the editor of the Society's journal, Copeland, a man of great influence and ability, who had an extensive practice in London.

Dickson's paper was published against the background of the *Edinburgh Journal* publishing[8] what they claimed was the first domestic, presumably Scottish, publication of progress with vegetable alkalis. They recommended quinine sulphate because of Dr Chomel's work but were reticent about other alkaloids. So they welcomed clinical results from a Scottish naval surgeon, who made two important points: the great advantage of a small dose for children and that quinine sulphate would be useful for treating fevers in tropical countries. The Navy, as much as any Britons sallying forth into the Empire, suffered from malaria and 'infectious fevers in the close confines of ships in the tropics'.

Dickson had had wide experience of disease aboard ship since starting his naval service in 1798. He was in Egypt in 1801, served in the West Indies, and was in the expedition to New Orleans. Then he spent time in the Leeward Islands before returning home. Soon after he was promoted to Physician to the Mediterranean Fleet. At the time he wrote his paper on quinine he was serving in HMS *Carnation* and spending time ashore as Physician to the Fleet at Clifton.

He used this period to investigate fevers and other illnesses familiar to him in the Service, publishing several papers in the *Edinburgh Medical Journal* and the *London Medical Repository* . These reveal that he read widely for he refers to the American and French journals.

Dickson used Morson's quinine to cure his five- year- old daughter Rose, who had been ill for more than a month with high temperatures and stomach upsets. She had 'morning paroxysms with the cold, hot and sweating stages distinctly marked'. She was given a grain of quinine a day for two weeks and was cured.

Dickson passed the medicine remaining from Morson's supply to a surgeon colleague in Bristol, Henderson, who gave it to a seven-year-old girl suffering from a 'quotidian intermittent'. She too was cured within a few days. It is hardly surprising that Dickson was quick to realise the implications for naval crews.

Dickson's reputation was such that he went on to run the Naval Hospital at Plymouth and before his career ended he was promoted, in 1840, to Inspector of Fleets and Hospitals; service in these posts led to his being knighted by King William in 1834.

Clinical results were being published in Italy; for instance Dr Mathaeis used quinine in 1822 and a Dr Martinet, whose practice was in a marshy plain near Pisa, was successful with cases of malaria, but not until he had doubled the dose. This is an aspect of the use of quinine which can explain failure – that an insufficiently large dose was given.

Throughout Europe, the demand for quinine grew rapidly. Being the discoverers, naturally the French were the first to be in manufacture, that is supplying the needs of others rather than merely making for the needs of their own pharmacy. Pelletier was in production soon after he announced his discovery, French professors being permitted to be in business; and he had the capital to invest in equipment, which was transferred to the factory he bought at Neuilly in 1826.[9]

It has been difficult to discover Morson's scale of production apart from his telling us that his batch size used two pounds of bark. His level of production was substantial to satisfy a large demand in Britain, but no figures are available. For France,however, it has been possible to discover what the production was. A lengthy search revealed a 'news item' in the *Medical and Physical Journal*, Vol. 49, 1823. In referring to the use of quinine, the editor reveals a conversation with 'one of the Edinburgh medical professors' who had been in Paris. 'The demand for quinine sulphate is so great in France that Pelletier is in the habit of using thirty-six pounds of bark a day, equivalent to 13–15 drachms of quinine, sold at 30 francs per ounce.'

When ounces are substituted for drachms, the yield is correct. Confusion may have been due to unfamiliarity with the new metric system which France adopted in 1795. Under one of the Napoleonic era's many initiatives, the French Academy of Sciences was directed in 1791 to address the chaotic state of French weights and measures. They defined the gramme as the weight of a cubic centimetre of water at its maximum density. There followed legal standards in 1799, although it was some years before the new system was in full use.

The yield achieved was representative of that recorded, for instance, in the *Revue Médicale* for May 1827 which reported the quantities of bark and sulphate of quinine included in Pelletier and Caventou's application for the Montyon Prize. It works out at 3.1%. Ure's *Dictionary of Arts* quotes the same yield, using calisaya bark, in 1860.

Pelletier and Caventou, in their letter of application for the Montyon Prize in 1827, stated that a total of 90,000 ounces of quinine sulphate were manufactured in France annually and that, of this, they made two-thirds. In May of that year the *Revue Médicale* published the details of how the amount was arrived at, with the comment that the large total would not appear exaggerated when the product was used throughout Europe, was exported to America and French and English commerce carried it to the Levant and the East Indies. The two main factories were those of Pelletier and of Levaillant in Paris; these treated bark for themselves and also for Delondre.

From all these sources, it is clear that Pelletier was producing 4,000 ounces in 1823; by 1826, he had increased this to 10,000 ounces, to which we can add the product of his bark-processing for his brother-in-law of 17,000 ounces.

Similarly, Levaillant made 32,000 ounces of which just less than half was for Delondre. The other manufacturers in France made 31,000 ounces, of which Henry's production and that of Thibouméry formed the largest proportion.

At the yield they were achieving, the French consumed bark at the rate of 107 tons annually.

Pelletier and Caventou were successful in obtaining the Montyon Prize from the Academy. It was worth 10,000 francs. At the same time the Academy awarded 2,000 francs to Henry, fils, together with a medal, for his process improvements. There is a mention of Pelletier 'preparing quinine on a large scale in 1820' in *Simmonds Commercial Products of the Vegetable Kingdom* in 1853. It seems very probable that Pelletier was the first manufacturer of quinine sulphate. He was its discoverer and he had considerable commercial skill; he would not have missed the opportunity.

Henry was in production almost as quickly as Pelletier. His production unit at the Pharmacie Centrale had the responsibility to produce pharmaceutical supplies for the Paris Hospitals and he published his process in July 1821. There was kudos to be obtained by publishing a paper and he would have done this as soon as possible. It is unfortunate that the records of the Pharmacie Central have been lost, partly by routine destruction of 'old' records and partly during the siege of Paris in 1871 when there was no other fuel;* otherwise it would have been possible to make a direct comparison.

With Morson in production in London, hard on the heels of his two French friends, these three competed for business. There is no evidence of export by Morson, which is not to say there was none, but there was much competition from the French in London. Horner, a merchant in the City, imported Pelletier's material to supply Allen, Hanbury & Barry.[10] In 1825 and 1826 they purchased from Thibouméry, who had been Pelletier's production controller and started a firm of his own, with whom Morson traded in other products for many years. In 1827, Howards commenced production[11] and started that year supplying Hanburys. As fellow Quakers it is not surprising that they traded as soon as Howards started up. Felix Garden manufactured in July 1823, reporting the same yield as Morson in the *Medical & Physical Journal.* He did not remain in production for more than a few years.

The first manufacturers in the United States were a firm started in Philadelphia by an Englishman, from Lincoln, who studied chemistry, probably finishing his learning in London before he emigrated in 1816. John J. Farr joined with a Swiss, named Kunzi, to start chemical manufacture[12] and in 1823, his order-books indicated a 'satisfactory demand' for quinine, the individual quantities varying from a fraction of an ounce to 'a few ounces', which he sold at $16 per ounce. Farr & Kunzi soon had a competitor when Rosengarten commenced manufacture in 1824, also in Philadelphia. These two firms expanded in spite of the French imports which at that time suffered from a 15% tariff.

---

* In common with other Anglo-French families, the Morsons by the time of the 1871 war had relatives, as well as friends and colleagues, in France. They were told of the awful conditions in Paris by letters sent 'par ballon monté'. Charles Lepac wrote to Thomas Morson, junior on 22 January 1871 that, 'apart from the noise of Prussian shells which we receive by the hundred, the most troublesome thing is the absence of good bread, of meat and of wood for burning'. I am indebted to Professor Jean-Claude Sournia, Membre de l'Académie de Médecine, who states in his letter of 16 October 1987: Nous ne disposons plus d'archives pour la période qui vous intéresse. Les administrations francaises qui aiment tous les papiers, n'aiment pas les archives et les détruiseux volontiers. Par ailleurs les incendies de Paris en 1871 du faix disparaitre d'innumerables documents administratifs, finianciers, hospitaliers, scientifiques etc. Je suis désolé de vous décevoir...

Before long this was increased and eventually reached 45%; meanwhile the two firms expanded their production of quinine and other chemicals until 1838 when they decided to combine.

They continued successfully in business, although the removal of the tariff in 1879 allowed imports to capture 75% of the American quinine business, much of it from Germany. Rosengarten's were incorporated into Powers & Weightman, another very successful Philadelphian firm, in 1905. Eventually Merck & Co. purchased Powers & Weightman, Rosengarten continuing the manufacture of quinine salts as a major business activity. Much later they found it necessary, during the period in the 1930s when the Germans, Dutch and British manufacturers formed a cartel, to grow cinchona trees in Guatemala.

On the European continent d'Ailly in the Netherlands was in production in 1823; this was short-lived as a year later they arranged to send their bark to Koch, in Germany, as he was now manufacturing.

Several makers started up in Germany a little later. Riedel, Obst, Zimmer and Böhringer, all commenced in 1828 and grew to substantial firms, which held the dominant influence on the quinine market in later years.

Merck[13] in Darmstadt started in 1833. A small outhouse just outside the city was Heinrich Emanuel Merck's first factory. He made morphine in 1827 and then extended his range of alkaloids by adding veratrine in 1828, codeine in 1832, atropine and quinine in 1833 and coniine in 1837. He established his scientific reputation in 1830 with a paper which earned him a gold medal from the Société de Pharmacie in Paris. In 1835, he was congratulated for his successes 'in one of the most difficult branches of practical chemistry, namely the separation of alkaloids from plant bases'. With so many process details and clinical results being published, there must have been attempts at production, not all of which were successful or lasting, in America and all the countries of Europe.

One of these took place in St Aubin, Jersey, and its story is revealing in a number of ways.

Alexander Low was the son of a Scottish army surgeon stationed in Jersey. He studied medicine in Paris under the famous Laennec and presented a thesis on quinine. It was published in 1822 while he was still in Paris and is entitled 'Recherches sur le principe actif du quinquina et sur son emploi medical.' The thesis was 'presentée et soutenue à la Faculté de Médecine de Paris, le 21 Mai 1822, pour l'obtenir le grade de Docteur en médicine, per Alexander Low, natif de l'île de Jersey, Bachelier ès-lettres de l'Académie de Caen'. The professors of the faculty included Vauquelin, Dupuytren, Orfila and Fouquier, all of whom made contributions to the chemical and clinical aspects of quinine. This clinical thesis does not refer to manufacture, but is interesting for its references to the contributions of the eminent men in Paris who took part in the chemical and clinical parts of the quinine story.

When he returned home he took with him what was said to be Pelletier's process, and set about making some quinine. It is fortunate for us that a descendant of his married H. Lloyd Howard and the process and some letters are in the Howard Archive.[14]

The process is detailed in French and includes a description of his apparatus. It is on the same scale as is described by Morson in his technical paper and yields 3% of quinine sulphate, as reported by a number of others subsequently. It took four days from the initial coarse powdering of two pounds of bark to the dried product. It was published years later in England's Workshops in 1867.[15]

The only indication of his making any product is a letter from Alexander's brother James, who wrote from Liverpool on 8 March 1824 that he had tried twenty shops and could not sell any quinine; 'it is little used here'. A second letter on 9 April, also from Liverpool, provides the interesting fact that James 'has not seen Mr Morson', without adding any explanation. We can draw the conclusion that Morson's commercial reputation was already well known outside London.

On 29 April, James wrote that he 'had disposed of your bark to Mr Morson, 19 ounces for 35 shillings an ounce; should you send any more, make it white. You will get five shillings more per ounce for it.' Indeed he would, for Morson's selling price was forty shillings. What is clear is that Alexander Low's operation of the process was not as skilled as was needed.

A quantity of 19 ounces, using Low's batch size, was 240 days' work, on the assumption that he did not do any of the stages in parallel with one another. He must therefore have started making it in 1823, a date which would be expected from the 1822 date of his thesis.

It is very interesting that Morson's business intelligence was good enough and that he decided to take off the market some inferior material, which he doubtless recognised as being recrystallisable.

James Low turns up again trying to sell quinine in Calcutta. He purchased some in 1828, only to find that Pelletier had sent 2,000 ounces with strict instructions that none was to be returned to France. This was a coup de grâce. The price of quinine in Calcutta fell below Low's purchase cost and he suffered a heavy loss. He subsequently became a bank clerk.

Both Morson and Pelletier used some of their undoubted commercial flair. It is possible that they shared some commercial intelligence. In the face of some technically second-rate competition, they decided to be ruthless.

Low's attempt at manufacture and the later Howard relationship had a sequel. The Wellcome Museum decided to arrange an exhibition in 1930 for the tercentenary of the first use of cinchona.

The Times reviewed the exhibition on 8 December 1930 and pointed out Morson's pre-eminence as the British manufacturer, something that Wellcome had failed to do. This article elicited a response from Howard's who had been approached for information and exhibits; and this is not surprising since Howard's were important manufacturers, having led the world in the nineteenth century, and more than one member of the family had made notable contributions to the botany of cinchona. The letter which *The Times* published on 11 December 1930 from H. Lloyd Howard claimed that Low had been in manufacture before Morson, the claim being based on Low's thesis. He did not refer to the correspondence from James which had probably been forgotten. The claim was noticed by the firm which was the successor to Pelletier's, Levaillant's, and Delondre's, called the Marque des trois Cachets of 1836 and which was renamed, in 1883, Société du Traitement des Quinquinas. This firm pointed out to Howard that Low's paper was a clinical one and did not refer to production. Howard then wrote to L. W. G. Malcolm at Wellcome and altered his date to 1823, but without explanation.

The yield of quinine achieved by Pelletier, Morson and, later on, other makers was close to 3%, the highest content recorded for South American bark being 3.5% although there would have been wide variations dependent on the bark used. In the early days, calisaya was preferred but, due to later scarcity, several barks of lower quinine content were used. They were achieving a yield, based on alkaloid content, in the region of 86%. This may be a figure flattering to their true achievement for we do not know how pure their product was, although the larger-scale operations with the recycling of mother liquors would produce higher yields.

The small-scale process, said by Morson to be more economical than Henry's, is an interesting one. First of all the bark had to be crushed, which was not altogether easy by hand for bark was purchased in 200 lb cases containing pieces 3 inches to 10 inches long. When the bark was stripped from the tree it was weighted down with stones so that it dried flat. Cinchona cordifolia, or yellow bark, was the variety containing most quinine. Morson's published process states that he used lancifolia, but his yield would suggest this is an error; additionally Dickson and Morson had some discussion about the different barks and their alkaloidal content and Dickson stated in his Edinburgh paper that he thought Morson had made a mistake and that cordifolia was used. After crushing, the bark was boiled for half an hour in water acidulated with sulphuric acid; the quinine salt in solution is then filtered off leaving the fibrous material to be discarded after a second boiling. The several decoctions are mixed and lime added to the solution until it is alkaline thus precipitating the quinine base which is washed and dried. The base is then dissolved in alcohol, boiled 'at a moderate heat', the liquid being decanted and spirit added again until it 'no longer acquires a bitter taste'. All the spirit liquors are mixed and distilled in a water bath. There remains in the vessel a brown viscid fluid covered by a bitter-tasting and very alkaline fluid. The latter is separated and treated with sulphuric acid concentrated by heating and mixed with charcoal, filtered while hot and the crystals of quinine sulphate form on cooling. The brown liquid is boiled in acidulated water to concentrate it and the crystals which appear are dried on filter paper. Morson does not mention temperatures nor tests for acidity, although he must have used thermometers and test papers then available for indicating if a solution was acid or alkaline. It may well be that he wanted to advertise his ability, but not to give away all details to competitors without their having to carry out experiments for themselves.

Low's process differs in several respects. He used ivory black (animal charcoal) for decolourising, and did not go to the same lengths as Morson in filtration, nor did he separate the two layers of liquid following the distillation. It is difficult to believe that what Low operated was Pelletier's process for such refinements would have been known, if not actually developed by Pelletier. The differences may well explain the whiteness of Morson's product when compared with Low's.

The thought of Morson operating on a 2lb batch size in the back of the small shop in Fleet Market in order to meet the increasing demand, reminds us of the long hours he spent at the laboratory bench as well as attending to customers and all the other necessities of a newly formed business, initially without any help for this could not be afforded.

In total contrast to these first operations in manufacture is the quinine extractor used by Roche in the 1930s in Switzerland; this was 50ft high, being continuously fed with ground bark, the aqueous solution being drawn off, thus leaving the bark free of alkaloids.

In between these extremes, the size of operations reached by 1850 was still a great advance on the laboratory-bench scale of the first manufacture even if the technology was virtually the same. Scaling-up, however, introduced problems associated with handling large bulks of material.

In the absence of protective clothing, operators wore aprons of materials like cotton twill and faces were covered with woollen scarves when dust or fumes were too much to bear. There was ignorance of the effects on the skin of all the materials used, except mineral acids and alkalis, until experience was hard won. Cases of workers being sensitised by contact with bark dust were documented. In an essay presented to the Académie des Sciences in 1850, Chevallier,[16] an experienced chemist in Paris and well known to Morson, noted that workers developed skin diseases which 'force them to stop work, sometimes for weeks, a few being permanently sensitised and leaving the factory for good'. He added the comment that abstemious workers suffered as well as those who drank excessively.

Zimmer, whose factory was in Frankfurt, called it quinquina fever. Both men recommended improved ventilation with hoods over boiling pans and avoidance of contact with both aqueous and alcoholic solutions. Zimmer pointed out that 'organic emanations' affected people living nearby. In England the passing of the Alkali Act in 1863* was the first legislation to effect improvements, although the devices suggested by Chevallier in 1850 were used quite widely long before the Act was passed.

The great popularity of quinine, due to its effectiveness and, almost equally important, to what today is called 'patient acceptance', led almost at once to a shortage of raw material. Even as early as 1826 the *Medico-Chirurgical Journal* complained of 'scarcity and dearness'.

Bark was the monopoly of Peru at first and they guarded their trees and seeds jealously in the hope of keeping their trade. They

---

*   26 and 27 Vic Ch. 124 came into force on 1 January 1864 and was designed 'for the more effectual Condensation of Muriatic Acid Gas in Alkali Works'. It required registration of premises, and set up an inspectorate. It stipulated that 96% of the gas evolved was to be condensed. The courts could impose fines for non-compliance.

granted monopolies to, for instance, Pinto & Co., an international trader, for limited quantities. Bolivia used the same method; their only agents were Alsop & Co. of New York, who supplied both the United States and Europe. Such attempts to keep control of harvesting over large areas in countries in which communications were primitive, were sure to fail. The increasing demand was followed by neglect of the tree- planting programme which in earlier times had been practised by the Indians very strictly; five cuttings planted for every tree cut down or stripped.

Bark trees were found in other countries of South America and soon the harvesting extended to areas in Colombia, Ecuador and Bolivia.

In this way, the situation was alleviated for many years but eventually worsened. In 1858, Richard Spruce[17] reported his conviction that the bark forests were becoming exhausted. Humboldt[18] had earlier reported that 25,000 trees had been destroyed in one year.

Britain had a special interest in all this; there were so many of her nationals in all corners of the earth and they included many of the places notorious for malaria. It was to be many years before the cause of malaria was discovered; in the meantime, synthetic production of quinine and growing cinchona trees outside South America were the only possible solutions. The former was impossible until chemistry had advanced a good deal, although in 1850 the Society of Pharmacy[19] in Paris offered 4,000 francs to the first chemist to discover the best synthesis; the Minister of War matching this out of his 'own budget' – another indication of the importance of quinine to Europeans serving overseas.

In fact, the prize was never claimed and it was not until 1944 that a successful synthesis was worked out – and acclaimed as one of the classical achievements of synthetic organic chemistry. It is not, however, a viable process.[20]

Attempts were made mainly by the French and British, to obtain seeds and seedlings for growing trees, either in Europe or, as Britain chose, in India. Curiously, attempts to extract the alkaloid in those countries where the trees grew, were unsuccessful. Delondre was in Cuzco in 1847 and set up a quinine factory in Valparaiso Chile using Pelletier's process. It was closed in 1849 for lack of work. In 1832, Babbage[21] had called attention to the apparent wastefulness of transporting bulky cargo of bark, when that of quinine would have been more efficient. In 1834, an attempt was made in Peru, according to Ledger[22] in a letter to H. E. Howard of 7 March 1881.

A large sum of money had been spent on equipping a factory, but for unknown reasons it failed.

Part of the difficulty at this time was ignorance of the botany of the species. Delondre visited South America, sending back via Guibourt an interesting account about various species. He and Henry made a chemical examination of several parts of the tree, even the leaves. Guibourt published a paper[23] in 1836, differing from Delondre as to which species the latter had obtained. Confusion was not surprising. Species of cinchona bark arrived in Europe from a greater variety of locations as demand increased and older forest areas became 'worked out'.

The three species of cinchona in commerce at the beginning of the nineteenth century were: a) C. cordifolia, or yellow bark, which was considered the best before chemists revealed that it had the highest quinine content; b) C. lancifolia, pale or quilted bark, containing a larger proportion of cinchonine; and c) C. oblongifolia, red bark, less digestible than cordifolia and containing equal quantities of quinine and cinchonine.

Yellow bark was sometimes referred to as brown bark because the best supplies were selected for the use of the Royal pharmacy in Madrid. It was harvested in Loxa and shipped from Payta, Peru. It contained 4%–5% of quinine. This was the original bark used in Europe and was named C. officinalis var Condaminea, Humboldt. Included in this species were the varieties C. uritusinga, C. chahuarguera and C. crispa.

In 1777, the Spanish government had organised an expedition to Peru when the Spanish botanists Ruiz and Pavon discovered seven new species. Other botanists followed, naming several other species, including C. nitida, referred to as grey bark.

C. calisaya became the main supply in the late eighteenth century, although the fact that it contained more quinine than any other species was not known until 1820.

In presenting specimens to the Pharmaceutical Society's Museum, John E. Howard in 1855 named them C. mutisic, C. calisaya, C. condaminia and included Rough calisaya bark, C. calisaya mondé of Guibourt and six varieties of C. lancifolia.

With increasing interest in cultivation in Nilgiri, India, and in Sumatra by the Dutch, further varieties were discovered. C.succirubra, a form of red bark, was found in Ecuador. Other varieties were named anglica, javanica, paludiana and carthagena. However, it is more than likely that there was duplication. Many of the newly named varieties belonged, in fact, to the original species C.

officinalis. A measure of the interest in this subject is that the *Index Kewensis,* by 1895, included 67 species.[24] By 1950, the number exceeded 150. The plant is heterostylous, a natural characteristic which prevents autopollination and is conducive to hybridism. 'It was this fact which was mainly responsible for confusion.'[25]

The complete botanical investigation had to wait until Howard and Hanbury did their work in the second half of the century.

Private and public attempts were made to collect seeds and plants. Delondre collected plants, but they died in transit. A Scottish botanist offered his services to collect seeds but no one would sponsor him; even though Christison[26] wrote to several people on his behalf, including Guibourt. The British Government became aware of the problem in 1835 as a result of the work done by John Forbes Royle,[27] who had recommended that cinchona trees be grown in India. However, it was more than ten years before the plan was carried out by the British Government who sent costly expeditions which eventually in 1860 managed to obtain, and send to India, seed which was viable. It was not long before great forests were planted and the supply of bark increased. Quinine factories were built and a new industry started based on Madras.

The Dutch sent a man named Hasskarl to Dutch America to procure plants and seeds, but he was inexperienced, both botanically and in not realising that his activities were watched by the locals, who discovered in June 1856 that he had 400 plants of C. calisaya and forced him to leave. All the plants, except two, died on the way to Java.

By far the most spectacular result was obtained by Ledger whose expeditions had the collection of seeds as a secondary objective, the primary- which failed- being to transport alpacas to Australia to grow their wool. On his return to Britain, he left instructions with his South American Indian helper and guide to collect seeds of a tree that they had both seen and recognised as better than any other variety. The British Government were offered the seed when, in 1865, Ledger received it; but with a successful business already in India, they refused the offer which was subsequently accepted by the Dutch, and for only £50!

The Dutch realised that Cinchona ledgeriana was an exceptional tree, for the quinine content of its bark was 8%. They soon put all their horticultural skill into growing plants, even having large seed trays on wheels to move from one set of growing conditions to another. The forests of trees sprang up in Java where climatic conditions were well judged to be right, and the highest bark content of their hybrid trees rose to 10%. The greatest ever production of quinine resulted. Eventually the Bandoeng Quinine Works[28] made 642 tons of quinine sulphate in 1919 to satisfy worldwide demand, at that time inflated by the needs of a world war.

Amsterdam had always had a thriving market for vegetable drugs, but by the beginning of this century they surpassed London, to become the greatest traders in bark and quinine in the world.

In the nineteenth century in London, the manner of purchasing supplies of bark, as well as of other vegetable materials, was to bid at auctions held at Garraway's Coffee House or by the East India Company. The method used was 'by the candle', a well-established one still used in Europe to this day. Bidding lasts while the one-inch- long candle burns. There were frequent disputes about who had made the final bid – candles flicker before the flame dies. From 1841, the English method came into use. This involves successively higher bids until the auctioneer 'knocks down' the item to the highest bidder.

London's pre-eminence can be gauged by the 1850s import figures: from 225,000 to 556,000 lbs were imported annually with some 120,000lbs. being retained for use by manufacturers in Britain. In addition, there were large imports from the Continent of quinine sulphate which reached nearly 9,000 ounces in 1850 with a value of £12,566. All kinds of other materials from cloves to tea were handled and the romance of it all is enshrined in a poem by John Masefield which he wrote in the visitors' book of the Cutler Street Drug Warehouse[29] in 1914:

> You showed me nutmegs and nutmeg husks,
> Ostrich feathers and elephant tusks,
> Hundreds of tons of costly tea
> Packed in wood by the Cingalee
> And a myriad drugs which disagree
> Cinnamon, myrrh, and mace you showed,
> Golden paradise birds that glowed
> More cigars than a man could count
> And a billion cloves in an odorous mount
> And choice port wine from a bright glass fount
> You showed, for a most delightful hour,
> The wealth of the world and London's power.

During the middle years of the nineteenth century, before new plantations in India solved the supply problem, scarcity caused rising prices and the sale of 'spurious bark' flourished, in spite of the chemists' ability to test before purchase, even Apothecaries' Hall was said to have purchased some and at a high price. Substitutes were also sought, the Americans using dogwood bark and the Italians the dried leaves of olive trees and also a substance called Phloridzine which was extracted from pear-tree bark.

Liebig's Annalen was reported by the *British and Colonial Medico-Chirurgical Review* in 1850 as saying that salicine had been used as a quinine substitute. Cases of admixing with sulphate of lime were also recorded. Liebig developed an easily adopted method[30] to detect cinchonine which depended on its difference of solubility in ether with that of quinine. Unfortunately it was only the more skilled and progressive buyers that employed such techniques.

The 'adulteration' situation deteriorated so much that the House of Commons set up a committee to investigate. Reading it now leaves one with an impression that science was of little concern; that the perpetrators of adulteration were solely responsible and no criticism should be levied against buyers of insufficient skill.

The House of Commons was told by Dr H. Letherby, who was an assistant to Pereira and a member of The Lancet Analytical Commission, that French sulphate of quinine was 'adulterated' with 50–60% of sulphate of quinidine and that French alkaloids were generally less pure than English.

Some twenty years earlier, evidence of greater interest and wider implication was given to the House of Commons Committee on Medical Education. In June 1834 several leading manufacturers of medicines were called. Both Morson and Daniel Bell Hanbury gave evidence, the latter recording in his diary that he went to look over his evidence given the previous day, 6 June[31]. Unfortunately, both men's evidence has been lost, either because Warburton, the chairman, did not think it worth recording or because it was destroyed in the House of Commons fire of that year, the assumption made by Jacob Bell. The evidence from Apothecaries' Hall about quinine is interesting. One is left wondering what Morson and his manufacturing friends thought of it. By this time, Howards, Morson and several others who would have known exactly what the situation was, both in their own factories and in France.

A Mr Field (he had been Master in 1825) was Treasurer at the Hall and did the buying and selling of medicines. 'We buy quinine. It comes from France. They prepare it better and cheaper than we can here.' One factor was the skill of French process workers, another was cheaper alcohol. He pointed out that he paid a penny per ounce in duty which was 'purely nominal' on a wholesale price of between six and seven shillings for an ounce.

Mr Field revealed that their laboratory, which was run by Henry Hennell under William Brande's guidance, (both Fellows of the Royal Society):

> would not be equal to the manufacturing of a thing of that kind; it requires a quantity of apparatus peculiar to itself of a very expensive description. There are not more than two or three manufacturers in England who prepare it. We attempted it once ... but the difficulties are so great that the manufacturers of it can do it much cheaper than we can. The article prepared in England is not very saleable for it differs so much in appearance.

The manufacture of quinine sulphate in 'considerable quantities' had been undertaken at the Apothecaries' laboratory. Brande, in a paper in 1823,[32] had used this phrase when reporting on his analysis of 'cinchouca' which had been prepared for him by Faraday and 'quinie', prepared by Hennell. In this paper, he referred to Elliotson's published clinical work in the Medico-Chirurgical Society's transactions. Brande suggested that quinine sulphate 'promises to come into general use'. Both Brande and Hennell appear to have been slow to exploit this first alkaloid whether as a medicine or in their task of manufacturing a substance needed by the Society of Apothecaries. It is significant that no mention is made of Morson whose own paper appeared in 1821. If they were ignorant of it, they cannot have been reading the literature. If they were also ignorant of Dickson's paper, the omission is even more serious because of the implications for their contract to supply the Navy, whose need for what Morson described as an elegant formulation had been confirmed by Dickson.

Hennell was at Field's elbow and occasionally answered a question. He must certainly have been embarrassed by the revelations, assuming he had read the published processes including the improvements by Henry & Plisson,[33] revealing that alcohol was not necessary, and that by Thibouméry,[34] for which he obtained a patent, to substitute turpentine for alcohol. Henry's work had simplified the tests which could be carried out on bark before purchase. If Hennell was not keeping abreast of such processes he was not contributing to the Hall's efficiency. From the phrases used by Field, however, it sounds as if he had taken a commercial decision. A well-informed and persuasive representative of one of the French manufacturers had perhaps been very successful in striking a deal with a large customer. It may even have been Pelletier himself, as he visited London for scientific meetings and business reasons in the 1830s. At all events, Field was shown up by the next witness.

The committee asked Robert Christison, Professor of Materia Medica at Edinburgh University whether alcohol was used for quinine. He replied, 'No, and I have reason to believe that processes not using alcohol are used in this country.' He believed most of Britain's needs were met here. Having examined samples from each country, he concluded that English quinine was equal to the finest he had ever seen.

Hennell's evidence concentrated on adulteration and malpractice, and his reference to 'printers who would sell you the labels and stamp of Delondre, Pelletier & Co.' is revealing. It is also a confirmation of how important the competition of this French company was to English manufacturers.

The business aspects of quinine sales provide some interesting figures. In the 1820s, Pelletier's sales reached 60,000 ounces at a price of £1 10s. 0d. per ounce. Thus he had a turnover of about £100,000 a year on this one product. That can be compared with Howard's figures[35] for later in the century. The earliest year for which figures are available is 1855, in which they earned £64,345 from quinine sulphate. It was their habit to record their sales after discounting them by 6%. Bernard Howard in a paper tells us that his firm then made 150,000 ounces for which they would have needed 130 tons of bark. So their average selling price, taking account of the 6%, was eight shillings and seven pence. In thirty years or so, the price fell from Morson's forty shillings in 1821 to twenty-four in 1827 and six to seven shillings in 1834, with a slight rise to 8/7d. in 1855. These prices are confirmed by printed price lists in journals like *The London Medical Repository* which obtained figures from George Waugh, a chemist in Regent Street, who was later to be a founder member of the Pharmaceutical Society. Competition, on a world-wide scale, had ensured that the price fell to about a fifth of Morson's original figure and was to fall further when the Dutch started up, and price competition from Germany resulted in Howards' price falling in 1886 to 2/6d. an ounce.[36] At these levels quinine was available to all and the price history exemplifies what competition can do, especially with ever-increasing demand.

By the time the Dutch had captured the bulk of the business, a broker in London saw his 1% commission shrink from £7 10s. 0d. in 1884 to 8/4d. on 1,000 ounce lots; by 1910 the commission was 7$\frac{1}{2}$ pence.

The price history in the USA was similar, falling from an initial $16 an ounce to $2.25 in 1830. It fluctuated around this figure until 1885 when it was less than $1 and dropped to 30 cents in 1900.

There is a detailed costing in the Howard papers which records expenditure, including packaging, in 1855 at £61,207, and gives a 10% profit before tax. The total sales of all quinine salts that year amounted to £71,872 with a profit of £10,664 or 14.8%.

There is a contrast to be seen with Howard's figures before they started quinine manufacture. In the seventeen years from 1820 to 1837, their sales increased from £32,000 to £34,000. It was their success with quinine which provided all the growth and the means of their establishing a worldwide reputation. This reliance on one product is confirmed for the period 1872-81 when quinine contributed 58.5% of their profits. This was a difficult time for business, including a recession in the mid-1870s and the gross profits on their business were halved, in spite of substantial increases in their price for quinine sulphate which rose from 7/9d. to 16/4d. in 1877, only to fall back again to 8/- in 1881.

Unfortunately, no figures of Morson's turnover or profits are available and such figures for a later period as exist are not helpful in in the context of quinine. As the first manufacturer of a new pharmaceutical, and taking account of what it did for his reputation, Morson appears to have been unable to exploit his position. The firm continued to manufacture, promote, exhibit and sell the range of quinine salts until the middle of the century but it was Howards and Pelletier, followed by the Germans, who captured the bulk of the business. Zimmer in 1851 was the largest manufacturer in the world and was at the centre of a cartel attempting to control bark prices, as well as allocations in the 1920s.

There are only two clues to Morson's situation, slightly contradictory, in correspondence in the 1860s. Morson was purchasing[37] his quinine from Böhringer, his orders totalling 5,000 ounces in 1866–7, so it would appear that by this time he had closed down his manufacture. On the other hand, he was purchasing bark in 1872, ordering 'another half ton' in June of that year. It is possible that his extensive contacts in the bark trade led him to find some opportunities for sales. The firm did not lose all interest in manufacture for they made 2,000 ounces of quinine in 1914. Perhaps this was taking advantage of the supply worries at the start of the First World War. It is certain that little manufacture took place after 1865 and that the firm was not in the top league of quinine makers from that date.

Notes

1. *Chemistry & Industry*, 23 December 1971, editorial, 'The quinine trade begun'.
2. *Annual Register* 1874, Obituary of T. N. R. Morson.
3. Battley, Richard (1770–1858), Navy surgeon and chemist and druggist of Fore Street, Cripplegate; later Battley and Maitland of St Paul's Churchyard. Founder member and Council member, Pharmaceutical Society. Generally the Censors, between 1815 and 1825, reported favourably on his premises but he was also criticised on several occasions for what nowadays would be termed quality control errors. He kept a Museum, exhibiting his products. He was said to be a first class druggist, making infusions from his own process. He taught at several hospitals in London.
4. *Pharmaceutical Journal*, 1 (1841–2), 218.
5. *Philadelphia Medical & Physical Journal*, Vol. 4, 215.
6. *Medico-Chirurgical Transactions*, Vol. 12, 1823, 'Illustrations of the Medical Properties of Quinina' by John Elliotson, M.D.; read 8 July 1823.
7. Dickson, Dr David James Hamilton (1781–1850), was educated as a surgeon in Edinburgh, becoming licensed in 1798. D.M. Degree 1806, F.R.S.E. 1816, L.R.C.P. 1823 (Gentleman's Magazine 1850). He was also an F.L.S., elected in 1816.
8. *Edinburgh Medical and Surgical Journal*, Vol. 18 January 1822, 151-62.
9. Boussel, Patrice, *Histoire de la Pharmacie et de l'industrie Pharmaceutique*, Patrice Boussel, Henri Bonnemain, Frank L. Bové, Paris Editions de la Porte verte, 1982, 172.
10. Pharmaceutical Society Archives; Ms. 22006, Allen, Hanbury & Barry Cost price book, 1822–44.
11. Miall, Stephen, *A History of the Chemical Industry*, London: Ernest Benn, 1931.
12. England, Joseph W., *The American manufacture of quinine sulphate*, Philadelphia College of Pharmacy, 1898; the paper was sent to me by Dr Jeffrey Sturchio, the archivist of Merck & Co. Inc.
13. E. Merck, Darmstadt, company publication, *A History of Chemical Achievement*, 1827–1937.
14. Greater London Library, Acc 1039, Howard papers.
15. *The Mechanics' Magazine*, ed. J.C. Robertson, published by Robertson & Co., Fleet Street, London.
16. Chevallier, Jean-Baptiste-Alphonse (1792–1879). From 1825, principal editor, *Journal de Chimie Médicale*. His paper was entitled:

'Maladies des ouvriers qui préparent le sulfate de quinine'; a
summary appeared in the *Journal de Chimie Médicale*, 11 (1850),
740–742.

17. Pharmaceutical Society Archives; Richard Spruce, letter to J. E.
    Howard ,5 July 1869; not catalogued.

18. Bastien, Joseph William, *Healers of the Andes*, Salt Lake City:
    University of Utah Press, 1987.

19. *Journal de Pharmacie*, Vol. 18, 1850, 57.

20. *Merck Index*, 10th Edition, 1983, Merck & Co. Inc., New Jersey,
    U.S.A. Synthesis: Woodward, Doering reported in J. Am. Chem.
    Soc. 66, 849 (1944) and 67, 860 (1945).

21. *London Medical Gazette*, 10 (1832) 515.

22. Pharmaceutical Society Archives (Howard archive), not catalogued.
    See also Charles Ledger, 1818–1905 by G. Gramiccia, MacMillan
    Press, 1988.

23. *Journal de Pharmacie*, Vol. 22, 1836.

24. *Medical Botany*, Vol. 1, 1819, 41–47; see Chemist and Druggist
    Special Issue, Vol. 112, No. 26, series 2629, 28 June 1930, 831-32;
    Pharmaceutical Journal 14, (1855), 395.

25. Dr Jaime Jaramillo-Arago, *The Conquest of Malaria*, London:
    William Heinemann, 1950, 83.

26. *Op. cit.,* Note 23 above, 614.

27. Royle, John Forbes (1799–1858). A pupil of Dr Anthony Todd
    Thomson. After qualifying joined the medical staff of the Bengal
    Army. Pursued his interest in botany and in 1823 became
    Superintendent of the East India Company's garden at
    Saharampora. 1831, returned to England and wrote his major
    work, *Illustrations of the Botany of the Himalayan Mountains,* which
    gave him a European reputation as a medical botanist. His work
    stimulated the growing of tea in India. 1837–56 Professor Materia
    Medica, King's College, London. F.L.S. 1833, F.R.S.1827.
    Hon.member Pharmaceutical Society. Commissioner for both the
    1851 Great Exhibition and the 1855 Paris one 1855. Published his
    work, *On the fibrous plants of India,* i.e. those used for clothing,
    cordage and paper.

28. *Chemistry & Industry,* 4 December 1937;
    'A hundred years of alkaloid industry'by Dr W. M. Wuest.

29. *Chemist & Druggist,* 108, 30 June 1928, 867.

30. Ure, Andrew, M.D., F.R.S., M.G.S., *Dictionary of Arts, Manufactures
    & Mines,* London, Longmans: 1860.

31. Diaries of Daniel Bell Hanbury; these small pocket diaries record,
    intermittently, details of his work, family, weather, holidays in cryptic

sentences and are also appointment books. They were very kindly
lent to me by Mr & Mrs S. N. Hanbury of Broxbourne, Herts.

32. Brande, W. T., F.R.S., 'Observations on the ultimate analysis of
certain vegetable salifiable bases', *Quarterly Journal of Science,
Literature and the Arts*, Vol. 16, 1823, 279.

33. *Journal de Pharmacie*, Vol. 13, 1827, 268 *et seq.*

34. Patent dated 19 August 1833 granted to Jean Blaise Auguste
Thibouméry in Paris.

35. a. Slater A.W., *Howards, 1797–1837 :a study in business history*,
London University, 1955.

    b. Howards, 1797-1947, company publication.

    c. Bernard, F. Howard, *Some Notes on the Cinchona Industry*,
Institute of Chemistry, 1930.

36. Hearon, Squire & Francis (wholesalers and exporters) produced a
graph of Howards' prices, 1867–86.

37. Personal archive; Morson's letter book, 1866–72, mainly orders to
overseas suppliers.

5

Opium

Morson's 'Price List of new Chemical Preparations, employed as Medicines' announced the first time that these substances were on sale in Britain, but the ready acceptance of quinine was quite different from that of morphine. Morphine had a competitor in laudanum; less expensive and less dramatic in its effect, it was so well established that the advantages of precise dosage and purity were outweighed. Another important factor was that quinine treated a disease, while morphine is a panacea for pain.

Opium has a long history, and medicines made from it were usually reliable and not unpleasant to take, whereas bark was unreliable, unpalatable and indigestible. Quinine was accepted as a replacement for bark whereas morphine was an alternative to opium. Since there was so great a need for quinine, the demand increased rapidly as soon as its advantages were pointed out in technical and clinical reports. The same could not be said of morphine.

The medicinal value of poppy juice – the source of opium whose active principles are mainly morphine, which is a sedative, and narcotine, which is a stimulant – has been known for thousands of years. The lakeside neolithic settlements of Europe have revealed poppy-seeds so it is likely that our ancestors used the plant, or parts of it, as a medicine. It was known in China 3000 years ago. The earliest recorded use of opium as we know it, the sun-dried latex from the unripe capsule of Papaver somniferum, is in the first century A.D. when Dioscorides distinguished between the juice of the plant and that of the seed capsule which contains the alkaloids, although the seeds do not. By the twelfth century, opium was an article of commerce for Venetian traders who imported it from Persia and perhaps Turkey; its use then spread more fully to all parts of Europe. In Britain, opium preparations became known as laudanum, or tincture of opium, containing 1% of anhydrous morphine; and paregoric, a camphorated tincture of opium with less than 0.1% of morphine, thus making doses quite small. The notorious Dover's powder, however, contained twelve times as much and patients needed to be warned about it, occasionally even being recommended to make their Wills!

Laudanum was prescribed by physicians for all manner of complaints: pain, diarrhoea, in surgery; but it was sold freely by several sorts of trader. The eighteenth-century medicine man or woman, grocer, druggist, apothecary and physician – all sold laudanum as prepared by the instructions in the pharmacopoeia, as well as the various patent medicines, some purely local, others more widely known; and occasionally used their own recipes. Consumption slowly increased, especially towards the end of the eighteenth century. This was partly the result of the famous seventeenth-century physician, Thomas Sydenham's opinion. He wrote that opium had been 'bestowed upon mankind' by a kind Providence and could be used 'for the purpose of lightening its miseries' because of its power 'to moderate the violence of so many maladies and even to cure some of them.' It was, in Pereira's words, 'the most important and valuable' of all medicines and the most widely used. In addition to clinical use, it was the only analgesic available for all minor aches and pains.

Its use was not confined to adults. It was given to children as Mother's Friend to make sure they slept, sometimes because the parents wished to go out either to work or for pleasure. The famous surgeon-apothecary, Samuel Frederick Gray, author of *Gray's Supplement to the Pharmacopaeia*, had his son John Edward, who was a close friend of Morson, trained as an apothecary. He was an assistant early in his career in 1816, in an apothecary's shop in Brick Lane, Shoreditch. John used to recall how he dispensed to mothers, who came from all parts of London, a treacly opium syrup which they made up and stored in a barrel. It became known to the customers as the 'stuff out of the barrel.' So popular was it that some of the more frequent customers called it only 'stuffout' for short. Gray used to finish his story by commenting: 'I fear it poisoned many children.' His fears were probably exaggerated because mothers would not have returned for more if they had been giving their children doses large enough to upset them, although reports of babies being left with baby-minders in Manchester in the 1840s include references to small children dying from overdoses of narcotics. The precise cause of death may not have been known in each case, especially as this was a time of high levels of infant mortality due to housing, disease and sanitary conditions. The use of the opium preparations was not exceptional, Pereira stating that 'we should be careful not to assume that the moderate employment of opium is necessarily detrimental.' There was nothing else available except alcohol. The use of opium was a part of normal living for all classes. As Virginia Berridge[1] has written, its use 'was not a problem. Lack of access to orthodox medical care, the as yet unconsolidated nature of the medical profession and, in some cases a positive hostility to professional medical treatment ensured the position it held in the popular culture of the time.'

John Savory in his Presidential Address to the Pharmaceutical Society in 1848 complained of the indiscriminate sale of 'Infants' Quietness' but did not wish to make it a prescription-only item or even restrict its sale to pharmacists, as was the case in Europe. In that same year, Chevallier,[2] one of the editors of the *Journal de Chimie Médicale*,[3] wrote that a Manchester chemist was selling twenty gallons a week of an opiate mixture to women for their children. He commented that he doubted if the English could be called civilised; he did not say if French pharmacists were doing the same thing – perhaps French wine was a good alternative.

In confirmation of countrywide use of opium for children, we can turn also to Benjamin Stubbs[4] in the Potteries in 1826. He made a sleeping cordial for children containing a dram of crude opium, sweetened with treacle after infusion in half a pint of water. The dose the child took was a fraction of a dram of opium, assuming that he was not expected to drink more than a small portion of the fluid prepared in Stubbs' recipe.

With such a large consumption by children and over a long period, it is interesting that there are very few instances of addiction among people who were given as babies what all described as an addictive substance. Perhaps it is less dangerous than the experts claimed, especially as parents diluted only small quantities of laudanum and discovered by trial how little they could give their infants to send them to sleep. In any case, it is probable that it was better than beer or gin whether in its immediate effects or for the stomach upset that usually follows the use of gin. Very importantly, in most instances, it was cheaper!

Opium was a 'source of cheap and effective relief'[5] from pain and the frequent gastro-intestinal problems from which many suffered as a result of their diet. There were also many men and women doing heavy work causing their limbs to ache and opium provided convenient relief. Constipation was probably the worst effect of frequent opium usage, excepting those addicts whose whole systems were deranged. A serious warning by one toxicologist stated that the regular use of opium 'shortened life expectancy through chronic poisoning.'[6] It was a question of degree. Adults and children openly used opium whenever the need arose.

At the beginning of the nineteenth century when the economy was improving, adults consumed large quantities of opium and there was extensive social use as an alternative to beer. A Mr Scruton, a chemist in Glasgow, stated that laudanum 'was much used among the lower classes' who took 3 or 4 ounces at a time, needing the stimulant effect of the narcotine. The fact that laudanum is mentioned as a stimulant is interesting. While it was well known that narcotine was a stimulant, the use of laudanum was generally as a sedative, the effect of the narcotine usually being initial and transitory before the effect of the morphine was felt. This and other references to the uses of opium raise the question of the degree to which the preparation of opium products was manipulated to produce sedative or stimulating effects long before the scientific explanations were known. The same point was made by a Mr Milner who saw some of his customers twice a day to supply them with an ounce and a half. There were those who voiced their objections to alcohol because there was so much drunkenness as a result; they rarely mentioned laudanum. One witness to a Parliamentary Committee in the 1830s, felt that taxes on beer were driving people to use laudanum instead and that it was a reason for the ever-growing imports of opium.[7]

These imports had been increasing for years and they probably doubled in the twenty years to 1840.[8] But it is difficult to be precise. London was the centre of the opium trade except for the huge quantities which went from India direct to China. A large proportion was re-exported as opium and some which was processed was also exported by the makers of opiate medicines. Until the 1820s, the majority of opium was sold as laudanum or one of the other similar medicines, but how much of this was used for social rather than strictly medical purposes it is not possible to say. There were also large variations in imports from year to year and these were affected by the sizes of the harvests, prices and stocks. Additionally, none of this takes account of indigenous production which was quite significant in the eighteenth century and well into the nineteenth century. The encouragement to local growing and the detailed methods published are powerful evidence for the importance and extent of opium-growing in Britain. There was parallel activity in continental Europe, especially France where Journals made as frequent references to this subject as British ones.

Many doctors grew their own poppy plants and made laudanum for their prescriptions. Philip Miller in his *Gardeners' Dictionary* of 1768 mentions plants growing 5 or 6 feet high with heads as big as oranges. Advice on growing methods appeared in several publications.

The Caledonian Horticultural Society awarded a Prize Medal to James Howieson's sample of 'British Opium' in 1814.[9] He presented a paper the previous December giving very full details of the soil, situation, species, planting method and harvesting 'as best suited to the climate of Britain.' His opium sample was given to Dr Duncan at the Royal Infirmary. From the beginning of February till the end of April 1814, Duncan prescribed it to induce sleep, alleviate pain and 'restrain looseness.' He said it was the equal of the best Turkey opium. Howieson had been employed by the East India Company as Inspector of Opium in Bengal and had studied the methods used in Bengal where '200,000 lb. of opium are made annually.' He preferred the double red garden poppy to the single white one which was used exclusively in India and which had been grown successfully only ten miles from London. He criticised the method used for the 'fields of poppies for the use of the druggists', maintaining that the drill system he employed encouraged good growth and easier harvesting, avoiding the trampling down of part of the crop and the time wasted when bleeding the capsules if they were not in orderly rows. He applied a great deal of thought and common sense to his methods, not least in the way the capsule was wounded for bleeding the latex, while not puncturing it which prevents it from ripening its seed. He scored it by using a small wheel with 'lancets' on it so that by drawing it over the capsule's surface holes were made to allow the latex to exude. The latex dried more quickly than if a knife was used to make an incision – the method used throughout the East. He gathered the juice immediately and dried it in a sunny room.

Dr Howieson felt that the amateur gardener could always make enough opium for 'himself and neighbouring poor' to provide the 'valuable medicine.' Anyway he felt that it 'constitutes a rational and delightful amusement.'

The same attitude was evident in England, although it was understood that haphazard methods resulted in widely differing crops and that the effectiveness of the resulting medicine was uncertain. There was also the rain which spoilt the crop at harvesting time. By the end of the eighteenth century, it was realised that improvements were necessary; so to encourage this, the Royal Society of Arts offered cash prizes and medals for home-grown opium. They published all the details of soil preparation, growing and harvesting.

Some of the methods especially of soil treatment are, of course, ignorant of the nature of soil and the bacterial activity in it. One experiment treated soil with coal dust in one patch to compare the fertility with rabbits' dung in another, horse manure in the third and 'mud from an old drain' in the fourth. Mr Parkes reported in 1823 that the rabbits had been the greatest help though he does not say whether they also ate his crop.

In 1819, two surgeons, John Cowley who was a member of the Royal College, and William Staines, who had a farm at Winslow in Buckinghamshire, had developed their growing and gathering even to the point of developing instruments for capsule cutting; and all their methods were closely supervised in the field. By 1821 they recorded everything and submitted a paper[10] 'in consequence of a premium being offered by the Society for encouraging Arts, Manufactures and Commerce.' They were awarded thirty guineas.

They had produced 60lb from four acres of 'white poppy' and it was said to be as good as Turkey opium. They were supported by six doctors who praised the quality of their product. In their submission in 1822, they went into every detail of cultivation and of preparing the opium, drawing on their own experience and that of others, including a Mr Ball* of Williton whose efforts had been welcomed by the R.S.A. in 1794. The scarifying of the poppy capsule was a great difficulty as, after a number of trials, they devised an instrument with a knife blade made from a watch spring, which protruded only one-thirtieth of an inch from its side. In fact, this was not so different from a device invented by a man named Young and which was used in Scotland.

The opium collectors were trained to make incisions by passing this knife horizontally along the top of the capsule once the petals had fallen and the capsule had a 'bloom' on it. The incision went only a third of the way round. After twenty minutes the latex had dried if the weather was dry and sunny. The opium was gently scraped off with a knife. Successive incisions were made round the

---

* This is the same William Ball, 'surgeon of Williton, Somerset,' to whom the Society awarded four gold medals between 1788 and 1794 for growing the rhubarb, rheum palmatum whose roots were used to make a gentle and effective purgative. It was imported in considerable quantities so the Society encouraged its production to reduce imports following the introduction of the seed from St Petersburg into Scotland. The scheme had limited success; the imported kind was prefered and by the beginning of the nineteenth century, it was no longer a commercial crop (Clifford M. Faust, 'The Society of Arts and Rhubarb', *Journal of the Royal Society of Arts*, March/April/May 1988).

capsule, a second ring being made below the first. They found that four incisions was the optimum, but some capsules could be cut ten times. A day's crop was collected to be dried in the sun in tin containers, the opium being stirred occasionally. When it became malleable it was rolled into balls, the size of coconuts, and these were wrapped in poppy leaves, the same way that the Turks did, but in a different shape. Cowley and Staines provided a costing for this very labour-intensive crop, including details of the wages paid to the men, women and children employed. They included the cost of threshing the dried capsules to obtain the following year's seed and of the turnip crop for which the land was used through the winter.

The women were paid a shilling a day and provided with beer.

The crop in 1823 was 196lb of opium of 'such quality that it sold for two shillings a lb more than the best foreign kinds.' They made a profit of £96 12s. 0d. on an outlay of £274, the opium fetching nearly £300 and the extract from the crushed capsules £28 11s. 6d.

They won the R.S.A. prize for three consecutive years.

The weather played an important part, all operations stopping for rain which washed the opium off the capsule. There were also late frosts killing autumn- sown plants, competition from weeds and hares eating the plants.

In spite of all this, the attraction of a market that they estimated at 40-50,000lb a year was considerable and at a time when the import duty was 8/8d. per lb. They felt justified in proposing that 5,000 acres should be planted. The consumption figure is confirmed by the *London Medical Repository* in 1825 when the editor also commented that indigenous opium commanded the higher price because of quality and reliability.

The year following the success of these two surgeons, another named Jeston was awarded a 'large silver medal' for his improvements in the method of collecting the crop. He had been growing opium for six years. In 1816, the weather was very wet; he collected only 9lb. per acre in comparison with Cowley's 15. In 1821, his crop was 20lb an acre. He employed boys who earned 8 pence a day with a penny bonus for every bottle of opium collected; he called it 'encouragement money.' The numbers employed were high. The end of July and early August was the harvesting time and up to 165 men, women and children were busy and all were given beer twice daily.

It is evidence of his interest in opium and in chemistry that Jeston had read in the *Medical Record* for June 1821of Robiquet's process for separating narcotine from opium, taking advantage of its greater solubility in ether. He must have been one of the first men in

England to try out the new process in his own house. This was the very process that Morson had observed in Paris and which he tried out in Planche's laboratory before using it to his own advantage on his return to Fleet Market in 1821 and announcing that he made morphine 'deprived of narcotine.'

The impetus given by these surgeons to opium production in Britain lasted many years in spite of the unsuitability of the crop to British climatic conditions and the consequent frustrations. In 1836, the *Cyclopoedia of Useful and Ornamental Plants* included a monograph on Papaver somniferum. This pointed out that the plant had naturalised itself. It was grown in great quantities at Mitcham in Surrey, thence it was sold in London at £4 10s. 0d. for a bag of about 3,000 capsules. Its cultivation must have been widespread for it was seen growing wild in Kent, Norfolk and Cambridgeshire. These plants grew 3 or 4 feet high with capsules 2 to 3 inches in diameter, although in Turkey they were described as of 4 inches diameter, some growing 'as large as a baby's head.' Crushed capsules were used in a cold infusion to produce a poppy extract with about an eighth of the strength of laudanum.

The attempts of British growers were matched by Continental ones. Areas of Germany especially near Berlin, Switzerland, Italy, Greece and Yugoslavia were used, with Italy exporting to Britain. France made the most determined efforts, areas of the Somme, Brittany and Provence all being used. The French resented the payment by Europe to Asia of 'an enormous tribute' which James Howieson, who ran the East India Company's Bengal Office, calculated at more than £200,000 in 1822. However, no European country became self-sufficient. In the North, climate was too uncertain and with such labour-intensive harvesting, costs were high. All over Europe costs were higher than in the Middle East and Asia and could not compete with a well-established 'cottage industry.'

In Britain the successive reductions of the tariff were a major factor. Until 1828, the duty was 9/- per lb whereupon it was reduced to 4/- until 1836; then it was 1/- until 1860, when it was abolished. The only cultivation to continue was in the nature of a hobby or in times of crisis; one was the 1939–45 war during which Ransomes[11] used part of their land at Hitchin to grow the poppy as well as their other medicinal plants.

Cultivation in the United States appears to have been on a relatively small scale, even in the warmer climate of the south, the market there being supplied mainly from London.

Medicinally and economically opium was an important crop.

Those concerned avidly inspected samples and learned as much as possible about its growing and harvesting. In the 1830s, both the British and French sent knowledgeable men to visit Persia, Turkey and Egypt who sent back detailed accounts of their discoveries for publication in learned societies' journals. Texier[12] was a Frenchman whose papers were published in the *Journal of the Société de Chimie Médicale*. The journal was first published in 1825 and is filled with contributions from all the famous men working in Paris in the second quarter of the 19th century. As was the habit of the time, they also published items from foreign countries including America.

Morson's attendance at this Society's meetings renewed his friendship with Planche (whose contributions continued until a year or two before his death) and his acquaintance with a long list of men: Robiquet, Pelletier, Guibourt, Henry, Thibouméry, Dorvault, Magendie and Boudet. Speaking French fluently and having earned the respect of all these scientists, Morson's attendance at a meeting was one of the important and most enjoyable occasions of his visits to Paris. He did not contribute a paper, but then there are few enough of these in the transactions of societies of which he was a member. It is clear that he preferred to discuss informally and listen to the news of his colleagues' progress. He had developed a profound respect and liking for the way in which the French organised their scientific lives.

Morson joined the Society at a time when interest in opium was very high. He had a collection of samples from various sources and so reports from men like Texier were of considerable interest and use to his business. Texier pointed out the importance of climate in harvesting the crop. A dry June with low humidity even at night made gathering easy in Turkey, where it was a family affair with the children being trained to incise the capsules and collect the latex. In about 1830, the Constantinople government created a state monopoly but a lively black market developed for about a third of the harvest in south-west Turkey alone and that allowed various methods of adulteration to be widespread.

Morson's friend Guibourt was an expert, examining samples under the microscope so that he could identify their source. He maintained, and used as an indication of purity, that the best Smyrna and Anatolian opiums were made up of fawn-coloured transparent drops, these having oozed from the capsule. They were collected up into balls of about ¹/₂lb, dried and wrapped in poppy leaves; then sorrel seeds were put on them to prevent the blocks from adhering to one another, although this was not always successful.

Guibourt examined samples also from Egypt and Persia and in

these the individual drops could not be seen because the opium was moistened with water, according to Kaempfer[13] who described the opium being kneaded like dough and rolled into a 4¹/₂ inches long sausage about ³/₄ inch thick. They weighed about 2lb, were wrapped in calico and several were then placed in a wicker basket before being packed in a wooden case. Such extensive packing explains the considerable difference between gross weight and nett in the only opium invoice of Morson's to have been kept.

A case of 343lbs of opium weighed 422lbs so about one-fifth of the weight was packing. Guibourt had obtained his sample of Persian opium from Béral,[14] who had brought it to him from London. One is left to speculate if this had been done in conjunction with Morson who, ten years later, was to send his son as an apprentice to Béral's pharmacy. This incident is also an example of the visits that Frenchmen made for scientific purposes to London just as Paris was visited, only more frequently, by English, Scottish and German scientists. In the absence of railways these journeys were lengthy and uncomfortable but the rewards made them worthwhile, although travel weariness had to be overcome.

Morson was in the fortunate position of being able to know what was going on in both London and Paris; but Paris had the advantage

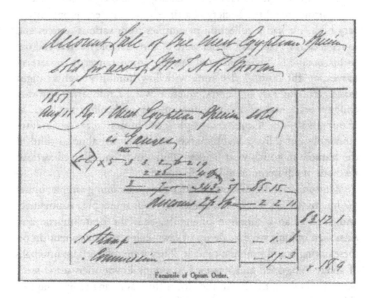

Figure 7: Invoice for a chest of Egyptian opium, dated 11 August 1851.

of several forums for discussion and debate whereas London had none until the formation of the Pharmaceutical Society.

As Morson was purchasing ever-increasing quantities of opium, he made many important contacts as a valued buyer among shippers and traders. He thus learned about the trade in all its aspects, including what was happening in India, only a little of whose production was exported to Britain, nearly all of it going to China.

He made use of his knowledge to write a long essay in 1840 on the 'Opium trade' for the Society for the Diffusion of Useful Knowledge.[15] The essay is anonymous, the clue to its author being the handwriting which is indistinguishable from that in his diary and letter book. Morson also knew many of those involved in the Society. These included Alfred Ainger, who was the Society's architect, other contributors of articles like Daniell and even the Professor of Arabic at Madrid University, Gayangos. Additionally, the aim of the Society was to benefit those who wished to improve their knowledge of literature and science by private reading of pamphlets, written by experts in their field and at a very low price indeed. There is no record of any payment to Morson, nor was his essay published. The views he expresses about Britain's part in the opium trade with China would not have been popular just as the opium wars were being waged.

He was critical of the East India Company and of the Government, revealing a number of figures from sources like parliamentary committees, which would not have been available to those for whom the S.D.U.K. pamphlets were intended. In addition, he strays from a description of the trade into suggestions of a rather naive kind concerning the reduction of opium addiction and the politics of the trade.

To write his essay Morson made use of several books as well as the parliamentary papers in the Library of the British Museum. He had met Richard Solly on the Chemical Committee of the Royal Society of Arts when he lived in Fleet Market. Now that he was in Bloomsbury, Solly was only across Queen Square, living in Great Ormond Street.

Solly was an influential man because he used his great wealth to benefit science at a time when support for scientific societies relied upon the rich for contributions, and help in management through service on committees. He was well educated, having obtained his degree at Magdalene, Cambridge, before studying law in London and being called to the Bar. He was about twenty years older than Morson. Their close friendship lasted until Solly's death in 1858 and they shared interests in the Royal Institution, the Linnean Society and in horticulture. Solly studied plant physiology and anatomy, so there were many common scientific as well as social interests.

Solly used his wealth to further his interest in science. His hospitality and friendliness made him many friends among scientists. They invited him to become a Fellow of the Royal Society in 1807 and of the Linnean in 1826. He took a greater interest in the Linnean, the Royal Institution and the Royal Society of Arts than in the Royal Society, leaving money in his Will to all three. His range of friends may be guessed from the list of those whom he proposed for R.S.A. membership.[16] Two earls, a marquess and a duke feature in the list along with W. T. Brande and Henry Hennell whose scientific achievements were notable as well as being responsible for pharmaceutical production at Apothecaries' Hall; J. S. Bowerbank and A. S. Taylor, who became famous – the one as an expert on sponges and founder of the Microscopical Society and the other as the greatest authority in Europe on medical jurisprudence – were also friends proposed for membership.

Solly typified the well-to-do Regency man, whose philanthropy and interest was founded on knowledge as well as wealth. When he died in 1858, one of his executors was a friend also of Morson – Alfred Ainger. His Will, valued at £80,000, stipulated large legacies, to his sister-in-law, nieces and nephews, totalling some £15,000. They must all have been grateful to their bachelor relative. Solly also remembered his first cousin Edward Solly who was a lecturer in chemistry at the Royal Institution in 1841 and was an F.R.S. Morson knew him when he was secretary of the Society of Arts and met him at the Linnean.

Morson spent a long time in the Reading Room preparing his essay, for he cites sixteen books and journals as references together with more than twice as many references to official papers.

The descriptive passages of the essay are interesting because the circumstances of opium production and trading in India over nearly fifty years are covered, including the means used by the East India Company to exploit the trade which involved huge sums of money, including very high payments to officials, some of them having incomes of £7,000 a year. India exported 4$\frac{1}{2}$ million lbs weight of opium cakes, with a tenth of that amount going to Britain, France and Holland, some of it for re-export to the Far East after processing; in addition one million pounds were used by the Indians themselves.

Calcutta was the centre of this trade and the port from which it was exported until 1830 when Britain extended its influence over opium production to the southern central region of India – Malwa.

The East India Company stimulated production, partly by increasing the price by 50% in the hope of preventing smuggling, but the Malwa region became the principal Indian producer. Even the sale of licences to transport the opium to Bombay netted £150,000 in 1831.

The steady increase in revenues to the Bengal Government culminated in their receiving an average of £1m annually at this time. Then the revenue declined because the quantities doubled and the price dropped from its peak in the 1830s. Between 1790 and 1835 consumption in China increased tenfold, the price increasing from 2¹/₂ Chinese dollars per lb to a peak of $12 in the early 1820s and falling to $4 in the mid 1830s but by then it was estimated that 20,000 chests each of 150 lbs were being shipped to China.

The Chinese officials at Canton also joined in to make money. They levied an unofficial $14 per chest as a fee for turning a blind eye to a banned import. Occasionally this was re-negotiated with the traders after the officials decided they had to confiscate shipments to pretend to their government that they were not idle in preventing illegal imports; at other times they reduced their fee to discourage traders from using small ports along the coast.

It is not surprising that the Chinese Government eventually took measures to reduce the imports and this led to war. They had attempted to persuade their people to give up smoking for a long time. The Emperors issued edicts at intervals from the middle of the eighteenth century onwards, but the habit became more widespread and was indulged in by Chinese in all the countries of the East. Local rulers made it a state monopoly, accepting its use by Chinese residents while forbidding it to their own people. The Dutch in Batavia netted a quarter of a million pounds a year from its sale in the middle of the 1830s.

In 1841, the Chinese built a prison specially for opium smokers providing solitary confinement for all. An ordinance of the Emperor was published: 'Can you, smokers of opium, listen to me without trembling with fright? I desire only your wellbeing in preventing you from the ravages of this frightful poison.' Anyone renouncing the habit could be returned to his family.[17]

By 1860, the two opium wars had ended with the Chinese Government paying compensation to the traders for their losses and cancelling the prohibition. It was a pyrrhic victory, for poppy cultivation in China increased to such an extent that they were soon exporting to India. In 1863–4, China exported over 4 million lbs of opium, about ³/₄ as much as India exported.[18]

The terrible effects of opium and morphine addiction are well-chronicled by the early travellers to the Near and Far East. A few tried it for themselves, describing its effects and the reaction in depression and headache especially when dregs from pipes were smoked and not the 'chandoo' prepared specially for smoking. The instructions for preparing chandoo were published in the *Pharmaceutical Journal* on 18 September 1880 by Hugh McCallum, who was the Government Analyst in Hong Kong. He pointed out that opium smoking was a social habit among the workers in the factories preparing opium for smoking. It was indulged in occasionally when any of their friends paid them a visit. McCullum thought that the process eliminated most of the morphine from the opium. He raised the question of which of the constituents of opium produced the observed effects when inhaled.

Opium smoking was a social habit among Victorian writers and their friends, as it was also in Paris. In the 1860s Morson wrote to a friend in Australia and in passing states that a recent visitor 'knew nothing of opium smoking.' That Morson smoked a little of the substance, which had been a main part of his business and scientific life since his days as an apprentice, is not surprising. We should remember as well that tasting raw materials and medicines was a standard quality check for all pharmacists. It is inconceivable that Morson did more than smoke with his guests occasionally, rather like having a cigar after a good dinner. He had no need to 'drown his sorrows' for, with a successful business and happy family, addiction could be left to those like de Quincey with his low threshold for pain and his intellectualising of his dreams. What is more, Morson had all the knowledge necessary to prepare his 'chandoo' deprived of narcotine. Thus prepared, it was a mild sedative producing a feeling of well-being which is what a good host would wish for his guests. It must not be assumed that there was any secrecy or shame in indulging in this social habit.

Morson exhibited his opium-smoking apparatus at the 1870 British Pharmaceutical Conference. As a precaution against temptation, or most likely because they are interesting and artistic, Morson had in his house the series of twelve Chinese pictures which tell the story of the degradation of a rich young man who takes to opium smoking and slowly ruins himself, becoming poorer as his addiction continues, eventually needing to be supported by his wife's earnings and becoming emaciated, with a parchment-like skin, his head sunk between his shoulders, slinking away from his wife and child.

That Morson was a recognised authority on opium, was consulted widely, with his comments at scientific meetings treated with respect, is exemplified by the frequency with which his views were reported in the *Pharmaceutical Journal* from the very first volume and for many years after. In 1841, when Dr A. T. Thompson was the Professor of Materia Medica at University College, he gave one of the first papers to the Pharmaceutical Society and this was on the subject of opium. It was Morson who was asked to take the chair, not any of the other well known men who had official positions in the Society.

By this time, Morson had twenty years' experience of purchasing and processing opium. He had his own collection of samples for reference purposes, both as a matter of general interest and in particular for checking quality. As a large buyer he was not only entitled to a 2.5% discount on the market price, he had to make sure that the opium brokers were being honest with him over the quality. He exhibited some of his samples at an early meeting of the Pharmaceutical Society; in August 1841 he showed opiums from Smyrna, Constantinople, Egypt, India, Benares, Patna; presumably the Indian was from Malwa.

His expertise was in use, even at the end of his career, when the Australians wanted to market opium in Europe, the price having risen to make it a good proposition. Trade generally had also followed the people who had migrated to Australia and Morson was in the van of those who took advantage of the opportunity. The volume of exports from the U.K. in 1859 of 'Drugs and Chemical Preparations' had reached about £100,000.

Most of Morson's business was done with Hood & Co. of Melbourne.

Hood was born in County Antrim, Ireland and arrived in Australia on 18 June 1840, aged 20. He was still alive in 1877 but his date of death is not recorded.

He joined the firm of R. Wilson & Co., Collins Street, Melbourne and became a 'provisional director.' The firm had been started by Dr Barry Cotter, a surgeon, and was the first chemist's shop in Melbourne; his partner was a Dr O'Mullane. Their partnership was dissolved in June 1840 when the business was purchased by Wilsons.

In 1847 the business was moved to Elizabeth Street. The settlement which became Melbourne grew quite quickly but when gold was discovered at Ballarat and Bendigo the rush to join the digging left many places deserted even of doctors and lawyers. It was serious enough for the Governor to send a despatch on the subject to London.

Hood prospered, becoming a prominent citizen and member of

the Legislative Council. A son became a judge .[19]

The business covered retail pharmacy, wholesaling and trading in gold as well as the opium-growing venture. An advertisement in *The Argus* of 23 January 1850 lists 'Aconitine, emetine, Collodion, Iron quinine citrate, and cod liver oil, potassium bromide and quinine sulphate among the imports of drugs, chemicals, patent medicines and perfumery', all of which were imported quarterly from a 'respectable house in London.' This was certainly T. Morson & Son from both the list of products and Morson's correspondence; his letter book refers to trading between the two firms, with one letter mentioning a credit note for £800 being sent in June 1869.

There is also a letter to Hood's son in the same year expressing the opinion that a tabletting machine referred to in an advertisement was a waste of time!

At the Pharmaceutical Society's Conversazione on 18 May 1869, Morson exhibited photographs of Melbourne and of tobacco grown in Victoria.

When Hood's son visited England in 1867, soon after his marriage, he and his wife visited Dublin to see her uncle who gave her £100. She decided to speculate in opium and bought a number of 14 lb. tins which she asked Morson to ship among goods going to Melbourne. They did not know that in addition to duty, there was a limit on the size of shipments. Unfortunately Hood junior did not reveal that there was more in transit when the Customs found the first consignment. His lying led to great embarrassment, a copy of the Melbourne *Argus* being sent to Morson's son with the report underlined and anonymous comments added! It was also sent to the editor of the *Pharmaceutical Journal* which upset Morson very much. His letter to Hood of 23 December 1867 also mentions other problems. It seems that a large quantity of morphine salts 'with our name or MacFarlans has been sent to Melbourne or Sydney as we have been swindled out of a large quantity.'

He assumed that the same export house was responsible as had purchased Davenport's chlorodyne 'obtained in like manner.' He was very depressed, writing: 'with such commerce it is impossible to compete. It is the story of the Morsons.' Quite what was meant by this last statement is a mystery for there are no indications that the firm suffered from frequent frauds. Perhaps he was depressed by the news that John Hood had been declared insolvent with a debt of £4,000, due to his being surety for 'one Pierce Jones Williams on insufficient security.' The letter ends wishing his friend well and hoping that he would soon overcome all his difficulties.

This recovery appears to have occurred because Morson displayed six samples of Australian opium for Hood at the 1870 Pharmaceutical Conference.[20] He made a particular request that they should be returned to him for further examination and then deposited in the Society's Museum. He was not manufacturing opiates at this time but still kept a close watch on the market perhaps out of habit, or because he knew he could either use it in later manufacture or re-sell the opium. The market in March 1870 was 'in the hands of speculators who rig it.' The price had risen to nearly £2 per lb. whereas for the 'last 30 years it has been about 14/-'. Even though he was seventy years old, and had his son helping, especially on the commercial side of the business, he felt the need to take part, both technically and in the possibility of a bargain.

An early example of his knowledge concerns the sample of British opium submitted to the Society of Arts in 1822. Henry Hennell, who was also on the Chemical Committee, had been asked to test it and obtained a result of 7.57% morphine. He had not, however, kept abreast of Robiquet's work and his analytical method did not distinguish between morphine and narcotine. Morson pointed out[21] that the true result was 4.4% morphine and 2.53% narcotine, making the opium a poor alternative to imported materials.

These results were published by *The Lancet* as part of their comments on British opium by its Analytical Sanitary Commission in 1854 and they also quoted from Morson's and Pereira's reports in the *Pharmaceutical Journal*. *The Lancet's* review of the sources and methods of production of opium is a very interesting and detailed account, making use of reports from all producing countries, in Asia and Europe, and discussing the analyses and opinions from French, German and British chemists. It is significant that the samples from Egypt, generally thought inferior, included one which contained no additions, being categorised as 'genuine'; it contained 14% of alkaloids, a figure twice as high as any other Egyptian one. As this is what Morson was buying in 1851, he was getting very good value for 5/-per lb, when most of the trade papers at that date were recording prices nearer 15/-. While he was not the only manufacturer analysing his supplies before purchase, he was selecting those that suited his needs for those opiates which he wanted for his customers both as pure alkaloids and as proprietary medicines in bulk.

One of the Analytical Commission's purposes was to draw attention to the adulteration of opium that could take place at all points in the chain of supply from harvesting to warehouse. They laid greater emphasis on the admixing of seeds, leaves, grains, stones, wood, sand etc. than on the available means of testing. *Caveat emptor* did not seem to be a principle which they wished to recognise. Undoubtedly adulteration was a problem, but it was not so severe that anyone suggested a return to the eighteenth-century practice in Nuremberg, last reported in 1764, when apothecaries were forced to prepare their medicines in public. The first use of inspection by hand lens probably occurred in the 1820s. In the 1840s microscopy used for detecting adulteration 'became more frequent' according to Ernest Stieb whose description of adulteration justifies the creation of the Lancet Analytical Commission.

Microscopical examination was in use by Robiquet and Texier in the 1830s and spread to more routine use by others in the following decade. A colleague of Morson's, Alphonse Normandy, was one of the first. Some analytical work was done by Richard Phillips. Morson pointed out the benefits of such purity tests in the 1820s. Attfield listed the official tests for impurities in *Pharmacopoeia* preparations. As chemistry advanced so did its use in analysis.

Physical and chemical testing became formally established later in the nineteenth century.[22]

An apocryphal story about Morson says that he carried a knife when inspecting shipments and pushed it into opium cakes to discover any that had wood or stones in them.

It is another example of the extraordinarily fortunate circumstances of Morson's stay in Paris that he arrived there the year after the German chemist, Sertürner, had contributed to a spectacular step in phytochemistry. He had isolated morphine in 1805, but it was the publication of his 1817 paper (more specific, though a repetition of much in the earlier one) to which everyone, especially in Paris, gave so much attention. He gave the base the name 'Morphium' and prepared several salts including the acetate, sulphate and hydrochloride. Just before Morson reached Paris, Planche had prepared the acetate pills, which Magendie asked for and tried in 1818,[23] and the sulphate pills which his trials showed were less active. The woman patient to whom Magendie gave morphine acetate had been ill for a considerable time with sleeplessness and other symptoms.

After four months, she was sleeping well and was generally so much better that the dose was reduced. After a further short period she agreed to try some narcotine pills which excited her, and gave her neuralgia. On resuming the acetate she was sleeping well again. Magendie concluded from this and other cases that both the sulphate and acetate were 'good narcotic substances.' This report in the *London Medical Repository* was translated from the first issue of the *Nouveau Journal de Médecine et Chirurgie,* one of a number of new journals published in Paris at that time.

By 1821, Magendie had done more clinical work and in May published his conclusions in the *Journal de Pharmacie.* He asserted that the 'variable effects of opium are due to the opposite principles of which it is composed.' He proposed the use of Robiquet's process for the isolation of narcotine, published in 1821 after he was asked to confirm Sertürner's work. Journals in London and Philadelphia were quick to recognise that here was a scientific explanation for their experience.

To arrive in Paris as a student of Planche at this very time was more beneficial than Faraday can have foreseen or Morson anticipated. Of all the eminent men to work with, the choice of Planche was extraordinary. One is left wondering what Dr Tupper knew of the chemical developments in Paris and of the individuals involved in them.

At the same time that Magendie was trying out morphine salts, Orfila, the Spanish toxicologist working in Paris, did some work on animals which he published in 1822. His work was academic and he concluded that opium extracts were more potent than the amount of morphine in them suggested. Opium preparations are absorbed more slowly than pure alkaloids so the effects take longer to appear. This persuaded doctors that the pure alkaloids were too powerful and, allied with a natural conservatism, it was many years before opiate alkaloids were included in the *London Pharmacopoeia.*

Robiquet's isolation of narcotine and knowledge of its effects was confirmation that the frequently observed initial excitement of a patient was due to this alkaloid in opium before the sedative effect of morphine took place. It is not surprising that de-narcotised laudanum remained a first choice. It was less expensive, so the use of alkaloids spread slowly, in spite of Magendie's work.

Morson made all the morphine salts available on his return to London, including the one recommended by Magendie in the first edition of his *Formulaire –* the solution of morphine acetate. It was Morson's first supply of any alkaloid to Allen, Hanbury & Barry in 1822.

Arguments about the effectiveness of laudanum versus the pure alkaloidal salts were confused by the continuing discussions about the amounts of alkaloid in opium. Only slowly was the variable content attributed to growing conditions in the different countries. As late as 1851, Garrod discussed the variable strength of tinct. opium in a paper to the Pharmaceutical Society.[24]

Prescription books of around 1830 confirm physicians' preference for laudanum in spite of the reliability and convenience of the alkaloids; it was mainly cost which controlled the choice. The situation is also made clear by the absence of any entry for morphine in a prescription book of T. & W. & W. Southall in Birmingham dated 1828. Books covering the period from 1821 to 1834 at Savory & Moore in Bond Street contain hardly an entry until 1833 when Drs Prout, Brodie and Elliotson were prescribing 'Morph.Mur' (morphine hydrochloride) and Sir Charles Scudamore had two patients regularly taking the acetate in 1834. Assuming these books, from two different places of differing social status, to be representative of general practice, it was more than ten years after they were first available that regular prescribing of opiates started. By 1840, every month includes an entry for acetate and muriate.

Morson's close friend, John Savory, who was so extremely successful as senior partner in Savory & Moore, wrote *A Companion to the Medicine Chest* whose first edition was published in 1836 by John Churchill, who was to become the publisher of the *Pharmaceutical Journal* in 1841. Savory wrote of morphine acetate, muriate and sulphate, that 'these preparations exert a very powerful narcotic influence on the system, without acting at the same time as a stimulant like opium. They are therefore preferable.'

The Savory & Moore and Southall prescription books indicate the difference between the use of opiate alkaloids and opium on the one hand and of quinine and bark on the other. The frequency of prescriptions for quinine in 1829 in the Southall book is seven times that of bark. Savory's *Companion* comments that 'patients often die of malignant fevers because they cannot swallow the necessary quantity of bark in powder' to obtain an effective dose.

These figures and comments summarise the differing circumstances that Morson had to confront in recommending 'his new chemical preparations' to doctors and patients.

In spite of the interest in and use of morphine, it did not appear in the *London Pharmacopoeia* until the 1836 edition. There had been many proposals for its inclusion and the elder Dr Babington, whose lectures at Guy's Hospital Morson had attended as an apprentice, had been given the task of producing the new edition. He arranged for five alkaloids, iodine and bromine to be added. This had taken twelve years, for the 1824 edition had been criticised for failing to include morphine, quinine and iodine. The timing was very different from creosote, which Morson introduced in 1834 and was included in the

1836 *Pharmacopoeia*. Even though the latter included morphine, the Lancet Analytical Commission decided to make the recommendation that pure alkaloids should be prescribed in preference to crude opium because preparations of them could be of 'ascertained strength.'

The early 1830s was a period of academic activity with opiate alkaloid processes. In 1828, Henry & Plisson of the Pharmacie Central had published[25] a method of eliminating narcotine from opium without using alcohol. In 1831, Gregory developed a process in Edinburgh[26] which had the additional advantage of a higher yield.

Robiquet reviewed[27] Gregory's work, giving him credit for making an important advance in attracting attention to morphine hydrochloride. He pointed out that the process did not isolate morphine at any stage, but produced the two hydrochlorides, one of which was Robiquet's new discovery – codeine.

It is significant that Henry stated that one of the aims of his work was to 'bring this precious medicine within reach of the less well-off.' Robiquet stressed the importance of avoiding the use of alcohol, 'always very expensive, above all in England' where the price was exceptionally high.

He now accepted that his 1822 process, which was the one he and Morson had used, did not completely eliminate narcotine from morphia. He had not suspected this previously. The most important feature of the process was the elimination of alcohol which the alternative processes required. This was also a prime factor in the success of Edinburgh firms in manufacturing morphine salts.

The academic activity in Paris was also stimulated by work in Germany by Merck, who began his alkaloid factory in 1828 and drew attention to his process improvements in 1830.*

Gregory was a doctor, therefore concerned with pain, but as a practising chemist he was concerned about the variable strength of

---

* Merck built an alkaloid factory at Darmstadt, Germany. The French, and then Morson in 1821, were thus followed by the production in Germany seven years later. MacFarlan in Scotland started in 1831. These firms probably supplied many wholesalers who had large export business in addition to their domestic markets. Savory, Allen & Hanbury and Corbyn all exploited the markets opened up by the expansion of Empire. According to the Philadelphia Record of 22 April 1918, a Swiss and a German started a company called Seitler and Zeitler in St John's Street in that city and were the first to manufacture opiate alkaloids in the U.S.A. producing morphine sulphate in 1823. The firm was bought by George D. Rosengarten in 1832, but the name was not changed to Rosengarten until 1845.

laudanum. He provided a solution to the problem which meant also that a dose of 'Gregory's Salt' was no more expensive than laudanum.

The small community of medical men in Edinburgh were soon talking about Gregory; he had never practised medicine, preferring chemistry which he studied under Liebig at Giessen. He was later to lament the fact that nearly every chemist of importance in Britain in 1842 had had to go to study in Paris, Berlin, Giessen or Göttingen.[28] He and another Scot, Lyon Playfair, were subsequently to translate Liebig's works into English.

Morson's friend of 1822, and the first to use his quinine, Dr David Dickson, was at this time in charge of the Naval Hospital at Plymouth. He wrote a *Report on the Effects of the Muriate of Morphia* on 8 February 1832 which Gregory's friend Montgomery Robertson saw and mentioned in a clinical and chemical paper[29] which did much to publicise the clinical successes with morphine hydrochloride and Gregory's salt by doctors all over the country. Dickson had only a small quantity of the hydrochloride 'put into his hands' and used it all in five days on sailors in the Plymouth Naval Hospital. He concluded that its cheapness, purity and permanence made it a 'valuable addition to the Dispensatory, and to the military and naval medicine chest.' It would be pleasant to record that this material came from Morson, but we cannot be certain, for Robertson includes only an extract from Dickson's report which would perhaps, like his quinine paper, have stated the source of his supply, but his report was a naval one and was not published in full by Dr Robertson.*

Dr Robertson's paper starts by drawing attention to the fact that the acetate and sulphate of morphine 'have made small progress in the estimation of the British practitioner.' This was due to so much that was produced by chemists being impure, even adulterated. He quoted an instance in Paris, of a young man who swallowed 24 grains of morphine acetate in a suicide attempt, but it was so impure that he survived. The failure of physicians to use these salts was due to 'the carelessness of the manufacturer and the knavery of the vendor.'

Up to this time, Morson was the only manufacturer of morphine in Britain. Now, however, the Scottish chemists seized a chance which created a new industry in Edinburgh.

---

* A search at the Public Record Office did not reveal the presence of this report in the Admiralty Records; amongst the *Reports of Medical Officers* nor in the *Reports of the Physician-General* of the Navy for the period 1822-52 (ADM 105).

Gregory's paper states that medical practitioners, 'who may wish to satisfy themselves of its [Gregory's Salt] efficacy, may procure it in a state of purity at Messrs. Duncan & Ogilvy, or Messrs. Cheyne of the Apothecaries Hall, Edinburgh.' He had helped friends to operate his process, so this reference is not to material he had produced himself. Besides, Duncan & Ogilvy, two years later to be Duncan, Flockhart, were both competent chemists and had set up a pharmacy at 52 North Bridge after creating a successful business in Perth. There is a reference to Duncan's sale of morphine in Robertson's paper of 1832. It would appear, therefore, that Duncan prepared small quantities of Gregory's Salt, probably for sale to physicians who were clients of his pharmacy, early in 1832.

The only early paper published by T. & H. Smith was an article detailing a 'Process for preparing a pure and concentrated solution of opium, free of narcotine', and this was published[30] in August 1841. It makes the assumption that opium 'will continue, in all probability, to be preferred by medical men.' The process produced a solution much paler than laudanum and Smiths claimed that it was freer of impurities than a similar extract made by Robiquet.

MacFarlan is said to have given Gregory's paper to his partner, David Rennie Brown, who was a chemist and who wrote on his copy that it was 'all the instruction I got.' It was Brown's skill that enabled MacFarlan to be the first Scottish manufacturer soon after publication of Gregory's 1831 paper.

Now that there was available something which showed a real advantage over laudanum, sales increased and by 1834, MacFarlans were making it regularly and in 1836 established a factory specially for opiate alkaloids. They were followed in 1837 by T. & H. Smith, also in Edinburgh, which was now to become one of the greatest centres for the processing of opium, retaining its pre-eminence for a very long time.

The medical men had still to be convinced of the superiority of the pure alkaloids and use increased only slowly. It was at a much lower level than after Wood's work on intravenous injection in 1853. Alexander Wood was the first to use a hypodermic syringe, a development which caused a huge increase in the demand for pure morphine hydrochloride, so helping the business of his fellow Scots.

Nearly all the records of Morson's, MacFarlan's and Smith's production have been lost. In Morson's case none has survived. We have to fall back on the ledgers of his account at the Bank of England, opened in 1841. They are only a partial record, since he used other bank accounts whose records are lost. A further difficulty arises over the conversion of the money figures to quantity of opium. The trade prices published in various journals are either retail or standard trade ones; Morson's reputation and the size of his consignments would have ensured that he purchased at a considerable discount. The only extant invoice for Egyptian opium charges him 5/-per lb and shows that he got a 2·5% discount on the price, without revealing if this was due to quantity or was for cash. Such a discount was negotiated also by Smiths, who forfeited it when they resold to firms making their own laudanum; an indication that it was a quantity discount. They, as well as MacFarlan for instance, supplied Ransomes at Hitchin. Presumably this was an assurance of quality for Ransomes as well as avoiding the need for them to visit London for auctions which would have required expertise only learnt by regular attendance over a long period.

In the 1850s opium prices were very stable, an examination of published prices showing that they remained so until the sudden increase fifteen years later. In 1858 there is a report of Egyptian opium being delivered at 6/8d. per lb before it rose towards 17/- by the late 1860s. If Morson could negotiate a price of 5/-, that is, some 25% lower than the published price of a few years later, and for only one case, it is reasonable to conclude that purchasing power was used effectively by the larger buyers. MacFarlan's and Smith's ability to negotiate lower prices need not be doubted so their profitability in opiates was somewhat higher than the available records suggest.

Besides, they soon accumulated enough experience to purchase opiums whose proportions of the main alkaloids suited their purposes, just as Morson was using Egyptian. This also had an important effect on the cost of production.

When calculating volumes, therefore, all we can do is use the trade price and bear in mind that it causes inaccuracy; it is also no help that Morson's ledger record of purchases applies to one supplier only. Since the ledgers cover the time when manufacture was at the factory in Hornsey, we can only be sure that the calculation produces minimal figures and that the possible error may be as high as 50%. It is unfortunate that we cannot know what Morson's consumption of opium after 1860 was, beyond the fact that it was described as 'huge.' It must have increased steadily before declining later in the century. By 1870, the effects of competition from Scotland and Germany, difficulties in his own firm, reduced profits and more variable market conditions had led him to be selective about which alkaloids to manufacture and which to buy-in.

Unlike the Bank of England, who have never destroyed a ledger record, MacFarlan's records, on the death of a partner, were burnt, or in Smith's case, put down a well which was then sealed. Presumably this had some advantage when excise or estate duties were negotiated. Fortunately, a few items missed this ritual destruction, including opium purchase quantities, yields and prices of products, but only for short periods after 1857.

MacFarlan* kept a chart of opium consumption and of alkaloid and opium trade prices. The quantities purchased are recorded, case by case, from 1864 to 1904, with other information going back to 1855, on graph paper that covers some 8 feet square. The opium purchases would have been the total ones, that is, they were used for galenicals, resale and processing. It is believed that these latter were about half the total and this was confirmed for the early years of this century by their own process records.

According to a former director of MacFarlans, the last quarter of the nineteenth century saw their production reach a quarter of a million ounces of opiates per year. By the yardstick in use by the companies for their early operations, this would mean that 55 tons of opium were processed. The records indicate only around 30 tons, but variations of yield and alkaloidal content of opium could explain large discrepancies; there may also have been differences due to the mix of the different alkaloids that were being produced.

· T. & H. Smith's figures show they were processing twice as much opium as their rivals, thus contradicting the opinion that they processed four times as much opium as MacFarlans. Perhaps rivalry exaggerated the difference. Smith's records are for process only and were supplemented by a summary extracted by Ken Reid.[31]

They can be cross-checked in some years from output of alkaloids using their standard yield of 2 ounces of products from a pound of opium – an improvement from Duncan's day, when he only continued 'so long as he got the price of a pound of opium for an ounce of morphine.' With all these uncertainties, the figures are only a broad guide.

The table comparing these three firms' usages, however, illustrates two points: Morson's manufacture increased twenty times

---

* I received help from Dr Marshall Smalley, managing director of MacFarlan Smith, and from Mr K. C. Reid, formerly in charge of research and development, who worked on the firm's archives after his retirement. Many records were made available. My appreciation of their efforts and kindness to me is recorded with much gratitude.

in as many years and was continuing to increase until the 1870s: and the much greater use of opiates through the century. It clearly shows how the Edinburgh firms' grasped their opportunity, part of it at Morson's expense.

Opium Purchase in Tons

Years	Morson	Macfarlan	Smith
1821-40	n/a	None	None
1841-44	¹/₄	n/a	n/a
1845	2	n/a	n/a
1850	2	n/a	n/a
1855	2	n/a	¹/₂
1860	5	n/a	2
1865	5 ¹/₂	36	9
1870	n/a	34	5
1875	-	40	27
1880	-	32	19
1885	-	35	24
1890	-	31	30
1895	-	32	n/a
1900	-	-	n/a

Source: Macfarlan Smith Archive and Morson's Bank of England account; one supplier only.

Note: It is probable that Morson divided his purchases between brokers; thus his usage could have been at least double the figures shown.

The two Edinburgh firms imported their opium very largely from Smyrna, where sales averaged 3,000 cases per year in the period 1857–66[32]. At that period the average usage in Edinburgh was 564 cases or some 19% of the output of Europe's largest supplier. The cost of this was probably a maximum of £70,000.

Using the ratios mentioned, the sales value of the opiates produced was at least £90,000. The proportion achieved by each firm is not known but the total shows how substantial this business had become. If estimated from the available records, Morson's sales in the middle of the century, and before the substantial rise in the use of opium after 1850, may well have been in the range of £15,000 to £25,000. Opium-related products must have been one of the largest contributors to overall business for about thirty years starting around 1830.

Profits must have been earned on at least a satisfactory level even if they were small when trading problems were severe. MacFarlan's chart reveals the wide and sometimes sudden fluctuations in both opium and product prices. Both firms used the yardstick that the alkaloids were profitable when they sold for twice the cost of their opium content.[33] Even though labour and equipment costs were low in the last century, the expense of selling all over the world in a competitive market would have been high. That profits were slim at times can be calculated from records of early this century when MacFarlan's expenditure on opium reached nearly £300,000 and the income, calculated from their morphine hydrochloride and codeine sales only and at the prices in the chart, was only £50,000 greater; this is a small return and ignores all the outgoings except their raw material.

From about 1855 competition became intense, so prices fell. The eighty years following Morson's 1821 Price List show a progressive decline.

In 1821 and 1825, records show Morson charging 144/- per ounce. Two years later Morson agreed with Barry for Allen, Hanbury & Barry to have 'a further supply' at 45/-. Competition from France was the cause of this, for the A., H. & B. price book shows imports from brokers in London who were known for their contacts in Paris. The years 1830 and 1835 show further reductions to 30/- and 20/- respectively.

The competition from Scotland halved the price again by 1837, but in 1838 it rose to 12/-; only to fall again to 8/- in 1840. After a further fall of 1/-, these morphine salts rose to 10/-, the stock at Clay & Abraham in Liverpool[34] being valued at that figure in 1845. Prices rose again to 12/8d. the following year. In 1848, they fell, Morson invoicing Allen & Hanburys in February at 9/6d., a figure quoted by Herrings[35] in their catalogue of 1853. Morson issued a price list in 1878 and listed the three (acetate, hydrochloride and sulphate) at 8/6d. an ounce.

Over nearly sixty years the price had fallen to 1/17th of what Morson charged when he first made it available; and most of this reduction took place by 1840. The French and Germans were the main competition to Morson until MacFarlan entered the trade. MacFarlan's first sale to Allen & Hanburys was in 1838, 12 ounces being sold at 11/- per ounce, undercutting Morson by 1/-. The competition did not affect Morson's sales of either pure morphia or the hydrochloride and acetate, so Allen & Hanbury's business was expanding. In 1840, Morson sold them 50 ounces and 64 ounces in 1841, getting the lion's share of their purchases.

MacFarlans had the advantage of the lower cost of alcohol in Scotland. This was very significant as the prices mentioned by Apothecaries' Hall in their evidence to the Parliamentary Commission in 1834 shows 2/6d. per lb in England and 1/9d. in Scotland. Paying only two-thirds of the price was advantage enough but by 1847 this had increased to just under a half.

One of MacFarlan's records of 1851 shows that they made a trial purchase of Morson's opiates, but unfortunately there are no details. Morson's ledgers show purchases from MacFarlan on an infrequent and minor basis until late in the century.

The three firms continued to expand their business and, as the opiate side would not have been subsidised for long, so their processing efficiency was constantly improved as selling prices fell, but this trade did not provide the profits that many other pharmaceutical chemicals achieved.

It must not be overlooked that all three firms had a profitable trade in proprietary products. In his 1825 catalogue Morson lists Paregoric Elixir and Lozenges besides the established Godfrey's Cordial and Braithwaite's Black Drop. By the 1830s he was supplying Tinct.Morph.Mur.(Morson) to, among others, the Highgate Pharmacy.[36] By 1850, his wholesale and retail trade in these kinds of products was increased with the introduction of his chlorodyne whose sales continued until about 1930; labels of that period stated that the 1850 formula was still in use.

Whatever the economics of the opiate chemical trade , the chemistry fascinated a large number of scientists. All over Europe discussions about opium and its sources continued while chemists sought new developments in processing, much of it kept as trade secrets, and in working out the formulae of the alkaloids they discovered. Morson was directly involved in both aspects throughout his life.

One of Morson's friends was Alexander Williamson,[37] described as one of the most influential chemists of the century, who succeeded Fownes as Professor of Practical Chemistry at University College. He had a protégé at St Mary's Hospital and arranged for Morson to supply narcotine for their researches into its chemical composition.[38] Matthiessen[39] worked with Foster on the structure of narcotine and cotarnine, work which had started about 1830 with Pelletier and had been followed up by Liebig in 1832 and continued with the publication of a paper for the new Chemical Society in 1844 by Blyth.[40] This work was taken further by Dr C. R .A. Wright, also at St Mary's who discussed his work with David Rennie Brown at

MacFarlans in 1875–6 because they supplied him with various alkaloids for his work, among them codeine, papaverine and narceine. Wright was continuing Matthiessen's work, receiving a Royal Society grant; part of this was a search for derivatives of some of these alkaloids for which he asked for a supply of crude narcotine to 'break up' into opianic acid and cotarnine.[41]

Williamson noted in 1863 that Morson had prepared for Matthiessen the nine samples of narcotine 'with scrupulous care' and that they had resulted from the 'huge quantities of opium' that Morson was processing, the residues used for this having accumulated during the preparation of very large quantities of morphine and codeine from opium of various qualities and sources. He arranged for Dr G. Merck, and Hopkin and Williams also to supply samples, three from the former and two from the latter. Both Hopkin and Williams* were apprenticed to Morson, who had passed on to them his 'scrupulous care' in the preparation of pure chemicals.

It is not surprising that so much academic work was done on opiates. Their use was increasing significantly; competition for greater purity at a lower cost caused an emphasis on process development. To permit this an improvement in the knowledge of chemical structures of opiates was needed. It is an interesting comment on the complexity of these structures and the state of chemical science at the time that, although Kop[42] in 1825 had forecast that alkaloids would be synthesised, it was 127 years before an American would find a synthesis for morphine, albeit one that is not viable.

That MacFarlans were the first manufacturers in Scotland is confirmed, at least to the extent of what he admitted was a less than perfect memory, by D. B. Dott,[43] who wrote on his retirement in 1934 that his firm was reputed to have precedence over Smith's and that they had started by using what Dott termed the Gregory-Robertson process. This was in use for many years and made a

---

* William King Hopkin and John Williams were assistants at Morson's Southampton Row pharmacy in the late 1840s. (There was also an assistant named P. T. Heys at this time.) Hopkin and Williams left Morson's service to set up on their own at the premises that Hopkin occupied at 5 New Cavendish Square, London, in 1849. They quickly earned a reputation for quality and for the purity of the chemicals they made similar to Morson's own reputation. At the 1851 Exhibition, they showed samples of aconitine in direct competition with Morson. Their other exhibits included chromic acid, ammonium benzoate, tannin and mercury biniodide. They were one of the first firms to market a range of analytical reagents.

product 'of a greyish colour.' Dott made very important improvements in the opiate extraction processes and took out a patent for preparing codeine 'artificially' – a reference to the conversion of morphine into codeine, which Robiquet discovered in 1832.

The greyish colour must have been eliminated, even if specially recrystallised samples were used, by the time of the Great Exhibition. Both Morson and MacFarlan were praised for their exhibits. While there is no clue to the purity of their routine production, both firms were jealous of their technical reputation. Some samples of Morson's other exhibits,* which certainly date from late last century and may be considerably older, were tested in 1990 and were of the current standard of purity for analytical reagents. The only indication about the colour of their routine morphine production is provided by occasional references in both French and British journals as early as the 1830s to samples which were 'snow white.'

Morson and MacFarlan cooperated in technical matters. In 1849, the latter sent Morson a letter accompanied by samples so that he could have confirmation of his results before publication in the *Pharmaceutical Journal*.[44] MacFarlan believed that morphine hydrochloride adulterated with salicine had been sold in Scotland. His analysis resulted in his writing that the material contained 54.73% of morphine instead of the 76.15% for the genuine salt. Morson confirmed that a large quantity of cheap material had been sold in London, writing that 'this sophisticated preparation is not distinguishable in appearance from the genuine'. His greater expertise, however, enabled him to report, three weeks after forwarding MacFarlan's letter to the editor, Jacob Bell, that his tests showed that sugar was the culprit. He knew that several hundred ounces had been sold over a period of twelve months so there were many doctors wondering why their patients had not benefited as they should. The report was repeated in the *Journal de Pharmacie*.

As the two most important manufacturers, the commercial aspects were vital, the sale of spurious material having depressed the price. The incident might have implicated Smiths had Bell not been at pains to point out in an editorial note that MacFarlan had written to exonerate Smiths of any participation in such a fraud, adding that the 'real offenders are known and do not reside in Edinburgh.' Three

---

* The samples were from the special glass jars used for exhibitions and were Potassium Iodide, Potassium Dichromate, Potassium Sulphate and Nickel Sulphate. It is remarkable that the iodide contains no free iodine after a lapse of at least a century.

months later, accusations by a London chemist against his supplier were published in the journal in the form of their exchange of letters.

Throughout this incident, Morson's opinion was sought first by MacFarlan and then by I. & J. Wright, who asked him to test the morphine which was the subject of their dispute with Heathfield & Burgess, their supplier.

I. & J. Wright, who were druggists in Holborn, were customers of the firm of Heathfield and Burgess of 8 Wilson Street, Finsbury. The latter complained that their customer would not tell them what the impurity in their morphine acetate and hydrochloride was. Wrights sent a sample to Morson who, they wrote, confirmed that the acetate was not pure. Heathfield & Burgess wrote asking Morson to tell them what the impurity was. Naturally all that Morson was prepared to tell

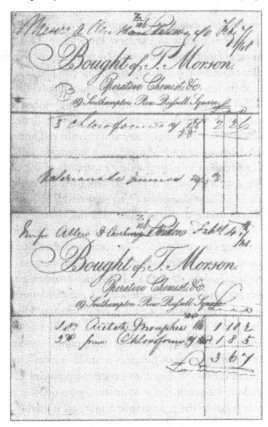

Figure 8: Firm's invoices for morphine acetate
and chloroform, 1848.

them was that he had examined two samples for Wrights, to whom he referred Heathfields for the details. Wrights refused to reveal them so the incident ended inconclusively with Heathfield complaining about Wright's attitude.

Bell's editorial comment pointed out that those making criticisms should support them with conclusive evidence.

Morson was being consulted for his ability and reputation as a chemist and not as a manufacturer.

The incident draws attention to the extent of fraud being practised, but also to the failure to test supplies, a practice that was not to change for many years, the reputation of wholesale suppliers being the criterion for relying on products being up to standard.

Incidents of this nature did nothing for the standing in which pharmacists were held, especially as they were recurrent and, in some instances, revealed ignorance of well-published processes. Even well known men were reluctant to use new knowledge. In 1824, the *Monthly Gazette of Health* raised the issue by pointing out that Battley had found that two hundred grains of morphine had had little effect – and this was at the very time that Magendie had reported that three grains had killed a dog! Battley was invited to publish his analytical method; meantime, the editor appended an anonymous letter from 'a most able philosophical and pharmaceutical chemist of London.' This may well have been written by Morson, with its references to French chemists and prices and including a clear expression of the chemistry involved. The author points out that Battley used a method which dissolved out the morphine before he prepared his laudanum and finished with a warning that true laudanum did contain morphine; without criticising Battley, he most especially wanted to discourage anyone from taking pure morphia 'as the result would be fatal.'

There was another occasion when Morson's skill was used to good effect. When the Society of Arts in 1834 had awarded a prize for English opium, Morson repeated Hennell's tests. His letter provides another example of the reasons for his great reputation. His opinion was that the opium was not unlike the bad varieties of Egyptian opium and inferior to that from Turkey: 'it contained codeine and a larger proportion than usual of meconic acid. 20 ounces avoirdupois of the dry opium contain 384 grains of pure morphia and 220 grains of narcotine. Mr Hennell in his examination gave 662$\frac{1}{2}$ grains – a quantity nearly equal to the narcotine and morphia united.'[45] Morson repeated Hennell's analysis and did not agree with him.* This incident

---

* See page 136, for further details of this incident.

had interest for French chemists, particularly Magendie, who referred to it in his *Formulaire* of 1836. He recognised Morson's ability by writing that he had no confidence in Hennell's results.

Hennell's test method had been published and reveals that it was out of date, not utilising the improvements in chemical technique that had been made in France and Germany, techniques which Morson not only read about but could discuss with friends ,particularly Robiquet who was the one making the most progress at that time.

The discussions about opium, of necessity less precise and scientific, were no less voluminous than the chemical work.* The French, German and British journals are filled with papers, comments and speculations about this fascinating plant and its harvesting, trade and variable alkaloidal content. Morson played a large part in this too, the *Pharmaceutical Journal* being peppered with his opinions. In a few instances he worked with John MacFarlan, their views being repeated in the French journals after publication in the *Pharmaceutical Journal*. Before this time, Morson's reputation was recognised throughout Europe. The *Journal de Pharmacie* reported in October 1845 his comments in the *Pharmaceutical Journal* about a new sort of opium without referring to the latter journal nor did they feel it necessary to include any personal details about him. The Dutch journal, *Berigten des Nederlandsche Mautschappij ter Bevordering det Pharmacie* (1845) – No.3,.23-4, one of the first pharmaceutical journals in the Netherlands, also referred to Morson's work in opium. In this instance they refer to his carrying out both chemical and microscopical examinations to determine how the opium had been treated and revealing 'die bij uitstek arm aan Morphine is, en daarentegen de aanzienlijke hoeveelheid van een derde berat, van eene veerkrachtige stof, uit Was in eene naar Caoutschouk gelijkende stof bestaande.'

As a well-recognised expert, Morson's experience was used by the Pharmaceutical Society from its inception. In the first volume of its journal, there is a report of Morson's opinion of some spurious

---

* Robert Christison worked on different opiums not only to attempt a means of identifying the different working types and sources but to improve the tests used to determine morphine content. He sent a long letter to Guibourt (*Journal de Pharmacie*, Vol. 21, 1835, 542–8) describing his work. The letter also had the purpose that his observations 'puissent être regardées comme un titre pour être admis au nombre des correspondans de la Société de Pharmacie.'

opium which had been sent 'a few hours before' by Lescher who, in turn, had been sent the sample by a general practitioner and who read to the meeting a letter published in *The Times*. Members asked Morson to say how he examined opium and he described his method which owed something to Guillermond and other European scientific colleagues for the development of chemical tests. This was the first of many occasions on which Morson's expertise was shared with his colleagues.

Being a natural product, processed locally by methods handed down from one generation of peasants to the next, the alkaloidal content and mix in opium varied widely. Even after fifty years of alkaloid extraction this variability could cause problems. Morson led discussion[46] in 1869 about Liquor Opii. The question of its strength arose and he remarked: 'the quality of opium should be made the basis of any good process for while differences occurred in the amount of morphia in different samples to the extent of 200%, there could be no uniformity when this was overlooked.' Morson concluded with typical modesty; he had had something to do with opium during his lifetime and it was never the same twice.

Some of this caution born of great knowledge would have prevented Battley and many others, who were so mistaken in their views and ignorant of the chemistry in spite of the published work of French chemists and later of Morson, Williamson and Matthiessen, from spreading false information.

Morson's interest in and his reputation with opium and opiates continued throughout his career. At the last British Pharmaceutical Conference that he attended in 1870, he was involved in presenting the paper and six samples of Australian opium, which had been sent by his friend Hood, who was encouraging opium-growing in 1869.

Morson had found very little morphia and a great quantity of the other alkaloids. Hood wrote that 'an opinion from so well known an authority on all concerned with opium' discouraged the Australian farmers. The next year further samples were sent from those who had persisted with growing opium and, Morson's opinion being so much thought of, he was asked to analyse samples from six areas which showed 8–10% morphia. A trial shipment to London was then made. Hood added that it would be some years before they would have a surplus for export because local consumption was enormous due to the large numbers of Chinese in the colony.

The discussion after this report was made included a comment from H. B. Brady[47] about opium production in Norfolk. So it was still the case that local needs were being met partially by local production, although it may not have been used for laudanum, but for the poppy-heads to be made into an infusion, popular as a means of getting rid of a headache. That it was grown locally is also a factor which makes estimating British consumption of opium based on import figures quite misleading.

Estimates of the consumption[48] of opium in Britain in the nineteenth century based on the difference between the official figures for imports and exports of opium are bound to be misleading. Firstly they disregard the significant volume of indigenous production. Secondly, there was a substantial export of pharmaceutical products derived from opium, especially from 1840 onwards. These products ranged from those containing opium to opiate alkaloids and medicines containing them.

MacFarlans, Smiths and Morsons all made direct and, via other pharmaceutical firms, indirect exports over many years; one example being Morson's chlorodyne, which from 1850 onwards was widely used as more British people travelled to European countries. As the century progressed, MacFarlans, developed a very large export trade in opiates.

We should take into account that indigenous growing of opium is another factor whose size is completely unquantifiable, even though it was actively encouraged from the late eighteenth century. This was partly an import-reduction exercise until the climatic and labour-cost advantages of the Middle Eastern countries were recognised; afterwards, duty abolition finally made encouragement unnecessary.

Morson's expertise, gained early in his life, was supplemented by the knowledge acquired in processing the 'huge' quantities of opium at his Hornsey factory, once the premises at Southampton Row had been outgrown. His production was of a size that the sales contributed a large proportion of the firm's income. It is surprising that his knowledge was never the subject of a published scientific paper, but he seems to have avoided that means of enhancing his reputation, though he made good use of the academic work of his friends in Europe.

His achievement was to start an industry which flourished and to maintain his business and scientific reputation for half a century, contributing to raising standards both in product quality and in his profession.

Notes

1. Berridge and Edwards, *Opium & the People,* London: Allen Lane, 1981, 37.
2. Cf. Chapter 4, note 16.
3. *Journal de Chimie Médicale,* founded 1825, publication ceased 1876; Guibourt, Henry, Pelletier, Planche, Robinet and Robiquet were frequent contributors. Alphonse Chevallier was *rédacteur* of this journal from its inception. In 1850, Morson was appointed the only Briton among six collaborators and remained so for more than ten years.
4. *Pharmaceutical Historian,* Vol. 20, No.1, March 1990,6.
5. Parsinnen, Terry M., *Secret Passions, Secret Remedies, Narcotic Drugs in British Society, 1820–1930,* Philadelphia: Institute for the Study of Human Issues, 1983, 35.
6. Christison, Robert, 'The Effects of Opium-eating on Health and Longevity', *Edinburgh Medical and Surgical Journal* 37 (1832), 123–35.
7. Select Committee on Adulteration of Food, Drink and Drugs, 1854, Vol. VIII, para. 2073; evidence of P. L. Simmonds.
8. Public Record Office, *Annual Statistics of Trade in Opium,* 1800 – 50.
9. Caledonian Horticultural Society *Memoirs* 1813.
10. *Transactions of the Royal Society of Arts* Vol. 42, 9.
11. William Ransome & Sons, established 1846; famous grower of medicinal plants. His huge range of galenicals was known countrywide. The firm still operates independently.
12. Texier, French botanist/chemist; made several journeys to Middle East for French learned societies; see *Journal de Chimie Médicale,* I (1835), 267.
13. Kaempfer, Engelbert, (1651–1716). Born at Lemgow, Westphalia. Ph.D. Cracow University. Famous for his journey via Russia, Persia and the Dutch East Indies observing plants and local medicine. Left Batavia in 1689 for Japan where he spent two years, enabling him to write a book on the botany of Japan. Returned to Europe in 1692.
14. Béral, founder of important pharmacy in Paris; an editor of the *Journal de Chimie Médicale* in 1850.
15. Society for the Diffusion of Useful Knowledge, 1836–48. Its object was to 'impart useful information to all classes of the community, particularly to such as are unable to avail themselves of experienced teachers, or may prefer learning by themselves.'
16. Royal Society of Arts; membership records.
17. *Journal de Chimie Médicale,* II (1841), 145 – 50.
18. *Ibid.,* III (1867), 96.

19. *Australian Journal of Pharmacy,* 30 September 1957,1037 – 39 and April 1968, 225 – 9.
20. *Transactions of the British Pharmaceutical Conference* 1870, 377 and 465. Interest in Australian opium continued, with the receipt in 1871 of a sample 'as good as Smyrna' by J. Bell & Co.
21. *Transactions of the Royal Society of Arts* 50, 25.
22. Stieb, Ernest W., *Drug Adulteration, Detection and Control in Nineteenth-Century Britain,* Madison, Milwaukee and London: University of Wisconsin Press,1966.
23. *London Medical Repository,* 9 (1818).
24. *Pharmaceutical Journal,* 11 (1851–2), 250.
25. *Journal de Pharmacie,* 14 (1828), 74.
26. *Edinburgh Medical and Surgical Journal,* 35 (1831), 331.
27. *Op. cit.,* Note 25 above, 96.
28. Pamphlet, *On the state of the Schools of Chemistry in the U.K.,* published by the author, 1842.
29. *Edinburgh Medical and Surgical Journal,* 37 (1832), 176.
30. *Edinburgh Monthly Journal of Medical Science,* VIII, August 1841, 284.
31. Personal communications; K. C. Reid to A. F. P. Morson, July 1987.
32. *U.S. Drug Reporter,*1907, Sources of Opium.
33. *Chemistry & Industry* ,4 September1976, 701 – 8, 'The development of alkaloid manufacture in Edinburgh 1832-1939,' by Deric Bolton, Technical Director, J.F. MacFarlan & Co. Ltd.
34. Pharmaceutical Society Archives; stock valuation of Abrahams of Liverpool. The firm of Clay & Abraham was founded in 1839 at 81 Bold Street, Liverpool. Robert Clay had been manager of the Liverpool Apothecaries' Company and John Abraham the head of its dispensing and retail department. He was President of the Liverpool Chemists' Association in 1856/7 and 1870/1. Both men had been assistants at Allen & Hanbury's Plough Court pharmacy. The firm was taken over in 1920 by Evans, Lescher and Webb, later Evans Medical Ltd.
35. *Ibid.*; Herring's catalogue, 1853. The firm of Thomas Herring of 40 Aldersgate Street, London, E.C., consisted of three brothers: Thomas, Edward and William. They were well known for the consistent quality of their products. Thomas was a Council member of the Pharmaceutical Society.
36. *Pharmaceutical Journal,* 185, 4th series, Vol. 131, 1960, 208.
37. Williamson, A.W., Ph.D. (1824–1904). Studied in Heidelberg with Gmelin, in Giessen with Liebig and in Paris for three years studying mathematics. He presented Matthiessen's paper on the structure of alkaloids to the Royal Society in 1860.

Professor of Practical Chemistry, London University; 1849,
F. R. S. 1855;
Foreign Secretary 1875–89.
President Chemical Society.
1862, Royal Medal of the Royal Society for his paper on
etherification, 'his most important' paper.
Retired 1887 as Professor Emeritus.

38. *Proceedings of the Royal Society,* 1863, 'The chemical constitution of
narcotine', Dr A. Matthiessen and Mr G. C. Foster, 345 – 67. In
1869, Matthiessen exhibited at the 18 May Conversazione of the
Pharmaceutical Society a specimen, made by MacFarlan, of chloride
of apomorphine, which he and Dr C. R. A. Wright had discovered.

39. Matthiessen, Augustus, Ph.D., F.R.S. (1831–1870). Started his study
of chemistry at University of Giessen, 1851–3 obtaining his
doctorate. Studied under Bunsen, 1853–7 at University of
Heidelberg.
In 1858 he began his considerable studies into the chemistry of
narcotine and other opiate alkaloids. His discovery of the
composition of narcotine is probably the earliest determination of an
alkaloid's structure and preceded by at least twenty years that of
coniine in 1884.
Cf. The Royal Society's catalogue of scientific papers, 1800–63 and
1864–73, 295/6 and 356; *Proceedings of the Royal Society,* 18
(1869–70), 111–12; *Nature,* 27 October 1870, 517–8; *Journal of the
Chemical Society,* 24 (1871), 615–7.
F.R.S. 1861 and later a councillor.
Lecturer in chemistry, St Mary's Hospital Medical School, 1862–8.
Lecturer in chemistry, St Bartholomew's Medical School, 1868 and
Professor from 1869, working with Professor Odling.
A man of world-wide reputation. He had a large practice as a
consulting chemist. He published 38 papers alone and 23 in
conjunction with others; the opiate alkaloid ones being with Professor
Foster and with Dr Wright at St Mary's Hospital. There were six
major publications on opiates published between 1860 and 1871.
The Royal Society awarded him its Gold Medal in 1869 for his
researches firstly into the electrical properties of metals, one result of
which was the improvement in the conducting power of the copper
wire used in submarine telephone cables (1860); and secondly into
the constitution of narcotics. One result of this was the process to
convert morphine into codeine which MacFarlan used.
Aged 39, he was accused of an indecent assault upon a young man.
'Although innocent it blights all my future prospects and, therefore, I

have resolved to resign all', he wrote before killing himself with prussic acid in his room at St Bartholomew's. His staff and brother stated, as witnesses at the inquest, that there could be no foundation whatsoever for the charge. The verdict was suicide while in a state of temporary insanity. It is an interesting reflection on Victorian attitudes that no mention was made in any obituary of the circumstances of his death. It was only in *The Times* of 8 October 1870 that details were reported.

40. *Chemical Society, Transactions,* 1845, 'Narcotine and the products of its oxidation' by Dr Blyth.
41. MacFarlan Smith Archive; correspondence between Dr C. R. A. Wright and Mr D. R. Brown.
42. Cavendish Society, *Chemical Reports & Memoirs,* 1848, 297, quoting *Revue Scientifique et Industrielle,* 1825.
43. MacFarlan Smith Archive; Letter, D. B. Dott to Mr Johnston, 18 May 1934.
44. *Pharmaceutical Journal,* 9 (1849–50), 483–5.
45. *Transactions of the Royal Society of Arts,* 50, (1833–5), 25.
46. *Pharmaceutical Journal,* 10, 2nd series, 1868–9, 390.
47. Address by H. B. Brady; *British Pharmaceutical Conference,* 1870.
48. Berridge, *Op. cit.* (Note 1) 274, table 2.

6

A Famous Pharmacy

The speed with which Morson's reputation spread among physicians and scientists was impressive.* His introduction of the alkaloids was quickly known among them as well as among pharmacists. He was very accessible to all and followed the precepts of his French colleagues in talking freely about his new medicines. Any forward-looking member of the medical professions found it easy to discover what he had introduced and could discuss possible applications.

His business and scientific interests combined to make the move to Southampton Row a logical one. Many of the people he met as a result of his work became friends and were entertained at Southampton Row where Charlotte added her skills as a hostess to enhance the fame of their home and pharmacy.

The move from the Fleet Market in April 1824, was advantageous from all points of view. Southampton Row was very

---

* As early as 1829 Morson's scientific reputation resulted in a letter of 25 April being addressed to him from a John Bywater in Liverpool. Bywater refers to his sending Morson 'two memoirs for your friend and yourself [because] you will do more credit to the investigation than what has been done to it already'. No details are included so what Morson and his friend (Captain Bagnold) were doing is unfortunately not revealed. The letter added: 'the time is not very distant when some active and general agent will be more clearly and satisfactory [sic] recognised by actual experiment than any of those occult agents to which we now refer so many phenomena', implying that the investigation was probably chemical and that some ☞

much part of Bloomsbury 'spiritually as well as geographically and its Georgian houses were to be compared with the most beautiful in the district; it had a quiet and scholarly air'[1]. Being far enough from the noise of Holborn, Bloomsbury was sought after as a place to live by lawyers, doctors, churchmen and scholars – all of them likely to be good customers and to appreciate the skills of their neighbour.

The countryside began a little north of Bloomsbury at this date when the population of London was barely a million. Bloomsbury felt itself separate from Holborn which was noisy and smelly, though every part of London suffered from smuts, with coal fires burning at all hours.

There was plenty of space and many of the houses had gardens, allowing views of other parts of London. Bloomsbury Square was mainly residential and the gardens, after a period of neglect, had been laid out anew after the erection of the statue to Charles James Fox in 1806. The area was kept tidy because the residents paid for the roads to be washed down by water carts filled from the roadside pumps.[2]

This was very different from the conditions described by Edward Osler on his arrival in London to study at Guy's Hospital: 'In dry weather the dirt suffocates me, in wet weather I am covered with mud from coaches and waggons. It requires very little rain to make the streets ankle deep. I am smothered by the smoke, deafened, jostled and impeded by the mob, sick of being run against by sweeps.'[3]

The Morsons made several friends who were at the British Museum, then new, with its King's Library being completed in 1825. The first of these was undoubtedly J. J. Bennett with whom Morson shared the experience of a medical training leading them to turn away from surgery and to an interest in botany which Bennett made his life's work.

---

science had been employed. Even Bywater's mention of his 'Physiological Fragments' being obtainable from Mr Hunter of St Paul's Churchyard has not helped in discovering any details about him.

However, the *Monthly Review or Literary Journal* (Volume LXV, London: Becket and Porter, 1811), comments on his essay on the History, Practice and Theory of Electricity that he 'fails to substantiate his opinions and his experiments are not always applicable'. In 1814 he wrote an Essay on Light and Vision. The only reference to Bagnold other than those at the Society of Arts is in the Allen, Hanbury and Barry Cost Price book which records a supply of Ammonium Chloride from 'Bagnold, Birmingham' in 1833. No record of such a firm has been found.

The immediate neighbours in Southampton Row included a surgeon, a confectioner and a 'medical electrician'.[4]

Morson's interest in the theatre, in literature and the arts was reflected in his circle of friends. His collection of playbills was huge and his library included volumes of eighteenth-century plays as well as Shakespeare's and other classics. The theatre had always been an especial interest: the references in his diary to his visits to the opera and plays in Paris as a young man make that clear.

Little is known of Morson's literary connections beyond a reference to Thackeray who may well have been introduced by Elliotson (see Appendix). Thackeray was one of Elliotson's patients and expressed his thanks to his physician by dedicating *Pendennis* to him. This was an age when recreation was created in the house and Morson's home, located in Bloomsbury, had many advantages for social contact among literary people.

The reading habit was passed on to his children. In 1861 Isabelle wrote to Elizabeth Masson asking for advice and received a reply[5] regretting the contemporary dearth of good literature: 'so little to recommend to your attention – of novelty none. We are obliged to fall back upon the old writers who are still the best ... '

This is a surprising comment since authors who were already known were publishing 'good literature,' e.g. Dickens (*David Copperfield* and *Dombey & Son*); Trollope between 1857 and 1860 published six books, two of which were Barsetshire novels; George Eliot published her first novel in 1859. Elizabeth Masson may have known that Eliot lived with George Lewes and would have taken a moralistic attitude towards a woman who 'lived in sin'.

The relationship between the Massons and the Morsons was a close one, the letters referring to all members of both families. In January 1861 Elizabeth Masson had been given a 'charming and much appreciated present' and, in thanking Isabelle, commented that she had received 'so many beautiful specimens of your skill in the use of the needle' that she was sending some 'little boxes from over the sea'. This is a charming reminder that the pair of fire screens worked in tent stitch, though separated for a time, survive together to exemplify Isabelle's skill. They were worked about 1850, the needlework being so fine that it could only have been done with the use of a magnifying glass.

Morson's musical evenings were attended by most of his visitors who brought their own contributions, like Nicolai Witt from St Petersburg. There are several acceptances and notes referring to 'your musical evening' among surviving papers.

During the 1840s Morson's children, with the exception of Robert, reached their 'teens. Thomas junior was sent to University College School before going to the Institut Mathé, in the Rue St Honoré in Paris; this was followed by an apprenticeship at the famous Pharmacie Béral in the Rue de la Paix. During his years in Paris, the funeral of Napoleon took place and he made sure of a good place from which to see the cortège and treasured the funeral programme as his souvenir of this occasion.

Morson encouraged his daughters to be interested in science as well as household and craft matters. Charlotte and Isabelle were 'subscribing' members of the Royal Institution in 1839, attending lectures and demonstrations. While they never became scientists their lives were to be spent among such men, Charlotte as Theophilus Redwood's wife and Isabelle as housekeeper and companion to Morson himself.

Languages were not neglected either for the whole family could speak French. With so many visitors from France, a second language was almost a necessity and certainly made life easier, especially when Thomas junior married a French woman.

Their French was also used for the visits of Morson's friends from Berlin. Heinrich and Wilhelm Rose, Poggendorf, Mitscherlich and Liebig are all mentioned as having enjoyed hospitality at Southampton Row and Queen Square.

The family thus lived a cosmopolitan and culturally varied life, with contributions to household and social duties from everyone.

The census records show that three servants (one a nurse) were kept in 1841 for the family of six with three assistants living-in; in later years two servants were kept. With such a busy social life, and with the living-in assistants and apprentices, the household required the competent guiding hand of Charlotte and help from all her children.

One suspects that this was willingly given because of the encouragement to be involved in all the activities. Filkin asked after his 'little favourite' and Witt in 1840 referred to Morson's 'amiable family'. In his letter of condolence to Thomas junior following Morson's death, Abraham[6] made a point of recalling the 'charming hospitality' he had received. Victorians were shy of reference to a man's home but the writer of the article in the *Chemist & Druggist* in 1870[7] included this reference to Charlotte: 'We may not lift the veil that shrouds home life, yet in the present instance our notice would be incomplete indeed without passing allusion to a house in Queen Square whose very atmosphere is unostentatious hospitality: nor can it be wrong to add one word in grateful recollection of the lady who till so recently resided there, whose gentle courtesy and kindly welcome live in the memory of so many, and whose removal left so large a circle of mourners beyond her own household.'

Charlotte died in 1863 having suffered for years from poor circulation. There were plenty of opportunities for Isabelle, therefore, to assume the role of hostess under her mother's guidance. Certainly she continued to entertain her father's friends. Acknowledgements from George and Eliza Cruickshank,[8] who enjoyed a long friendship with both Morson and his son, include reference to their busy lives with public appearances both in London and elsewhere. John Winter Jones, who was Keeper of Printed Books at the British Museum,[9] enjoyed a musical evening so much that he forgot to return some borrowed copies of *The Lancet*. Parties continued at Hornsey, Alfred Ainger[10] regretting that he could not 'join your family party at Dinner', with the comment that dinner engagements come 'fast and furious' at this season (June).

The Grays came to dinner and returned the hospitality by inviting Morson to meet new-found friends at their house.[11] Thomas Graham, whose sister Mary looked after him, lived in Gordon Square,[12] so they had only the short walk through Russell Square to reach their friends in Queen Square for a dinner engagement.

These occasions were not exclusively social, as one of Daniel Hanbury's letters tells us.[13] There was some discussion over dinner in 1872 about St Ignatius' bean fruit, an important source of strychnine, which Morson produced in quantity. Morson showed him a specimen that was globular and similar to that in the Jardin des Plantes. Hanbury points out that the one sent to Ray, which figured in the *Philosophical Transactions* for 1699, was oval. He expected that Morson's specimen was immature. He suggested, in the letter written a few days after the dinner, that the way to establish if it was a true Saint would be to do some trepanning to examine the seeds as this would not spoil the specimen. Hanbury later noted in his *Pharmacographia* that this was the only specimen he had ever seen. He did the trepanning on 15 January and recorded that it contained seventeen mature, well-formed seeds. Ignatius beans are the seeds of Strychnos ignatii. The beans may contain up to thirty seeds which, like the fruits of Nux vomica, contain brucine and strychnine. A different opinion was expressed by Magendie in his *Formulaire*. He stated the St Ignatius bean contains strychnine but very little brucine.

The scene conjured up is of the experienced Morson producing a specimen from his collection for discussion with the younger, highly expert botanist whose work had earned him an F.R.S. and great renown. They had many contacts from the days when Hanbury was a student. Neither was to live long after this meeting; Morson dying two years later and Hanbury three.

Morson moved to his house in Queen Square in late 1850, leaving the apartment above the pharmacy for his son, soon to be married to the daughter of a French pharmacist from Boulogne, Héloise Dagomet. The house was visited frequently by Isabelle's nephews and nieces; she was also remembered affectionately by her great-nephews and niece because she took an interest in them and enjoyed family gatherings even in her seventies. The sitting-room at Queen Square was on the first floor and overlooked a small garden. It was well furnished, some of it Georgian which seemed old-fashioned to the youngsters at the turn of the century. They enjoyed the pictures and prints, the collections of ornaments and the books which, with many French and German scientific journals, added an academic touch. Morson had his own laboratory with an assistant. It continued in use at least until 1900. The house was pulled down in a mid-twentieth-century redevelopment.

Queen Square[15] was open on the north side in Morson's time and when he emerged from his front door in the south-east corner of the square he could look to his right and see the hills of Hampstead. A few steps along Great Ormond Street was Solly's house and a stroll past the water pump at the southern end of the garden brought him to the Church of St George the Martyr and a few steps farther on to the bustle of Southampton Row. Familiarity with the square and its garden went back a quarter of a century before his move there. Its garden was a playground for the children who must have felt that Bloomsbury was their 'village', since they had been born and grew up there, and knew so many who lived in the squares of Bloomsbury and adjacent streets.

They were lucky in health too. All five children grew up fit and well – due not only to genetic factors but to the skill of their parents in matters like hygiene and diet. In addition to the epidemics of childish illnesses, there were serious outbreaks of cholera especially in the 1830s and '40s. Tuberculosis was a menace together with smallpox and other infectious diseases. In spite of this they all survived to live long lives, although Robert died in Huelva in 1865, when working for a construction company, probably from malaria-which must have raised some ironical thoughts in Morson's mind. The eldest sister died the same year from consumption, having had too many babies too quickly.

Progressive in many ways, we may be sure that Morson encouraged his family to have a balanced diet, and take exercise in the fresh air. Health and hygiene were matters of increasing discussion from the 1830s. Daniel Bell Hanbury went so far as to leave his house in 1860 while it was spring-cleaned. The house was 'thoroughly cleaned and white-washed'. His diary records that he and his daughter Anna (he was a widower) visited a small house in Richmond on 6 May to see if it was suitable for them to rent while the cleaning was completed. In 1865 Hanbury had arranged for 'Weeks and Co' to install 'the hot water apparatus for warming our house', recording on 7 November that it seemed to 'answer tolerably well'.

An incident which impressed itself on the memory of Morson's family came in 1848. The Chartists decided to hold a demonstration in Russell Square. There was much local concern which spread to the Government. Shops and houses were boarded up and everyone stayed indoors. At the British Museum, all the staff were recruited as special constables, troops joined them and they barricaded themselves in, taking enough food for several days. All were armed and waited inside the Museum expecting an attack. If this had occurred it would have been very worrying for Charlotte Redwood and her very young children in Montagu Street: their house faced the Museum. It was only a hundred yards or so from the Pharmaceutical Society's House at the corner of Bloomsbury Square, so perhaps they took refuge there. Fortunately Fergus O'Connor persuaded the demonstrators to disperse so the episode was marked by noise and threats but no damage was done. The residents must have been thankful that their neighbourhood could return to its usual calm.

Charlotte and Tommy Morson, as he was known within his family, had created a settled and cohesive background to their lives. Morson made firm friendships among as wide a range of people as can be imagined. In his biography of Muller, N. N. Solly, [16] Richard Horsman's cousin, put Morson's character succinctly when he wrote that he had 'unusual intelligence and pleasing good manners', the latter perhaps expressed today as genuine charm. His friendships would not have lasted as they did, if the charm had been of the opposite kind.

One of the first of these friendships was with his fellow apprentice, Thomas Gale, who gave him the four volumes of *Chemical Essays*,[17] written by Dr R. Watson and dedicated to his pupil, the Duke of Rutland, who was at Cambridge in 1781. The object of the book was to stimulate interest in chemistry, not merely to provide a textbook. It seems to have succeeded!

The first decisive step along Morson's road was Morley's permission for him to attend lectures at Guy's Hospital and to listen to Brande at the Royal Institution; these being the first formal parts of his chemical training. Immediately following was his joining the City Philosophical Society. Founded in 1808 by the silversmith John Tatum, who gave lectures which Michael Faraday attended, the Society met at Tatum's house at 52 Dorset Street, which was off the Strand and therefore only five minutes' walk from 65 Fleet Market. The importance of the Society to Morson was its twin objects of spreading scientific knowledge and as an aid to self-improvement. The former was satisfied by the inspiring lectures of Faraday in 1817 and the latter by private discussion among members.

Faraday's lectures took place in the two years following his return from his Continental tour with Humphry Davy and were the beginning of his success as a lecturer. This early success continued and his technique developed until he became a popular and famous lecturer. It was written in his obituary that he was 'capable of exciting enthusiasm among his audience'.[18]

The obituary of Morson points out that it was Faraday who 'helped him in his early efforts' in chemistry. Once it was clear that Morson, eight years younger than Faraday, had decided to become a chemist, discussions about where to study can only have been short. Faraday had seen for himself that Paris was the place; nothing could be achieved in London, and Germany was some years away from setting up schools as good as those in Paris.

The second object of the Society may have made its contribution to Morson's self- improvement. Dr Frank A. J. L. James[19] has pointed out that Faraday and Magrath, who was a young lawyer, 'set up a mutual improvement plan particularly as regards their use of language'. Did Morson take part? Perhaps this was one of the reasons for his ability to write well in his diary and elsewhere.

Dr James' paper reviews the membership of the Society and how they had difficulty in persuading the authorities to accept their registration under the Seditious Meetings Act of 1817. The application was made on 14 April and refused with a request for evidence of their non-political nature. After questions in the House of Commons, the licence was granted without question on 2 May. The refusal was probably more the result of the authorities' nervousness after Waterloo than a judgement about the members' politics. Their general attitudes were almost certainly progressive but they were young men interested in science, questioning and developing hypotheses; that is certainly not sedition.

The members realised that offending the law during the post-Napoleonic War repression resulted in many heavy fines. 57 Geo 3, Chap XIX was *An Act for the more effectually preventing Seditious Meetings and Assemblies*. Contravention meant fines of £100 a day on the owner of the premises and £20 for each offence for anyone lecturing, acting as Chairman or collecting money. It came into force in London within a day of enactment. Perhaps the severity of the Act is put in perspective by the fact that it was another three years before an Act was passed to stop the practice of whipping women for certain offences. Jumpiness and harshness went together.

Two years of attendance at Philosophical Society meetings resulted in Morson becoming acquainted not only with Faraday but with several others who influenced his life. The Society was a small one of 30–40 members. This size would have suited Morson who cannot have been full of self-confidence when so young and having had a difficult start to his early adult life without family or guardian. As the author of one of his obituaries wrote: 'he was thrown back on his own resources'. Fortunately he had some small financial resources but much more relevant to his subsequent career were his resources of character.

The company of at least three of his fellow members was congenial. Faraday, Solly and Ainger became intimate friends of his. Though their backgrounds were different, they found science and a progressive attitude as common interests. They seem to have preferred discussion, informally in small groups, to larger formal gatherings although each was capable of addressing large meetings effectively. Faraday especially developed his technique to the point where it was a performance anticipated with relish by those lucky enough to attend the Royal Institution. Henry Deane said that Faraday 'could not be forgotten for his simple eloquence and unfailing success in all his experiments'. A formative influence on Faraday's technique had been his Philosophical Society colleague, Edward Magrath, who had coached him as part of their mutual improvement plan.

Another tribute has lain unseen among Isabelle Morson's papers probably for over a century. It is her description of her father's friend lecturing on 31 January 1845 on the condensation of gases. Although Isabelle wrote the date wrongly, nothing can detract from her little witticisms and descriptive skill in conjuring up the atmosphere of this occasion. Perhaps this was partly due to some familiarity with the great man, partly her fortunate position as the daughter of one of the active members in being familiar with her surroundings. As a subscribing member in 1839 together with her elder sister Charlotte, she had attended lectures and demonstrations at the R.I. for some years.

Following meticulous preparation, Faraday used his pleasant voice to hold the attention of his audience. His technique is best summed up in his own words: 'A lecturer should appear easy and collected, undaunted and unconcerned, his thoughts about him and his mind clear and free for the contemplation and description of his subject. His whole behaviour should evince respect for his audience and he should in no case forget that he is in their presence.'[20]

Isabelle records the evening thus:

Friday Evening Meeting 30 January. 1845 Royal Institution Albemarle Street.

'At a quarter past eight the stairs of the Royal Institution were crowded with eager aspirants for a seat in the theatre where Professor Faraday was about to deliver a discourse on the condensation of gases into the liquid and solid state. The library was overflowing and the Secretary the Revd Mr Barlow, in answer to the numerous entreaties for admission into the lecture room stated that the doors would be opened at half past eight. In the meantime the pressure of the crowd increased and the condensation of the solid forms of the victims into the liquid state was rapidly taking place when Mr Barlow gave the word of command. The doors were opened and a rushing forward commenced which resembled what takes place at the pit entrance of a theatre when a star is taking a benefit.

'Ladies and Gentlemen eagerly pressed forward and in a few minutes the ladies' gallery and the theatre itself were nearly filled. A pause ensued; during which interval some of the company who were less particular than the rest about their seats walked into the library.

'On the table were displayed a few plated and gilt goods and other works of manufacture with the names of the makers as an encouragement to industry. Queen Elizabeth's watch in a glass case attracted some notice.

'The clock struck nine and Mr Barlow gave the signal for the committee who were already marshalled in due order to follow him into the lecture room.

'The door opened and Mr Barlow came forward clapping his hands and looking around in every direction as if inviting the audience to do the same. But the audience did not take the hint, for Mr Faraday followed and hastened to his place at the lecture table apparently desirous of cutting short the clapping.

'The lecturer began by attending to the various discoveries in chemistry which had been made during the present century and quoted a letter from Professor Liebig in which it was remarked that the English were generally but little interested in any discoveries except those which are calculated to fill their pockets. The truth of this assertion was responded to by all present but Mr Faraday proceeded to give an instance in which he hoped to awaken the interest of his audience although he could not promise them any pecuniary advantage from it.

'It was formerly supposed that water and air were two distinct elements dissimilar in all their properties, but it is now well known and understood that they differ only in degree not in reality – that water may exist as an air and that gas or air may exist as water. Again water may exist in the solid form as ice, so may some of the gases; and here comes the discovery. By recent researches Mr Faraday has succeeded in condensing several gases hitherto supposed to be permanent in the aeriform state and this he has effected by a new method of reducing the temperature to 160° below zero. Carbonic acid is a compound of carbon or charcoal and oxygen one of the constituents of water. It is generally known as a gas – the fixed air of soda water or the choke damp of a well. But when disengaged under great pressure at a low temperature it becomes a liquid.

'Mr Faraday placed on the table an iron vessel containing several pints of this liquid and on opening the stop cock received some of it in a tin box. The intense cold produced by the evaporation of a portion of this fluid when relieved from pressure, froze the remainder and by this means the tin box was filled with a white snow consisting of carbonic acid.

'When some of this carbonic acid snow was placed on mercury and melted with ether the cold which it produced was so intense that the mercury was instantly frozen into a solid lump. By passing gases under great pressure through glass tubes plunged in this freezing mixture Mr Faraday mentioned that he had condensed the following which had hitherto been known only in the gaseous form: Olefiant gas, phosphoric hydrogen, hydriodic acid, hydrobromic acid, fluoroboron and fluorosilicon.

'Mr Faraday gave some idea of the progress of science when he stated that hydrogen which is a gas, the lightest substance known is supposed to be a metal! Mercury is a solid metal at a low temperature, at ordinary temperatures it is a fluid but by the aid of heat it may be distilled in the form of an invisible aeriform gas. In like manner it is supposed that hydrogen might under certain circumstances exist as a solid metal the difference between the two metals consisting merely in the temperature and pressure at which they respectively evaporate, melt or freeze.

'If the progress of science should enable us to produce a sufficiently low temperature and high pressure, to effect this change in the physical state of hydrogen, we may yet live to see spoons and forks made of this new metal which will probably rival silver in brilliancy although not in cheapness. Such articles however could only be used at the North pole and if held in a warm hand would instantly evaporate.

'Mr Faraday concluded with a few remarks very delicately expressed in which he requested the gentlemen who habitually visit the Royal Institution not to incommode the ladies in the gallery, not to usurp the seats appropriated to the managers, and not to wear their hats in the library – the latter idea was hypothetically alluded to as he knew that no gentleman could do such a thing.'

If a public lecture excited so much interest in one who already knew him, a visit to Southampton Row by Faraday must have also been eagerly anticipated. The facilities for an enthralling demonstration of chemistry were at the back of the shop where the children could watch the magic of changes of colour and precipitation, and also be shown how to grow large crystals. In between such occasions they had their father to fascinate them with his own versions of chemical entertainment.

Faraday was one of the first to visit Morson in his new house in Queen Square.[21] He records in his diary that this was one evening in September 1850; he saw a balloon which had just risen from Vauxhall Gardens. These were to the south-west and he says that the sun was so bright that he could not see the basket, and that when ballast was discharged, the sun's rays were deflected leading him to speculate what experiments might be conducted by pouring sand or brick dust out of the basket and observing the subsequent dispersion of light.

By the time that Morson met him at the City Philosophical Society, Henry Hennell was already well established under Brande at Apothecaries' Hall. Whatever conclusions may be drawn from his rather inadequate performance before Warburton's Committee at the House of Commons, his inaccurate analysis of English opium, or the circumstances of his awful death, he impressed Faraday who had considerable regard for his chemical skills.

A paper by Hennell, 'On the production and nature of Oil of Wine',[22] discusses the reaction between sulphuric acid and alcohol. Earlier he published a paper 'On the mutual action of Sulphuric acid and alcohol' in the *Philosophical Transactions* in 1826, and in another in 1828 Hennell showed that when alcohol is mixed with sulphuric acid the first reaction produces 'sulphovinic acid, the starting point for numerous important researches',[23] and that ether can be produced by its distillation. This theory was later fully adopted by another friend of Morson's later years, Alexander Williamson. The importance of this synthesis was not lost on Faraday who abandoned his work because he recognised that Hennell had priority. The implications were, however, overlooked and then forgotten, until a paper outlining the history of this first preparation of alcohol from ethylene was published in 1935.[24]

Richard Phillips was lecturer in chemistry at the London Hospital when Morson met him at City Philosophical Society meetings. He was a Quaker aged 39 and one of the older members. He had been employed at Plough Court under William Allen.[25] He was already well known and he used his chemical knowledge to criticise the pharmacopoeias. By the time Morson returned to London and was manufacturing the alkaloids, Phillips was even more critical of their absence from the *Pharmacopoeia*. The 1836 edition was improved by his attention to it. After more than ten years' neglect of 'new' medicines, the alkaloids, some inorganics and even Morson's creosote were included, the latter having been available for only two years. The encouragement of higher technical standards, in the production for instance of mineral acids, was a contribution to better standards in the making of medicines generally.

Phillips was described by Bence Jones[26] as Faraday's 'especial friend'. The link between all these men was forged early in the century. Phillips who was a founder of the Cavendish Society and of the Chemical Society, died when President of the latter, in 1851.

Although Thomas Lott was not a member of the City Philosophical Society, he was a close friend of Morson's at this time. Otherwise Morson would not have complained in his diary when first in Paris, that he had had no letters from Lott. This young lawyer was Morson's solicitor and family friend, becoming godfather to Thomas junior. Lott married the daughter of a pharmacist, Stephen Darby,[27] whose widow made Morson an executor of her Will, the other one being Alfred White with whom Morson shared similar interests in botany (both became F.L.S.) and chemistry in the Cavendish Society.

It was a wise move to go to Paris, but Morson left behind him friends who would be the first to welcome him back into their circle on his return. Dunn & Morley, Faraday and other members of the City Philosophical Society, had given him a good start and his departure for Paris was a logical step in the process of learning his chemistry. The auspicious circumstances that then led him to Planche meant that he worked for an eminent man who was to become his mentor. A prolific contributor to medical chemical literature, the author of 45 papers between 1802 and 1841 on an extraordinary variety of subjects, Planche worked very hard himself and his young English apprentice learnt that he was expected to work from 7 a.m. to midnight on six days a week. Perhaps there was no time left for continuing his diary.

As soon as he returned to London, Faraday and Morson renewed their friendship. By March 1822 Faraday had proposed him for membership of the Society of Arts, leading to a further widening of Morson's contacts and experience.

Joining the Committee of Chemistry,[28] he was an assiduous member, the respect in which he was held leading to his election as chairman in 1834, a duty shared with Faraday until 1838 and for three further years with Henry Hennell. The committee had an important function: it reviewed a wide range of subjects and devices in applied science, all submitted by individuals hoping at least for approval and perhaps a 'premium' or cash prize to encourage further work as well as recognition of achievement. These prizes were reviewed from time to time in order to encourage efforts on subjects the committee felt would enhance industry.

They considered new chemical processes for industry; considered the means of preventing dry rot; wine produced from English grapes (which they felt was very indifferent); pigments for paint and cloth; equipment such as filters; and a wide range of instruments: barometers, hydrometers and alkimeters. The committee shared some members with the Agricultural Committee and those of the Mechanics and Polite Arts.

Some of the most regular attenders at Committee of Chemistry meetings were Solly, Varley, Hennell, Ainger, Lott, Winsor and Faraday himself. Cornelius Varley had an intense interest in instruments, development of which it was one of the Committee's functions to encourage.

We have seen how Morson's expertise with opium was almost immediately used by the committee, but it is a mystery why he was given for analysis 1,000 grams of British-grown and made opium in December 1824, was reminded of it in November 1832 and reported on it 26 April 1834. His results were far too late to affect consideration of further premiums for encouraging indigenous production. It is probable that Morson convinced the committee that our climate and wage rates precluded effective competition with Middle East opium, for prizes were not given much after 1825. There may also have been some embarrassment because his results and method revealed Hennell's ignorance of Robiquet's paper of 1822 and he had no wish to chance giving offence to Hennell. As co-chairman in 1834 perhaps he felt that the lapse of time made the matter unimportant.

Morson was one of a number of City Philosophical Society members who joined the Society of Arts and its Chemical Committee. The interesting paper by Dr James[29] points out that the number of people proposed by Faraday and a few others was quite significant and that it was this group who were to play the important roles in the committee. The Society of Arts had successfully claimed that the Seditious Meetings Act did not apply to them. More than a dozen City Philosophical Society members joined the Society of Arts and they took an active part in several committees. There is no evidence that their activity was co-ordinated but subsequent events suggest that they shared a view of the importance of science and its contribution to industry; in addition, it would appear that they also shared views about the training and education of scientists and disliked the barriers, especially religious ones, that acted against entry to the universities. Most helped the S.D.U.K., London University and acted in scientific societies so that membership was broader. It was probably no more than the stirring of the middle class and its consequent assertiveness. The eventual results were seen in the removal of religious and other barriers as their affluence and, therefore, influence grew.

One of the only two extant letters from Faraday to Morson is in the New York Public Library.[30] Its style is typical of the short note that is passed between friends. It assumes a trust in the other's judgement that only a close friend would have. Written from the R.I. and dated 23 November 1823, it requests Morson to vote for 'a very worthy man, a friend of mine', Mr Chater, in the election for the post of Collector to the Society. The position was responsible for all membership fees so was quite central in the administration of the Society. Faraday adds: 'do all you can for him and me by influencing others also'. The postscript says that he believes Morson can do 'a good tune' with Mr Winsor and through him with Mr Pollock. Faraday was certainly keen to see his friend get the job and his lobbying was successful. Chater occupied the post until his death in 1838.

Dr James has pointed out that at least five new members were nominated as part of this campaign and all by former City Philosophical Society people. Gladstone[31] concluded that the latter were a caucus within the Society of Arts. They had acted together in this instance but scientists were few in London at this time and so knew one another and met quite frequently at Society meetings which were held weekly during the winter and spring months. It seems more likely that through so much contact they had developed broadly similar views about the way they wanted the Society to achieve its aims.

Morson worked for the Society all his life and brought some influential friends to be members. These included Jacob Bell and his brother James, both of whom he introduced in 1847.[32]

The famous achievement of the Society was its support for the Great Exhibition of 1851. Major contributions were made by Lyon Playfair and Richard Owen,[33] who was very proud of the part he played, as a Juror. He was also a Juror at the 1855 Paris Exhibition, another event at which Morson won a prize. At the early age of 25, he was a lecturer on anatomy at Barts, becoming Hunterian Professor for twenty years at the Royal College of Surgeons where he was conservator of the Museum for over thirty years. Humboldt described him as the greatest anatomist of the nineteenth century.

He was a tall man 'with great glittering eyes', an impression which even his photographs show, including the one that Morson had in his album. As Fullerian Professor of Physiology at the R.I. from 1859 to 1861, there were further opportunities for these two to meet.

The exhibitions of this period provided the opportunity for Morson to meet Lyon Playfair who was made a special commissioner of both the 1851 and 1862 Exhibitions to help ensure their success.[34] Their contacts ranged from nitro prussides that Playfair worked on, and Morson manufactured, to a mutual interest in the education of scientists for which, with Government encouragement, Playfair did so much. The year that he became F.R.S. was also the first year Morson was the President of the Pharmaceutical Society, Playfair making a point of attending the Reception held to celebrate that occasion. They were both founder members of the Cavendish Society which initially met in Thomas Graham's house in Gordon Square. As a Juror for the 1862 Exhibition Morson made his own contribution to its success even if the earlier one outshone it. Their social contacts are confirmed by Morson arranging for Playfair's second wife to be a member of the R.I. in 1858, being joined by Mr & Mrs Barlow, Bell and Faraday.

While there are no papers presented by Morson to the R.S.A., there are not infrequent references to his presence. Two meetings[35] attracted interesting comments from him during the discussion of the papers. Dr Edward Smith lectured on *The Nature and Action of Alcohols as Food* in January 1861 and put forward the idea that the bitter taste of ale was due to the addition of strychnine rather than hops. Morson's rejoinder was that he would be sorry if the paper were the means of promulgating a false idea. The same assumption had been made by a Frenchman of Morson's acquaintance. He pointed out that the large consumption of strychnine in both England and Australia was due to its use in killing vermin. In his reply Smith said that the use of strychnine in beer was safe, giving the figure of its dilution, but he did not state the basis of his assertion.

The other occasion was the next year when iodine was the subject of a paper by Morson's friend Stanford. The meeting was chaired by another of his friends, Alexander W. Williamson, who was Professor of Chemistry at University College. This was also the time when he had assisted Matthiessen in obtaining pure narcotine from Morson for the work on the structure of alkaloids.

Stanford, the son of a founder member of the Pharmaceutical Society, was an expert in the extraction of iodine from kelp and had managed enterprises for this purpose in Scotland and Ireland. Morson reminded the audience, during the discussion of the paper, that iodine was of considerable commercial importance. It had originally been introduced at £1 per ounce, was later sold by Dr

Andrew Ure at 7/6., and the price declined until it was then fourpence an ounce. It is worth interpolating that Morson's 1821 price was 7/- and that by 1844 his resublimed material was 1/3d. an ounce for the 16 ounces he sold to Allen & Hanburys. The continued success of the firms in this trade, and there were at least four, had been due to their selling potash salts also extracted from the seaweed. Dr Ure[36] was at Glasgow's Andersonian University as Professor of Chemistry and was the first to market iodine in Britain in 1817. Morson also knew that Faraday had experimented with resubliming iodine in 1824.

Ure became an F.R.S. in 1822 and was described as one of the founders of the Industrial Revolution. He came to London, living not far from Morson in Keppel Street, where he practised as an analytical chemist. His analysis of water from Foxhole Colliery, Swansea in 1852 was carried out on Morson's behalf. He stated his conclusion that if the water were evaporated the residuary sulphate of iron 'would fetch some money in the ammonia manufactures from coal gas liquor', an expanding industry at the time.

There are many indications of the range of Morson's interests in the industrial chemical field. Faraday's reference to his contacting Winsor is due to his and Morson's interest in the use of coal gas for lighting. Winsor[37] had seen demonstrations of gas lighting by the French chemist Le Bon who had patented his coal gas process in 1799. He and his chemist Clegg erected gas lamps in 1807 to light the south side of Pall Mall after they had had the new idea of carrying gas from one house to another in pipes. Winsor was a prime mover in the Bill presented to Parliament in 1810, when the Gas, Light and Heat Company was formed; Morson became a shareholder.

The use of coal gas lighting spread throughout large towns, but not without incident. Morson's friend A. S. Taylor, whom he was instrumental in inviting to be an Honorary M.P.S., wrote a paper in the *Medical Gazette*,[38] after a large explosion had killed a person in Albany Street. His paper points out the dangers of gas lighting and lists simple safety precautions, the most important being ventilation.

Taylor's brilliant career covered an extraordinary range of subjects, outside his activities in medical jurisprudence of which he wrote an important textbook. For his book *On poisons in relation to medical jurisprudence and medicine*, he was awarded, by the Society of Arts, the Swiney Prize. A committee of the Society with members of the College of Physicians gave him the prize in 1859. It consisted of a silver goblet spherically designed into which 100 sovereigns were put.

One of the greatest contributions he made was his evidence to the Privy Council concerning poisoning. His experience over so many years as Professor of Medical Jurisprudence and Chemistry at Guy's Hospital resulted in his being convinced that poisons were too easily obtainable. He was asked by the Privy Council what could be done to control the sale and storage of poisons, and his report led to the inclusion in the 1868 Pharmacy Act of proper controls, a process started with the Arsenic Act of 1851.

He was the author with Brande of a chemistry textbook in 1862. He suggested the use of hyposulphate of lime as a fixer in photographic development, an interest which led him to make other improvements. He lived in St James's Terrace, Regent's Park, and was a tall and imposing figure, which he found useful when giving evidence in court.

Morson's interest in photography probably started with meeting Antoine Claudet, who was a glass merchant before he took up photography. The Pharmaceutical Society's library and windows used glass supplied by Claudet and Houghton.[39] For their specimens of various kinds, the glass domes with which they were covered were also supplied by Claudet. As Morson spoke fluent French, Claudet found it easy to talk to him. Though he had been in England since 1829 when he opened his warehouse for sheet glass, he used French even as late as 1840, writing to Lubbock at the Royal Society[40] concerning his use of Daguerre's patent; a letter of 1851 is, however, written in English. The association of Claudet and Morson continued for many years, Morson supplying him with his chemicals. Claudet's son, Henri, credited Morson with the suggestion made to his father of substituting formic acid for acetic in photographic developing solutions. At the time of the 1862 Exhibition, Henri was using the 'fast' exposure time of seven seconds and describes his process, stating that he used Morson's formic acid. When collodion was introduced for coating glass to make photographic plates in 1851, Morson was already aware of the need to manipulate the proportions of ether and alcohol to control the physical properties of the collodion – toughness and flexibility – because he had been making it for surgical purposes since 1849. His trade extended as far as Australia whence he received a complaint[41] in 1869; his reply was short and pointed: 'It was tested by one of our foremost photographers Mr Claudet, who now uses no other. Tom's portrait sent you in my last was taken with it. I may say that he finds it improves by keeping. He uses none that is not months old.'

The collodion process enabled exposure times to be reduced to 15 seconds from 3 minutes by Fox Talbot's process. It is an amusing sidelight on the conditions under which photographs were taken in the 1840s and 1850s that Claudet's opinion was that the English were far easier to photograph than his fellow Continentals because they were better able to sit still long enough for him to obtain a sharp image.

One of the best portraits of Morson is one by Claudet made about 1850 and hand-coloured. There were many taken of the family as well and Henri took photographs in the garden at Hornsey in 1870, also entering the factory to record the scenes there with managers and a few staff standing stiffly by, for the exposures inside the buildings would have been of perhaps half a minute.

Claudet published papers in the *Transactions* of both the Royal Society and the Society of Arts. At the time of the 1851 Exhibition he was taking stereo-daguerrotypes which he displayed at the Pharmaceutical Society. He also exhibited portraits of the famous visitors like Heinrich Rose, whom Morson took to evening meetings.

Morson's last official duty at the R.S.A. was on 23 December 1868 when he took the chair at the 6th Ordinary meeting when a paper was given on the electric organ. His work for the Society thus spanned his entire adult life.

Morson never forgot that his business required that he should keep in touch with physicians and surgeons. His contacts started early for he is recorded as a member of the Medico-Chirurgical Society in 1826, along with Filkin. They enjoyed discussing medical politics which reached a fever pitch in those years; he found the experience useful in the middle of the century when he was in the various delegations of the Pharmaceutical Society in its contacts with medical bodies. The Editor of the *London Repository*, James Copeland, a fellow Scot and friend of Playfair, was a member of the Medico-Chirurgical Society. He had had extensive experience of fevers in Senegal and Gambia when he had a medical appointment with the Africa Company before returning to England in 1821. This experience was much in his mind when Morson introduced quinine. The dermatologist Gaskoin, whose prescription for the Bishop of London Morson dispensed, was another member; he shared Morson's interest in botany and had two of the same sponsors as Morson when he was proposed for Fellowship of the Linnean Society. Dickson, Roots and Elliotson were the other colleagues in the Medico-Chirurgical with whom Morson worked. The first named, as already described, carried out the original clinical trial of his quinine sulphate. Roots became the Morson family doctor. He was famous at St Thomas' Hospital for his clinical teaching. He lived close to Morson in Russell Square. A little note dated 7 December, but unfortunately without the year, suggested that Morson should buy that week's *Lancet* because he knew of his friend's love of science. The two families continued a close friendship marked at one time by the gift to Thomas junior of a fifteen-volume set of *Pennant's London*, a collection of nearly 1,500 prints depicting London in the eighteenth and nineteenth centuries.

Although Coindet, a physician in Geneva, is credited with the introduction of tincture of iodine for goitre, William Prout, the English chemist and physician, stated in 1834 that he was the first to use potassium iodide as a remedy in 1816. It was he who told Dr John Elliotson about it. Elliotson was the first President of the Royal Medical and Chirurgical Society of London in 1834; this was the predecessor of the Royal Society of Medicine. With such eminent medical friends, Morson had certainly impressed an influential section of the medical profession. Iodine was in Morson's original list just as potassium iodide was, although it had to await Phillips' 1836 amendments before it was included in a *pharmacopoeia*. His contribution to the discussion at the R.S.A. in 1861 was, therefore, supported by forty years of experience in its manufacture and use.

In 1831, Morson's application[42] to join the Royal Institution was supported by Faraday, Brande, E. R. Daniell and W. R. Basham.[43] By this date Faraday was Director of the R.I. Laboratory and was to become Professor of Chemistry two years later. Brande, the oldest of the four, was in charge of the chemical operations at Apothecaries' Hall, was famous for his lectures at the R.I. which had started in 1813, and had been Secretary of the Royal Society for ten years until 1826 – an established and eminent figure in European science. Daniell, a relative of J. F. Daniell, was a barrister living in Russell Square. These three were all Fellows of the Royal Society. The youngest of the group was Basham, born in 1804. He enrolled as a student at Westminster Hospital that year and became well known as a lecturer in botany and medicine. A man of wide culture, he illustrated his medical works with his own watercolours. He was an early advocate of fresh air and exercise, bathing in the Serpentine at all seasons.

Morson was admitted as a member on 7 March. He remained at

the centre of the R.I.'s affairs for a quarter of a century.

Clearly his friends wanted the benefit of his views and prestige as a scientist in the Royal Institution. At this time, there was a move to replace the aristocratic and landed interest by scientists and those who would help to guide the R.I. towards the application of science to industry and the education of all in a knowledge of science. There was great interest and the popular lectures satisfied the objective of spreading knowledge of science among adults and young people alike. The courses of lectures, which were well established by Brande some years before, continued with invitations being extended to, for instance, George Fownes.[44]

Fownes had been Assistant to Thomas Graham at University College and in 1842 was Lecturer in Chemistry at Charing Cross Hospital, whence he wrote in March 1842 in reply to the invitation to lecture at the R.I. from the Managers' Secretary, E. R. Daniell: 'I shall be happy to give, after Easter, a short course of six lectures on Organic Chemistry considered in relation to vegetable and animal life.' This was the year that Morson obtained agreement for the Pharmaceutical Society to appoint him Professor of Chemistry. His 'brilliant, disconnected sorties into organic chemistry' had marked him out as one of the best chemists of the day. His association with Morson was such that he looked round Morson's laboratory quite freely, on one occasion finding a bottle of a dark viscid fluid on a shelf. It had been given to Morson by a chemist named Jones and was the result of digesting bran in sulphuric acid. Fownes was given the sample, determined its formula and named it Furfurol. He went on to do further work on this and identified an alkaloid to which he gave the name Furfurine. He thus anticipated a great deal of work on the synthesis of alkaloids. In his papers to the Royal Society describing his work, he gave credit to the source of his original material. He was awarded a Gold Medal by the Royal Society in 1847.

Morson's knowledge of what was happening in the world of chemistry and who was working on particular subjects was unrivalled. He was, therefore, making a contribution to encourage the R.I. to be more professional – the dilettanti were being replaced by experts.

Faraday understood the need for such changes but his interest in research made him dependent on the support that the R.I. had from its members. His popular lectures and fame for his discoveries were a huge contribution at a time when there was no habit of endowment of research by government. Faraday was critical of the English disinterest in discoveries which 'did not fill their pockets' and of trade generally which he found distasteful. He was nonetheless dependent on the proceeds of trade for funding his research. Even Morson's contribution was not insignificant for he had made a deposit of £100, the equivalent of over £3,000 today.

In the early years of the century, the R.I. had had financial problems, loans and gifts from wealthy members allowing it to survive until the mid-1830s when the Visitors could report that it was out of debt thanks to those who excused it from making repayment of their loans and, also, to a sinking Fund which had been set up, so that by the time Morson was a Visitor a substantial sum had been invested in 3% 'consols'. The Committee of Visitors had the responsibility of inspecting the premises at least every six months and of auditing the accounts annually. Thus they reported on the state of the R.I. Morson was the Presiding Member in 1858.[45]

Brande led and Faraday supported what he called 'attracting the world' – a world of better-educated people who had an interest in science and technology. Increasingly, the audience for the Friday Evening Discourses and funds for research were provided by the new group of the professional middle class.

Morson proposed a number of people for membership of the R.I., the first being John Taylor in June 1836. Taylor had been apprenticed to him in 1831 and remained working at Southampton Row and Hornsey until 1838, some two years longer than his apprenticeship. These dates are interesting for there is an engraving of a young boy entitled 'Morson's First Apprentice', 1835. It is by S. S. Gent and is referred to in the *Pharmaceutical Journal.*[46]

While it is possible, from his dates, to assume that the apprentice is John Taylor, it seems unlikely that Morson did not have an apprentice before 1831. Besides, the details of the engraving are unsatisfactory, with a metal siphon on the floor when it would certainly have been practice to hang it up; and the two glass alembics are so small as to belong on a bench and not in the furnace room depicted with very industrial equipment. The young man depicted in the engraving is too good-looking and bears no resemblance to the *carte de visite* portrait of Taylor in Morson's album, making allowance for fifteen years' difference in date. Artistic licence must be the explanation.

John Taylor's dates were lost until the details of the Hornsey site were researched and by chance provided information about him. In 1880, the property was sold to Edwards and Tindall, who occupied the premises next door and operated it as an ink-making factory. It is an important detail that on this site was made the ink for printing the famous Penny Black stamps. A problem had arisen over the question of land tax, and John Taylor, re-employed by Morson since 1871, was asked to make a Statutory Declaration stating that no such tax had been paid. Since his employment went back to a date prior to Morson's purchase of the first parcel of land in 1834 and he had always 'been familiar with' Morson's business affairs, his statement was needed by the new owners, who still occupy the site, having been in business there for over 200 years.*

John Savory and Alexander Williamson were two other friends proposed for membership together with Thomas Hyde Hills, and much later on, Joseph Ince. The first three men were close friends of Morson, Savory because of business done between the two firms over a long period and because of their mutual interest in pharmacy. At the time of his proposed membership, Williamson was Professor of Pharmaceutical Chemistry at University College. Hills became Jacob Bell's partner and assisted Morson at the time of Bell's death with the transfer to the Pharmaceutical Society of the Journal. He was a frequent visitor to both Morson and his son.

Morson's involvement with aspects of Faraday's work, and with visitors to him and Faraday from the Continent, is indicated by the letters that both men kept. The earliest is from Heinrich Rose to Morson in May 1838. Rose[47] was helping Poggendorf with contacts for his tour of Europe to investigate chemical production. Poggendorf was accompanied by a Professor Weber from Göttingen. Rose finishes his letter with a reference to Morson's recent short stay in Berlin, which 'gave much pleasure', and with an assurance that Poggendorf and Weber would bring his good

---

* As with so many facts concerning Morson's business there are no surviving papers. The invitation received from A. C. D. Kay of Shackell Edwards & Co. Ltd. to inspect papers from the archive was generous and revealed all the facts concerning the site itself. What was also interesting was being allowed to visit the site where Morson's original buildings are still in use, the only ones which he occupied to remain following redevelopment, in turn, of Farringdon Road (Fleet Market), Southampton Row and Queen Square. The evidence of chemical manufacturing operations in these buildings is clear – the brickwork is stained and continues to effloresce. My gratitude to Mr Kay is acknowledged for his courteous response to my enquiry and the trouble he took to ensure that I reviewed all the relevant papers.

wishes.* Poggendorf published Morson's process for aconitine in his *Annalen* in 1837[48] when the journal was first established. Rose's contributions to chemistry lay in his discovery of niobium, tantalum and other rare metals. He was an F.R.S. and addressed the British Association on several occasions. He was Professor of Chemistry and Pharmacy in Berlin from 1834 to 1864.

Faraday had a letter from Rose two years later. The style is quite formal and is very respectful towards Faraday, but it ends less formally, sending his good wishes to Winsor and Morson. The purpose of this letter was also an introduction: this time of Bunsen, who was Professor of Chemistry at Marburg. Bunsen became a Foreign Fellow of the Royal Society in 1858 and had had Matthiessen as a pupil, the two working on the 'electrolytic preparation of metals of the alkali earths'; he and Playfair spent some time in England investigating the chemical reactions that occurred in blast furnaces.[49] There was then, as now, no shortage of international cooperation in science.

Rose sent samples of niobium, 'pelopium' and tantalum to Faraday[50] in 1846, the accompanying note expressing thanks for 'so much kindness during our stay' and sending his own and his wife's compliments to Morson as well as to Faraday himself.

During one of his visits to London, Pelletier[51] sent a letter to Faraday enclosing samples of three new substances which he, Robiquet and Couerbe had found in opium. These must have been narceine, codeine and meconine respectively because they had been announced in 1832 and, from the place the undated letter occupies in Faraday's correspondence, it was about 1835. Pelletier was in London for a meeting of the Medico-Botanical Society in 1836 when he described his discovery of narceine. The paper[52] gives us the information that he had allowed the mother liquors from extensive opium extractions to accumulate so that he could discover whether they contained alkaloids not so far known. Pelletier's mention of the scale of his chemical operations is

---

* The letter says: Es ist wohl kaum nötig, dessich ihn meinen Freund Poggendorf empfehle, da sie ihn während irhem kurzen Aufenthalter in Berlin Kennen gelernt haben. Er hat, gemeinschaftlich mit meinen Freund, dem Professor Weber aus Göttingen eine wissenschaftliche Reise nach England unternammen, und wird während seines Aufenthalter in London sie besuchen, um Sie recht herzlich von mir zu grüssen, und ihnen zu sagen, dass wir uns Ihrer Reise mit vieler Freude erinnern. Berlin, Heinrich Rose 28 Mai: 38.

another indication of their considerable size and of the competition he provided not only for his French competitors but for the English as well.

Morson's skill in making very pure chemicals was much appreciated by Faraday. He records in his diary[53] that he obtained crystals of 'red ferro prussiate potassa' in 1848; he was testing the magnetic properties of all sorts of substances. These included quinine and morphine salts. In addition, solutions of these substances and a sample of creosote were used in experiments on polarisation and the effect that electricity had on them. The sample of creosote which was accepted by Faraday in 1841, was recorded in the *Minutes* as 'very fine'.

Morson's assistance to Faraday extended to his using the 'large magnet' which Morson had had installed at the Pharmaceutical Society. On 26 March 1850 Faraday went to the Society's house and experimented with various combinations of Grove's Plates, as a source of electricity, measuring the magnetic vibrations produced. This work continued through the summer with Faraday using pole ends and other parts from the Pharmaceutical Society's magnet at the R.I. The facility provided by his friend allowed Faraday to make better progress in his researches, which by this time were almost exclusively electrical.

One of Morson's closer friends was James Scott Bowerbank who was the instigator of the idea that a Microscopical Society should be formed. It was Solly's opinion that this was unnecessary as the microscope was an instrument and not a science; he thought the society would not survive. It has just celebrated its 150th anniversary! Bowerbank was a large man with a very extrovert personality. He and his brother ran a distillery, mainly of non-potable solvents, and he was, therefore, well known as an important supplier to chemists and pharmacists for turpentine, spirits of wine etc. Records of Morson's purchases are entered in his bank accounts which are available only from 1841, so we can safely assume an acquaintance started before that. The only surviving letter to Morson, dated 8 April 1872, refers to his visit to Bowerbank's winter home at St Leonards-on-Sea, when he was promised seed of 'our new variegated Marigold' and an open invitation to lunch. In London Bowerbank lived in Islington where he kept open house on Tuesday evenings for scientific meetings during the summer months. He was the greatest expert on sponges, making a huge collection which his wife helped to catalogue and mount.

It was Bowerbank's misfortune that one of his papers submitted for publication to the Royal Society was referred to Professor Busk of Linnean Society fame. Busk was slow and infuriated Bowerbank with his comments. Eventually he wrote to the Royal Society's Secretary, Sir George Stokes, pointing out that Busk was ignorant of the subject.[54] Busk was being deliberately obstructive because Bowerbank, in his capacity as Treasurer of the Ray Society, had accused Busk, Huxley and Lubbock of misappropriating £1,000 of the Society's money. He must have felt he was on firm ground to accuse three of the most eminent men of the day and write to Stokes saying that he had been 'in hot contest' with them.

Morson was among those who were invited to be photographed by Maull and Polyblank under one of Bowerbank's schemes; he was so widely known in learned societies that he knew all who mattered. He started in 1854 what he called the Literary and Scientific Portrait Club which invited eminent men to be photographed, paying a reduced fee to Maull, who had a very considerable reputation. Faraday was on his list but needed to be reminded in a letter of 12 March 1855, Bowerbank asking if he 'might add Faraday's name to the list before it goes to press'. He did include Faraday's name along with about 250 others so the list consisted of nearly all the famous men, which is not surprising as photographic portraits were very popular, if highly priced, and some men took great care to ensure their portraits were in suitably dignified poses. Morson's album includes many of those with whom he was associated in all his scientific work. Bowerbank presented complete collections to the Linnean, Royal and other societies and also to Prince Albert. While many individual portraits are in their collections, no complete one is extant.

Among Morson's collection is a photo of a lesser light in the scientific world but one who assisted Faraday with some of his experiments. John Peter Gassiot[55] was a scion of an Anglo-Portuguese family whose wealth came from satisfying the English penchant for sweet wines. He left the Royal Navy to indulge his scientific interest. In 1846 it was he who demonstrated to the Pharmaceutical Society Faraday's apparatus for the magnetisation of light. Faraday records in his diary that he made visits to Gassiot over a considerable period of years. He saw Gassiot's 'fine experiments', producing luminous striae from electrical discharges.

Morson's scientific life had a stronger social aspect than his business one, judging by the numbers of scientific men who enjoyed his hospitality. It was a preference for those of similar interests, not a rejection of colleagues among pharmacists. He ran a successful business but his bias was towards practical chemistry. It is not surprising, considering his background, that he had a sense of responsibility to others, including those of low income. His interest in education, which extended to women, high technical and professional standards combined to ensure that people of progressive views became his companions. His lifelong friendship with Bennett is not surprising as both were Liberals, as also was Bell; Gray was described as an advanced liberal partly because of his experience of visiting a friend in prison for debt and being appalled at the awful conditions in prisons which held people whose offences did not, in his view, deserve such punishment. Although Morson's interest in people primarily concerned their health, he extended his interest to their general welfare. He lived in an age of self-help, being a good example himself. His social conscience extended to his being a Vestryman for five years, being elected by the parishioners of St Giles & St George annually, starting in March 1846. He was made a Director of the Poor. Vestrymen decided on the property tax rate, saw that it was collected and spent it, partly on Poor Law relief.

He cannot have been eligible for this work without being a member of the church. Evidently he felt no inconsistency between his religion and his science, a subject of great controversy in the nineteenth century.

Witt's letter provides part of the evidence for Morson's social life. He had come to London from Russia to learn how pharmacy was being organised and taught. He went on to Paris before returning home. Morson assisted him with introductions as well as inviting him to join in his social life.

It was on his return to the then capital of Russia that he wrote to thank Morson for his help and let him know that a Government post was likely to be his; he was waiting for the Minister of Public Instruction to return from a visit to Germany. He invited Morson to visit St Petersburg the next spring so that he could show him the sights 'as I was conducted by you through your gigantic capital of the world'.

The geological samples that Witt sent, added to Morson's large collection and interested his friends at a time when geology was seen as such an important element in the introduction of scientific thinking. They interested particularly men like Morson's friend Tennant who had a very considerable collection and supplied Faraday with geological specimens for his work on electricity. He was among those who helped increase the interest of evening meetings, which Bell and Morson inaugurated at the Pharmaceutical Society, by exhibiting cases of minerals.

Witt's enjoyment of the social side of his visit is evident. 'What did your fair daughters think of the Russian Music?' He asks after the family. He points out that Morson had been in Paris just after he left and provides another indication of Morson's continuous contacts with his French colleagues when he writes that he had despatched a letter and journals at Pélouze's request from Le Havre to Morson at Southampton Row.

The reference to Pélouze is important not only as an indication of Morson's continuing contacts with eminent men in Paris but as a reminder that this 'young chemist of well-recognized merit', as Robiquet called him in 1833, was a professor when aged 23; and was to be President of the French Mint. Morson's contact with him continued for he was invited to be an Honorary member of the Pharmaceutical Society. He, too, was a friend of Liebig.

It is not surprising to find Solly's name mentioned in Witt's letter for this near-neighbour was a frequent visitor. Giles has not been traced;[56] White was a fellow chemical manufacturer in North London. He was a botanist and a Fellow of the Linnean Society. He was one of the two men who were executors of Solly's will, the other being Solly's brother. His business was absorbed by Burgoyne, Burbidges, a fine chemical manufacturing and trading firm which was important in the quinine trade.

Bennett was the John Joseph Bennett of fame in the Natural History Department of the British Museum. He had trained as a doctor but never practised. This was not uncommon in the late eighteenth and early nineteenth centuries. Such training was sometimes seen as a means and not an end in itself, rather as young people might study history today and then become accountants. In addition, medicine in the early nineteenth century was one of the few professions through which a man could alter his social status. It was also the means of obtaining a scientific education, the lectures attended ranging from anatomy, medicine, mineralogy and chemistry to electricity and magnetism.

Bennett was Robert Brown's amanuensis and later his executor. Robert Brown was Keeper of the Banksian Collection and President of the Linnean Society – being one of Morson's proposers. It was he who had investigated evaporation and it is to him we owe the discovery of what is known as Brownian Movement. After Brown's death in 1858 Bennett had to fight long and persistently in his gentle way for the retention at the British Museum of Banks' library and herbarium, preventing it going to Kew which he believed was too far from London. Morson's friendship with Bennett started some years before the foundation of the Pharmaceutical Society, which benefited in 1856 from the gift by Bennett of no less than 300 specimens from Brown's collection of materia medica.

There is an interesting mention of Morson in one of Bennett's letters to Sir William Hooker of Kew Gardens. On Brown's death, Bennett had to arrange for the transfer of the books from his library in Soho Square to the Museum. A photograph would have been a wonderful record and souvenir for Bennett of the hours he had spent there. Morson asked a photographer to see what could be done: the attempt was unsuccessful due to the lack of light and the slow plates of those days. Bennett writes as if Hooker knew Morson – a strong possibility, since Morson was interested in botany, in an age when attendance at scientific meetings was a social as well as a technical occasion and many men held scientific evenings in their houses. Those with large rooms did not bother with invitations, just letting it be known which day was theirs for holding open house.

One such very popular and regular function was held in their home by Mr and Mrs John Gray. Mrs Gray was an accomplished conchologist and algolist. She was some twelve years older than her husband who was the son of the great surgeon-apothecary S. F. Gray, famous for Gray's *Supplement to the Pharmacopoeia*. John Edward trained as an apothecary but turned his attention to botany and zoology. He was refused Fellowship of the Linnean Society, to its everlasting discredit, on petty grounds concerning his father not whole-heartedly embracing Linnean nomenclature. Years later when he was world-famous he accepted the Society's invitation – a remarkable act of forgiveness.

He was a prolific writer for there are about 1,500 papers which he published. In fact he went into print about everything, in contrast to Bennett who disliked writing papers for publication.

It is apposite to remind ourselves that in the 1840s chemistry was seen as a catalyst for change. Pharmacists particularly, followed quickly by the rest of the medical profession, led the use of chemistry to solve problems of health and hygiene. There were those who thought that it was being used as a lever for chemists and druggists to obtain professional status (and why not?). The setting of standards had the effect of improving practice and of advancing knowledge, but also of keeping out the many unauthorised and unreliable practitioners that existed in the 1840s.

In the first half of the nineteenth century, the advance of science made it possible for the first time for a man to earn his living from it, so the rich men who had treated it as a hobby and who had controlled institutions like the R.S.A. and R.I., many of them also F.R.S.'s, no doubt resented the rise of this middle class. The amateurs had also provided much of the money which had enabled such institutions to survive.

Science did mean something rather different in Georgian and Regency times than to us. Some reference in what was understood by the term is contained in a paper written by another friend, J. F. Daniell, who invented the electric cell of that name. He typified the privately educated man of independent means who took up science as a hobby. So successful was he that, in 1831, he was invited to turn his amusement into a job – as the first Professor of Chemistry at King's College with whom the P.S.G.B. had close contacts in the persons of Forbes and not least Bentley, who was the Professor of Botany and became the School of Pharmacy's Professor of Materia Medica. Earlier Daniell was a contributor to that wonderfully named Society for the Diffusion of Useful Knowledge for which he wrote the *Treatise on Chemistry.* He was one of the first Honorary M.P.S. Daniell thought that science consisted of three classes:

Numbers and quantity	–	Mathematics
Matter	–	Natural Philosophy
Mind	–	Moral Philosophy

He wrote of the 'objects, advantages and pleasures of science' pointing out that 'there is hardly any trade or occupation in which useful lessons may not be learnt by studying one science or another': that all sounds naive to us.

Daniell was the first to introduce some science into the management of greenhouses, an achievement recognised by the Horticultural Society with a medal. He was close to Faraday and also to Jonathan Pereira, who wrote to him saying that he was obtaining some chemicals they needed from France. Pereira who, in his biographer's words, deserves lasting credit for placing the knowledge and use of drugs, which had been chaotic and empirical, on an organised and scientific basis, consulted Morson on such matters ,writing on one occasion that he was waiting for Morson's views on potassium bromide from Normandy.

When Morson was first elected President of the Pharmaceutical Society in 1848, he held a Reception to celebrate the event. This was separate from the meetings and dinner held earlier as part of the Society's Annual Meeting at which his predecessor Savory presided. The attendance list has survived: some six sheets of signatures. We know from the list that 258 people attended to congratulate Morson. The list includes most of the Society's Council, even those from Edinburgh (MacFarlan), Exeter (Palk) and Liverpool in addition to those who lived in London. Most impressive of all was the presence of 18 men who were, or would shortly become, Fellows of the Royal Society, among them the most eminent chemists, botanists and medical men of the era. This was an impressive personal tribute to a respected colleague and, in most instances, a friend.

The paper is watermarked 1848. Confirmation of the date of the Reception comes from the presence of Captain Bagnold's signature. A letter advising Morson of his death on 2 October was received at Southampton Row and was written by W. E. Bagnold, his brother, from Essex on 24 October 1848. The details are of interest: 'seized with symptoms of a violent cold but which soon showed its seat in a severe congestion of the liver, his usual medical attendant took active measures but leeches would not act, blisters but slightly and mercury only on the bowels. This action, however, with venesection reduced all the hepatic symptoms. On the 15th I was sent for, since which he has gradually sunk though thank God without pain until the last three days. I had hopes that his iron constitution might bear him through it, yet always fearful that his lately increased corpulence, somnolency and a long suspected heart affliction would eventually render his further stay among us doubtful. 'The letter ends with a personal message.*

Although his family physician, Roots, was absent, Drs John Elliotson, Pidduck and Huxtable were there. The latter was a friend from thirty years before in the City Philosophical Society; and Pidduck was a neighbour from Montagu Street who was Physician to the Bloomsbury Dispensary.

Some people brought friends and two of the more intimate

---

* There is a reference to Captain Bagnold in Hudson and Luckhurst, *The Royal Society of Arts (1752–1954)*, (London: John Murray, 1954). He was awarded a large silver medal in 1812 for a gun and gun-carriage which 'could discharge 144 musket balls at every fire'.

acquaintances, his lawyer Lott and the artist pupil of W. J. Miller, Henry J. Johnson, brought their sons who were to find that Morson junior was among the guests.

The publisher, John Churchill, who included the *Pharmaceutical Journal* in his list, was also a guest.

There were a total of ten medical men headed by Elliotson and Golding Bird, who was Professor of Materia Medica at Guy's and an F.R.S. He had studied the chemistry of urine, of stones in the kidney and bladder; he had published, among other papers, essays on chemical pathology and clinical medicine. The others had special interests in forensic medicine, narcotics and the effects of particular substances on different organs of the body.

Five years after this Reception an epidemic of cholera spread to London. It provided the opportunity for one of Morson's guests to make a mark in the history of medicine since it was the first epidemiological study. The quality of water supplies in London was a subject of great concern to those who realised that much of the water supplied came from rivers and streams into which sewage flowed. John Snow studied medicine first of all in his house at Newcastle, no stranger to cholera. He qualified as M.R.C.S. when he was 25 and obtained his M.D. at London University when 33; he was L.R.C.P. in 1850 and died very young in 1858. He published an essay on the mode of communication of cholera in 1849, for which the Institute of France awarded him a prize of £1,200. During the 1853 epidemic in London he carried out a further investigation which showed the connection between outbreaks of cholera in Soho and the source of the water supply. By 1855, his conclusions were accepted and the actions needed to control the disease that had killed tens of thousands started to be taken. What pleased Morson and those who thought like him was that a scientific investigation resulted in altering established practice. Many had a vested interest in perpetuating the latter but the Government turned to scientists to serve on the committees, whose recommendations eventually led to water distribution throughout the capital by the Metropolitan Water Board. Morson's interest over a very long period was in water analysis. For instance, in 1842 he called attention in the *Pharmaceutical Journal* to illness caused by water containing free carbonic acid dissolving the lead in pipes.

Two years before Morson's Presidential year, Snow had demonstrated the use of ether at St George's Hospital Dental

Department. He worked with Liston who was the first to use it for a major operation in Britain and had accumulated considerable experience as an anaesthetist. His reputation was high enough to be asked to give chloroform to Queen Victoria for the births of her babies on 7 April 1853 and 14 April 1857. Since Morson had made chloroform for years, and in anaesthetic quality as soon as Simpson demonstrated its effects, he may well have supplied Snow with his chloroform.

Among the best-known men at Morson's Reception was Henry Bence Jones, whose textbook on the chemistry of urine published in 1857 became a classic. He wrote the first biography of their R.I. colleague, Faraday; he had studied under Graham and Liebig and worked under Fownes, whose *Manual of Chemistry* he edited after Fownes' death. As one of the first medical men to value chemistry as an aid in the explanation and cure of disease, it is easy to understand his interest in Morson's work.

The list of F.R.S.'s attending includes the names of a few, in addition to those already referred to, who reflect Morson's interest in botany and zoology. The Appendix lists these scientists and their main interests.

Ten years after Morson joined the R.I. saw the founding of the Pharmaceutical Society with its objectives of higher standards in pharmacy and of establishing a School of Pharmacy to educate and train pharmacists. Many, like Morson, had been forced to go abroad to learn their chemistry, there being no facilities in Britain. Among these was John Lloyd Bullock[57] who also went on to Giessen to study in Liebig's famous laboratory. It was here that he met Dr John Gardner, who had passed the examinations of the Society of Apothecaries in London. In 1843, these two developed a proposal[58] for a school of chemistry which they discussed with Brande. There had been much discussion about the establishment of such a school, Fownes being one who was convinced of the need.

On 6 November 1843, the proposal was formally presented to the Royal Institution's Managers by Brande; their reaction was favourable, the minutes recording that they felt the R.I. was the most suitable place for it. It was agreed to have a discussion on the 10th.

On 9 December, the minutes of the Managers' Meeting state that the report on the proposal was made by Brande and Faraday. So Faraday had been persuaded to support the proposal. A school of chemistry at the R.I., however organised, would have diverted attention and resources towards teaching and away from discourses and research. Moreover, it might have developed links with the medical schools and, for example, University College. Faraday's work would have been affected and at the very time when his discoveries in electro-magnetism were guiding him away from chemistry. 1845 was the year he announced his discovery of the action of magnetism on light. It is surprising that he was in favour of Bullock's and Gardner's proposal.

Morson will have seen it as competing with the work initiated to establish a school of pharmacy, which to him included chemistry, hence Fownes' appointment. His interest was as much in the scientific as in the professional aspects of the Pharmaceutical Society. The detailed proposals of Gardner and Bullock make clear their intention that the school should be capable of training pharmacists. Thus it was directed against the Pharmaceutical Society's interest, partly out of a genuine conviction that the Society should be a scientific body only, and partly because they did not wish Jacob Bell and the other leading men to be even more influential; these were the causes for Bullock's resignation from the Pharmaceutical Society in 1844.

As former students at Giessen, they knew that the application of chemistry to agriculture, started by Liebig, was of interest to the land-owning members of the R.I. Did they also wish to see industrial chemistry at the R.I. in a lesser role? If so, Morson would have been the first to argue against any proposal likely to produce such a result. What support such counter-arguments had from the managers is unknown. Faraday may not have realised the likely consequences of the proposal until after he had given his support to his senior colleague. Moreover, Morson may already have begun to realise what a strain on the Pharmaceutical Society their School of Pharmacy would become. He may have pointed this out and argued that two such schools meant both the R.I. and the Pharmaceutical Society losing money. In the event, the proposal was turned down. Whether this was due solely to the argument about the worth of the proposals is not recorded. In any case, Gardner and Bullock made a serious tactical error in promoting themselves as Secretary and, in Bullock's case, teacher of chemistry. No one in the R.I. was suggested, thus leaving the impression that the proposal was also a means of personal control.

In 1845, the proposal to establish the Royal College of Chemistry succeeded but it was not run by either of the two men by whom the initial proposal was made. Although the Pharmaceutical Society had opened its chemical school in 1842, the laboratory course did not start until 1844 and disappointed many who wished the School to become the leading chemical school. It was a lost opportunity although the Society was set up with other objectives of equal importance.

Much of the enthusiasm for the establishment of the Royal College emanated from those, Bullock among them, who had visited Giessen. More important may have been Liebig's visits to London, during which he expressed his opinions very freely about chemical education.[59]

One other incident occurred while Morson was taking part in the running of the R.I. In 1846 Fincher was dismissed for embezzlement. This led to an overhaul of the Institution's procedures.

Although the Institution was financially more secure at this time, it was not well-off. None the less, they proceeded with the work – the results can be seen today – of improving the façade of the building with the addition of columns. Morson contributed a guinea towards the expense, a sum which might reflect some doubts about the proposal; his friend Solly contributed £10.

Morson knew, and assisted in their scientific work, a significant number of the eminent scientists of his time. A man who could attract the presence at his celebration of such a wide circle of friends was himself an important figure in London's scientific life. This was recognised in the same year as his Presidency of the Pharmaceutical Society with a Fellowship of the Linnean Society.

At the time of his election, there were 520 Fellows of the Linnean Society. In the previous decade 157 elections had taken place; in the decade 1848–58, there were 149 elections. Fewer elections took place in this twenty-year period than at any similar period in the Society's history. In 1854, moves were initiated to rejuvenate the Society and to increase the number of Fellows, which had declined from 650 in 1834.

Morson joined many well-known men, a large proportion of whom were friends, a few of very long standing. Among medical men, there were Thomas Bell, later President of the Linnean and concurrently of the Ray Society for six years; Robert Brown, a Vice-President; Richard Owen; John Forbes Royle who was Professor of Materia Medica at King's College, London; Thomas Horsfield, Jonathan Pereira, Golding Bird and the Scottish naval surgeon, Sir David Dickson. In addition, there was Richard Solly, one of his proposers, a man always active in promoting those interested in science to be members of the Linnean and also of the Society of Arts, Royal Institution and Horticultural Society, the last two of which he had helped to form. The names were mainly of middle-class people but also included titled men – an indication that he held consistently to his opinions from the days when he joined the City Philosophical Society, to widen membership in order to promote science.

Other familiar names were Nathaniel Wallich, Alfred White, Jacob Bell, Edward Forbes, James Bowerbank and an intimate friend of many years, the long-serving Secretary of the Society, John Bennett; Edward Forster, a Vice-President, was one of Morson's proposers. Other faces familiar to him would have been those of Sudlow Roots, his doctor's brother; Edward Solly, lecturer in chemistry at the Royal Institution; Sir William Hooker, John Barlow and Professors Henslow and Henfrey, Professor of Botany at King's.

Morson was one of Robert Bentley's proposers in 1849. He was Lecturer in Botany at the London Hospital and was described as surgeon of 14 Bedford Square, Stepney. He was appointed Professor of Botany at the Pharmaceutical Society.

Henry Deane became a Fellow in 1855, the year of his Presidency of the Pharmaceutical Society. This was also the year of election of W.F. Daniell the surgeon with experience of West Africa; there was also Morson's young friend Daniel Hanbury who was proposed by Joseph Hooker and Robert Bentley.

His sponsors make an impressive list: two Vice-Presidents, his friends Robert Brown and Edward Forster, the latter a frequent visitor to Morson's home; and John Bennett, the Secretary. They were joined by Solly, Thomas Bell, Nathaniel Wallich,[60] and Thomas Horsfield – all of them F.R.S. There was only his friend and fellow manufacturer, Alfred White, who was not an F.R.S.!

Thomas Bell was a famous dentist with a large practice in the City. Morson's friendship with him included close contact when Bell was Reporter of the Chemical Jury of the 1851 Great Exhibition and also because Bell was one of the founders of the scientific section of the Zoo; he had been Professor of Zoology at King's in 1836 and became President of the Linnean Society from 1853 to 1861. He held a supreme position in the scientific life of the country when he became President of the Ray Society for six of the years of his Presidency of the Linnean. He was associated with two other friends of Morson, Richard Owen and Edward Forbes, whose short life of only forty years was remarkable for its contributions to marine botany and geology. His frequent visits to Southampton Row were a part of his love of social life, being an exceptionally genial character.

Both these men would have known of the story about Morson walking across Southampton Row and along the north side of Bloomsbury Square to reach the Pharmaceutical Society's premises. It was almost a daily occurrence and was just to see how things were and pass the time of day with the staff and any members who were there. On one such occasion, Morson was greeted by a friend and they stood in conversation. The weather was cool and Morson was wearing a light overcoat. To his friend's great surprise, there appeared through a hole torn in the coat first the paw and then the head of Morson's pet marmoset.

Thomas Horsfield became well known to the Pharmaceutical Society through the influence of Jonathan Pereira. Horsfield, born in Pennsylvania in 1773, worked for the East India Company and studied the natural history of the East Indies and India. He arrived in England and was responsible for arranging the Company's huge collection, selecting plants from the herbarium for the Company to present to the Pharmaceutical Society.

At the core of Morson's scientific interest, as the basis of scientific pharmacy, was chemistry; and botany, zoology and mineralogy were hobbies. It is not surprising, therefore, that his circle of friends in academic science, applied research and in medicine was drawn from men who had the same interests.

His importance had been recognised in the 1830s; a decade later he had become eminent, his home famous not only as the place in which so much had been achieved but for the wide interests of the company enjoying the 'kindly welcome' given to those who attended the Morsons' Sunday Scientific Evenings, events for which invitations were eagerly sought by young scientists as well as the established ones.

An indication of the extent of his contacts is provided by a letter that Faraday wrote to him on 17 November 1843:

Dear Morson

To the canvassings which I have already had (pretty close ones) I have given for answer that I am not on the council- do not mix with the managing part of the R.S. take no responsibility as to its conduct - and therefore must not interfere. I am constrained to give you the same answer as to Mr Williams.

Ever truly Yours

M Faraday

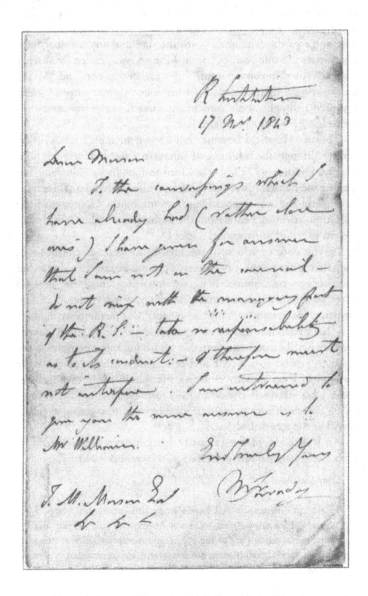

Figure 9: Letter of November 1843 from Michael Faraday.

This letter is reproduced in Volume 3 (letter 1536) of *Faraday's Correspondence* and Dr James points out that a replacement as Assistant Secretary for the Royal Society was needed following John Robertson's death.

It is extremely unlikely that Morson was interested in the post. He had a successful business to manage and was comfortably off. He was, moreover, very much involved at this date in establishing the Pharmaceutical Society. The most likely explanation for his writing to Faraday would seem to be that he was promoting the interest of one of his friends. He was part of the network of forward-thinking scientists eager to see an improvement in the management of London's scientific institutions among which they included the Royal Society as being in need of change.

Morson had secured for himself a recognised position among an élite but far from exclusive group dedicated to the use of science for the benefit of his fellow men. They all wished to raise the standards of their professions by replacing the old empirical ways with modern scientific ones.

Morson's reputation as a scientist was the prime reason for his eminence. His intelligence resulted in his making a contribution beyond the confines of his profession. His circle of friends, including the eighteen Fellows of the Royal Society at his 1848 Reception, was wide. He kept no record of those attending his Scientific Evenings, any more than there is a record of those he attended. We can be certain, however, that his scientific life included events at which Robert Brown was included, initially through Morson's friendship with Bennett. The contacts extended beyond this because of Brown's and Bennett's work with Sir William Hooker whose son, Joseph, married Harriet, daughter of Professor Henslow, an acquaintance of Morson's. Included in this group were Horsfield and Wallich, both honorary members of the Pharmaceutical Society and the latter a close colleague of Hooker père. The London scientific community was not a large one but was close-knit. There can have been few who were not acquainted with the eminent chemist of Queen Square.

Notes

1. *The Book of Bloomsbury*, London: Gordon & Deeson, 1950,58.
2. Jackson, Peter, *George Scharff's London; Sketches and Watercolours of a Changing City, 1830–50*, London: Murray, 1987, 76.
3. Wilkinson, Anne, *Lions in the Way*, London: MacMillan, 1957, 122.
4. *Boyle's Court Guide*, 1829.

5. Private archive; two letters, Elizabeth Masson, 53 Bolsover Street, London to Isabelle Morson, 2 January and 18 October 1861.

6. Private archive; letter, John Abraham to Thomas Morson junior, 26 March 1874. Abraham was a Council member of the Pharmaceutical Society and partner with Clay in the Liverpool firm bearing their names.

7. *The Chemist & Druggist*, 14 May 1870; 142.

8. Private archive; letters, George Cruickshank & Eliza to T. N. R. Morson and Isabella respectively; undated.

9. Private archive; letter, John Winter Jones, British Museum, to T. N. R. Morson, 6 July 1871.

10. Private archive; letter, Alfred Ainger to Isabelle Morson, 2 June, no year.

11. Private archive; letter, M. E. Gray to T. N. R. Morson, 3 September 1872.

12. Private archive; letters, Mary Graham to Mrs Morson, undated; Thomas Graham to Miss Morson, 2 July, no year.

13. Private archive; letter, Daniel Hanbury to T. N. R. Morson, 10 January 1872.

14. Trease, G. E., *Textbook of Pharmacognosy*, 4th edition, London: Baillière, Tindall and Cox, 1945.

15. Hamilton, G. H., *Queen Square*, London: Leonard Parsons, 1926.

16. Solly, N. N., *A memoir of the life of W. J. Muller*, London, 1874.

17. Watson, R. D. D., F.R.S., Regius Professor of Divinity Cambridge University, *Chemical Essays*, 4 vols, London:T. Evans,, 1784. This is the third edition, the first appeared in 1781.

18. *Pharmaceutical Journal*, 9, 2nd series, 1867–8, 204.

19. *Transactions of the Royal Society of Arts*, Michael Faraday, the City Philosophical Society and the Society of Arts by Dr Frank, A. J. L. James, 1991.

20. Bence Jones, H. C., *Life and letters of Faraday*, London: Longmans 1870, (8) 1:15.

21. *Faraday's Diary* Vol V, London: G. Bell & Sons, Ltd., 1934.

22. *Quarterly Journal of Science*, Vol. 19, 1838, 96.

23. Herstein, B., *Chemistry and Industry*, liv, 4 October 1935, 881.

24. *Ibid.*, 881–4.

25. Phillips, Richard (1778–1851). F.R.S. 1822, F.C.S. 1841, and President Chemical Society, 1849.

26. *Op. cit.*,note 20, (9) 1:13.

27. Darby, Stephen (1825–1911). Apprenticed to Lloyd Bullock, 1842 and later Assistant. M.P.S. 1853. With Ralph Stamper (a founder member) established business at 140 Leadenhall Street, 1856.

Examiner 1867. Translated Wittstein's *Chemical and Pharmaceutical Processes*. The Darbys were personal friends of the Morsons.

28. Society of Arts; *Minutes of the Committee of Chemistry*.

29. *Op. cit.*, note 19 above.

30. New York Public Library; letter, Faraday to Morson, 23 November 1823. My thanks are due to Dr James for telling me of its existence.

31. Gladstone, J. H., *Michael Faraday*. London: Royal Institution, 1874.

32. Society of Arts; membership records.

33. Owen, Sir Richard, M.D., F.R.S. (1804–1892); British Library Mss 33348 – letter to Benjamin Dockray 31 October. 1851.

34. Lord Playfair (Lyon Playfair) (1818–1898) F.R.S. 1848. Cavendish Society 1846. Studied under Thomas Graham 1835–7; Giessen under Liebig 1839. 1845 Chemist to Geological Survey and Professor, School of Mines, London. 1853 Secretary for Science in Department of Science & Arts. 1868–85 M.P. for Edinburgh University, and 1885–92 for South Leeds. Postmaster-General 1873–4.

35. *Journal of the Royal Society of Arts*, 9 (1860–61) 126 (Dr E.D. Smith, M.D., F.R.C.S.) and *Journal* 10 (1861–2), 185 (Edw. C. C. Stanford, F.C.S.).

36. Ure, Dr Andrew, F.R.S., Hon. M.P.S (1778–1856); author of *Dictionary of Arts, Manufactures & Mines* 1836.

37. Winzer, Fredrich Albrecht (1763–1830) was born in Brunswick. He came to England,adopting the name Winsor. I am grateful to Dr J.G.L. Burnby for calling my attention to 'The Crown & Anchor and Gas Lighting' by T. D. Whittet; *Pharm. Historian*,September 1984, Vol. 14, No. 3.

38. *Medical Gazette,* 26 August 1848, 'Gas Explosions in Houses'. Taylor became one of the greatest figures in medical jurisprudence. He was a pupil of Orfila, in 1828. He died in 1880: see *Lancet,* 5 June 1880 and *Medical Times & Gazette,* 12 June 1880, 642 and 653.

39. Royal Pharmaceutical Society archives; *Council Minutes,* 5 July 1841; 'Glass for Museum' approved £23 1s. 9d.

40. Royal Society; Lubbock letters.

41. Private archive; T. N. R. Morson's letter book' 134: Letter to Hood of Melbourne, Australia dated 16 June 1869.

42. Royal Institution; *Minutes* G.IV, 112.

43. Daniell, Edmund R. (1792–1854). F.R.S. 1828–50. Secretary, Royal Institution.
    Basham, W. R., (1804–1877), M.D. Edinburgh 1834. Visited China 1835–8. F.R.C.P. 1850. Member, Royal Institution; Lecturer, Materia Medica and Botany, Westminster Hospital 1849. Sole lecturer,

Medicine, 1855–7. 1858 published his work on dropsy. 1870 published his work on renal diseases.

44. Fownes, George, (1815–1849). Giessen, with Liebig 1839. Professor of Chemistry, University College, London: 1845. F.R.S. 1845; Royal Medal 1847. Died of pulmonary tuberculosis.
   Published: *Manual of Elementary Chemistry*, 1844. Furfurin, 1845. Benzolin from bitter almonds, 1847. Many others between 1842 and his death.

45. Royal Institution; *Minutes of Managers' meetings*, Vol. IX: 1799–1900.

46. *Pharmaceutical Journal*, 117, 1926, 773.

47. Rose, Heinrich, (1795–1864). Eldest of the four sons of Valentine Rose, Pharmacist and Assessor of the Superior Medical College, Berlin, who died in 1807. Brother of Gustav, distinguished mineralogist. Trained as a pharmacist. 1819 worked in Berzelius' laboratory. Gained a Ph.D. at Kiel, 1821. Taught chemistry at Berlin, University, 1822. Appointed Extraordinary Professor 1823. Member, Berlin Academy 1832; Foreign Member, Royal Society 1842. Wrote 200 papers on inorganic chemistry and chemical analysis making him unrivalled in this field. His publications included his *Handbook of Analytical Chemistry*, which went to five editions with a sixth in French in 1861. Honours were bestowed upon him by all European countries.

48. *Poggend. Annal.* XLII, 1847 175–6.

49. Bunsen, R.W. 1811–1849. Playfair married the daughter of an ironworks owner at Alfreton where he worked with Bunsen.

50. Royal Institution; Faraday Folio I.

51. Royal Institution; Faraday Folio II.

52. Medico-Botanical Society, 23 March 1836, *Minutes* 60.

53. *Op. cit.*, note 21 above, Vol. V, 65.

54. Cambridge University Library; Stokes Collection, RS260–368.

55. Gassiot, John Peter (1797–1877) of Martinez, Gassiot & Co., London and Oporto. F.R.S. 1840; Founder, Chemical Society 1847. His house on Clapham Common was filled with the best scientific apparatus.

56. The only Giles traced had a pharmacy in Bristol. He was a founder member of the Pharmaceutical Society: Richard Babbet Giles of 52 Royal York Crescent, Clifton, Bristol.

57. Bullock, John Lloyd, (1812–1905). Following an apprenticeship in Newtown, he became a pupil of T. B. Duncas in Paris and then of Liebig at Giessen. He returned to Paris to work in Orfila's laboratory. In 1841 he started his own pharmacy at 22 Conduit Street, moving to Hanover Street later. Analytical consultancy was developed.

Bullock was a founder member of both the Chemical Society and the Institute of Chemistry and was the last surviving founder member of the Pharmaceutical Society. His business was taken over by Savory & Moore. There is an interesting comment about Bullock in the discussion reported in *Pharmaceutical Journal,* Vol. 209,1972, 130. Dr W .H. Brock (of Leicester University) 'illustrated how Liebig, Hoffman, Bullock and Gardner had plotted to profit from Liebig's discovery that there were unexploited amounts of quinine present as quinidine in the waste products from the pharmaceutical manufacture of quinine sulphate. The plan was to market the quinidine as patented 'amorphous quinine' at an inflated price once Liebig had published his deliberately-delayed identification of quinine and quinidine. The plan, however, failed.'.

58. Royal Institution Archive; CG 4/4/14: the Gardner/Bullock proposal, marked 'early November 1843'.
59. Roberts, G. K., *Historical Studies in the physical sciences,* 7 (1976), 437–85.
60. Wallich, Nathaniel; Danish doctor working in East Indies, becoming Curator of Calcutta Botanical Gardens; F.R.S. 1828; wrote a famous book on Asiatic plants.

7

The Pharmaceutical Society

At the time that Morson's business was recognised as one of the 'most respectable dispensing businesses in London, enjoying the patronage and recommendation of the leading physicians', as *The Forceps*[1] described it, and with his scientific reputation at its height, the problems in the medical professions had grown to the point at which mutual criticism, jealousy and recrimination were a regular, if not continuous indulgence. The exchanges were ever more shrill and occasionally rude. A profession dedicated to the cure of disease found it impossible to discuss dispassionately the solutions of its own problems. Technical changes, like the availability of inorganic substances as well as new medicines like quinine; the surplus of doctors; the fear of a reduced income from dispensing if this were 'lost' to pharmacists; generally, failure to improve standards of expertise, all these played a part. Amid the arguments there was almost no discussion of patients' needs.

At the beginning of the century, general practitioners' charges excluded all but the middle classes from becoming their patients. The 'deserving poor' had to seek approval from local church wardens and receive a note allowing them to attend a Dispensary if the town was large enough to have one. That they were popular and successful is shown by the fact that early in the 1840s they were treating 50,000 Londoners a year.[2]

Technical changes, including the availability of inorganic chemicals for medical use, as well as increasing incomes among the public gave an impetus to a trend away from general practitioners, with the public using chemists and druggists. At this period, the chemists and druggists were giving medical advice, prescribing and dispensing their own medicines as well as those of physicians' prescriptions. General practitioners did their own dispensing, with some of them keeping 'open shop'. Dispensing had always been a lucrative part of a general practitioner's income, so much so that the Society of Apothecaries had set up the first large pharmaceutical manufacturing laboratory to supply its members and others; this operation was very profitable.

What Jacob Bell described as the 'G.P.'s shop' had a large business with the members of the Society who were proprietors, who bought their medicines at a discount and had a share of the profits. Sales[3] to these proprietors in 1820 were worth £16,700. Two years later they had fallen to £12,235 and dramatically to £7,000 in 1823, remaining at this level until 1835. Then there was another fall to £5,551. By 1845 turnover was down to £3,989 and to £2,992 in 1857. The same trend occurred with the retail sales from their shop counter in Blackfriars Lane. They fell from £14,385 in 1825 to £11,317 in 1830; a further fall had happened by 1840 when sales were £6,374. In 1850 they were £5,279 after which they recovered slightly to £6,162 in 1857. Although this affected individual members, the total business of the Society rose because of their monopoly of East India Company business and through government contracts for prisons and similar institutions. As a result their total sales rose from £26,796 in 1821 to £65,720 five years later and to £102,996 in 1855. Profits in these years were £7,872, then £10,054 and in 1855 £18,461. In all the years between 1820 and 1857, the profits never fell below 13.5% of sales and several times reached 30%.

The policy of the Society of Apothecaries in charging high prices rebounded on them; it 'led to the G.P.'s unpopularity with the public and also with physicians who turned to the druggists whose charges were lower'.[4]

As the Apothecaries' Society lost business, so private firms increased their turnover; slowly at first but climbing rapidly after 1840 as new products were available and there was more money about. Increasing trade at good levels of profit was a decisive factor in giving pharmacists the self-confidence to combine in the face of the attacks made upon them. From the general practitioners' point of view, it is not surprising that they tried to retain dispensing trade when it was at such a substantial level. The trend away from them and towards chemists could not be more clearly shown than by the Society's figures.

As the chemists' business increased so did general practitioners' resentment. More frequent accusations of quackery were made; they were accused of invading the prescribers' function, that is, of acting as medical men. However, one of the reasons for the public to turn to chemists for some of the medical advice they needed was because chemists were sensitive to changes in their customers' needs. After all, their clientele was local and well known.

The arguments about how the profession should divide the functions continued for many years. There was no real encouragement from government or the chartered bodies to raise standards. There was much discussion but no action because the surgeons, physicians, chemists and apothecaries could not agree. By the time of the Hawes Bill in 1841, which was an attempt to introduce comprehensive change in medical organisation and training, each group was holding its own discussions. The physicians, surgeons and apothecaries had their professional headquarters in which to hold their debates. The chemists held their meetings in one another's houses, partly because there was a large minority of Quakers among them and were in frequent contact as a result. D. B. Hanbury wrote in his diary that the Bill 'excites much of our attention'.[5]

Earlier, the chemists had been approached by their assistants who were concerned about the long hours they kept on every day of the week, Sundays included. Morson referred to this 'commotion' of early 1839, at the Benevolent Fund Dinner at which he took the chair in 1848, standing in for his old friend John Savory who had found the duties of President of the Annual Meeting quite enough and was spending the evening at home. His record of attendance as President would suggest that his health at this time was not robust.

Every aspect of the chemists' trade was discussed. Organisation, shop hours, skills and charges were matters on the agenda of a group whose services were more in demand than ever before but who felt threatened by the rest of the medical world. Those taking the leading part were the more successful London men among whom the far-sighted knew that they had to raise their standards so that their occupation became both a profession and a trade.

They took part in the belief that their services and products improved their customers' lives. They wished to raise standards by using science to increase skills and to maintain quality control at the highest level science permitted. There was, however, none of what today would be called a corporate culture. They were competitors who avoided contact. Those who knew one another best were the Quakers who met at their Society of Friends' meetings and those who had business dealings with one another. These were the contacts that enabled them to discuss the threat contained in the Hawes Bill.

Jacob Bell's part in this was first of all to stimulate discussion informally with individuals and in small groups. He had been brought up in a pharmacy whose good reputation had been created by his father. John Bell had taken part in trade politics with William Allen and John Savory in 1815 when their association was one factor in successfully opposing the attempt to place them under the control of the Society of Apothecaries. It is not, therefore, surprising that Jacob took an active part in the wider aspects of his trade. It might be said that he was born to pharmaceutical politics. His knowledge of his colleagues made him realise that gathering all competitors together might not result in anything more than noisy discussion. His technique was to persuade individuals that joint action was necessary and to bring them together only when the common aim was identified and the basic means agreed.

D. B. Hanbury records one of his visits to Bell on 7 March 1837 to discuss the new *Pharmacopoeia* on which Jonathan Pereira was working. Two men born into their trade needed little stimulus to discuss its condition, especially as they were both Quakers, who in the early nineteenth century were prevented from going to Oxford and Cambridge Universities, which accepted only members of the Church of England; equally other professions were barred to non-conformists and so trades like pharmacy attracted many Quakers. Within a few years, Bell, with management flair, had so arranged his business that he could afford the time and money to pursue a political career. He was only in his thirties when circumstances combined to give him the chance of leading his colleagues in defence of their businesses.

His persuasiveness stands out above all other characteristics. When he decided to bring the trade together, they were ready to agree to the formation of an organisation.

On 15 February 1841, a committee was formed following the first public meeting at the Crown and Anchor that day. By 8 March, Morson had been contacted and then co-opted to this committee. His good relations with physicians and European scientific reputation were needed. It seems probable that he was reluctant to become involved in politics and required some convincing that he should take part. Once convinced that the committee was serving chemists' true interests, he lent his energies to the project. Morson's attitude was that there should be a proper division of responsibility between the sections of the medical profession and improvements in standards of expertise. He believed that the interests of the medical professions were not served by exaggerating differences nor by ill-tempered argument.

169

He made plain his views in his first paper to the Pharmaceutical Society on 9 June 1841 in which he outlined the 'Rise and Progress of Pharmacy'. He concluded by saying: 'Let us ever bear in mind that all branches of the Medical Profession are dependent on each other, and that we are bound to render mutual assistance and mutual respect. The day has passed for one class to be subservient to another, but the day has arrived when the public demands from every department in the profession an equal degree of proficiency.'[6]

On 10 March a sub-committee met to which John T. Barry of Allen & Hanbury's contributed, having had experience of the problems and of parliamentary matters when attempting to get the law changed in regard to forgery which had been a capital offence. He would certainly have made a larger contribution had he not been absent from later meetings. The explanation lies in a short entry in Hanbury's diary for 29 April, that Barry had returned to work after being ill for nine weeks.

This sub-committee had a meeting with the Royal College of Physicians to test their reaction and also decided to publicise its actions and programme.

The Hawes Bill was counted out in the House of Commons on 20 March, leaving the way open for the committee to continue its work without the complication of parliamentary action. A meeting was held at Bell's house that day, the first of the Pharmaceutical Tea Parties and the start of the process of finding solutions to chemists' problems, requiring 'unwearied perseverance'.[7] On 25 March, a second was held when the formal decision to create an association was taken. On 2 April, the committee met again, having added Savory, Squire, Hudson and Alsop to their number. The momentum generated by Bell was beginning to bring results.

No time was wasted under Bell's energetic leadership. A General Committee met on 5 April which drew up a constitution; two days later at Bell's house, the decision to hold a public meeting was reached. The famous meeting at the Crown and Anchor on 15 April 1841 followed. Hanbury commented that it 'was a satisfying commencement'.

Morson moved the resolution that day requesting the committee to frame by-laws and regulations for governing the Society. It seems appropriate that Morson chose this item as his first public statement, for it indicates that he had overcome any doubts about the formation of the Society and his involvement in it.

Once the Society was formed, its early meetings also took place at Bell's house. The first was on 11 May and the second on 9 June.

They were followed by further meetings on 8 September, 10 November and 8 December, the November meeting attracting a 'numerous attendance'. There was activity during the summer, but of a different kind.

Bell's proselytising on the Society's behalf involved travelling wherever he could recruit support. Thus in August 1841 he wrote to Morson from Plymouth on a 'Tuesday night'. Their friendship had developed quickly into intimacy; Bell addressed him familiarly as 'My dear Morson' and signed only 'J.B.'.

He had visited prospective members with Mr May of Stonehouse[8] and had added six to the list, expecting to get as many the next day.

This journey is referred to in the *Pharmaceutical Journal* for September 1841 as 'a flying journey through South West England'. Bell's letter tells Morson that he was starting for Bristol the following day and expected 'to arrive there on Sunday afternoon – touch at Bath – cut away to Birmingham – leave a card at Wolverhampton – and slide home on Wednesday'. A flying journey indeed. He concludes by saying that he 'can't get over the two guinea subscription entirely. The leading article No 2 of the Transactions had satisfied several and in fact that ammunition is the only thing that helps me on.' The subscription was a contentious issue later. Nevertheless Bell was optimistic: 'there is a degree of interest in the concern. If I could get up a meeting, I think I should get a good list. As it is I shall be content with 10 or 12 and leave the rest to Mr May. I have done altogether as well as I expected – but I have had no fun at the association', a reference to the association of chemists and druggists who wished only to discuss matters of trade. Bell's success with recruitment resulted in there being 1,958 members after the Society's first year.

His telling Morson by letter of his progress is a reflection of what must have been joint work in drawing up a list of chemists to visit; they both had countrywide contacts. It is also evidence of their cooperation from the earliest days of the Society.

Bell's sense of humour surfaces when he finishes his letter: 'If I had not been absorbed in Pharmacy, I sh'd have been disposed to turn my attention to Natural History for there are some very pretty specimens of the genus Homo flitting about. They flock to the Geological Section – the stones and Professor Sedgwick attract them. However, I let em alone and stick to my text.'

Adam Sedgwick's lectures at the Geological Society were very popular at a time when interest in geology was at its height. He was Professor of Geology at Cambridge from 1818 until his death in

1873. He was very friendly with one of Morson's acquaintances at the Society for the Diffusion of Useful Knowledge, John Stevens Henslow, who was Regius Professor of Botany at the age of 31 in 1827. Sedgwick was godfather to Henslow's daughter and another daughter married Joseph Hooker, another point of possible contact for Morson. Henslow taught Darwin and recommended him for the famous voyage in the *Beagle*. He made an exceptional contribution to popular scientific education from 1835 to 1855 and published a number of treatises between 1835 and 1840. Even though he had been educated conventionally and entered the Church as a young man, always having his parish near Cambridge, he, like Faraday and Morson, was convinced that the pursuit of science was not incompatible with religion. This did not please the bishops who made sure that his clerical career was stunted. 'The professor gained neither the same respect nor advancement in church circles as he did in scientific ones in spite of his undoubted ability and sincerely-held Christian beliefs.'[9] There were those who resented the intrusion of science into their conception of the world. Henslow was among those who welcomed the intellectual challenge of scientific ideas. His failure to be promoted in the Church was to be an advantage for the promotion of scientific education, a matter close to Morson's heart. Henslow's energies were diverted to scientific education and understanding. At the height of the religion versus science controversy in 1860, Henslow was chairman of the famous debate between Huxley and Wilberforce arising from the publication of Darwin's *Origin of Species*.

Later in 1841, Bell's letters[10] to Morson are short and to the point, excluding almost all of the formality of the time. The relationship had settled down to an easy working one in addition to friendship. He asks for two or three 'handsome looking Cantharides with their legs, wings and heads on'. A part of one of his experiments was also sent, the object to be explained when they met. Bell finished, 'Yours everlastingly, J.B.'

On the date, 12 August 1841, Bell was writing to Morson, he was in Paris, 'awaiting your strictures on my leading article before I go any further with it'. He wanted 'a few lines' and hoped to have a letter so 'you need not pay the postage* unless you like'. Bell also

---

* Depending on the country concerned, prior to 1840s postage could be paid on delivery. In the middle of the century Roland Hill introduced pre-paid adhesive postage stamps, with a single uniform rate based on weight rather than distance.

asks what Boudet says – probably a reference to the invitation to Boudet to start a scientific correspondence between the French and British pharmaceutical societies, a move approved by Council on 2 December 1841.

Bell had not quite understood Morson's report to the Society about opium and asked for a few lines about narcotine 'and what you thought it appeared to be composed of'. The item was needed for the *Transactions*.

There had been a meeting which had lasted until 11.30 p.m. (the Society's meetings usually began at 8 p.m.) and Dr Thomson 'cut me up and exploded my theory beautifully – I shall turn it all to good account in the printed report'.

A little later Bell writes asking for Morson's opinion on two papers. The first 'might be published this month in the Journal' and the second was to 'amuse our next meeting for which we have as yet no paper in prospect except yours which is our sheet anchor'. The

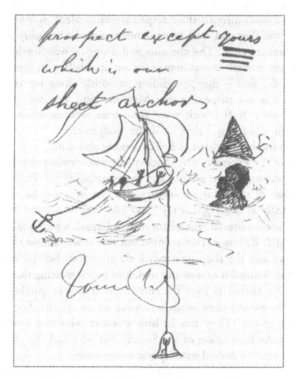

Figure 10: Jacob Bell's undated letter to Morson

173

last page is embellished with one of Bell's amusing sketches including a figure inside a bell, but whose head is on the right with the letter R behind it and a clown's cap above?

Morson's comments on Bell's articles were a regular practice. His influence was decisive on at least one occasion. Among Morson's papers is the draft of a leading article for publication in the *Journal* of 9 January 1845. It is entitled: 'The present position of Chemists and Druggists in reference to Medical Reform'. Morson has written on the back of the first sheet: 'a curious leader of Jacob Bell's intended to have been published 1848 – little of this original was published'. Although he confused the date there was published a leader on pharmaceutical legislation[11] in 1845 starting with the same first sentence. That the rest of the draft did not appear is not surprising; it is indeed 'curious', being verbose and filled with trite analogies. Reference is made to the battles being fought by the physicians, pure surgeons and general practitioners, neither party giving any quarter to the other, 'like sulphur nitre and charcoal combined according to their respective equivalent numbers are awaiting the flint and steel of parliament and will probably go off with a similar result'. The chemists and druggists were leaving 'the combatants to fight it out, remaining on the shelf with eyes open and mouths shut – they are gliding smoothly along the river of reform'. It is not surprising that Morson's 'attic salt' was poured liberally on a draft which must have been written when Bell's enthusiasm was stronger than his literary judgement.

Much has been written of Bell's energetic and skilful work in the creation of the Pharmaceutical Society. He was certainly the driving force in pharmaceutical politics and the organiser of the Society. He was a man of powerful personality. On one occasion he arrived unexpectedly at Ince's pharmacy[12] and said that he wanted Ince to join the small editorial committee of the *Journal*, which was about to meet at Bell's house. Ince pointed out that it was almost the end of the day and the shop demanded his attention. Bell picked up Ince's coat, handed it to him and took him to the meeting there and then! Bell's authority over his contemporaries was quickly and decisively established within a year or so of the Society's commencement. They saw in him a leader who had not only organised the foundation of the Society but who had the political flair to ensure it achieved stability and recognition.

However much his personality dominated his colleagues, there were a few whose opinions he sought and who influenced him. Jonathan Pereira's letters to Bell[13] reveal clearly that a strategy about the Society's aims was mutually recognised. Morson provided guidance and a check on any over-enthusiasm on Bell's part. When Bell did not have such checks, he sometimes made errors of judgement. In 1851 he was asked to talk to the Society of Arts about the chemical and pharmaceutical exhibits at the Great Exhibition. He used the occasion to make a political speech which was not well received.

Unfortunately, there are no letters of Morson's to provide documentary evidence of his attitude towards nor his opinions about these matters. He was not a good correspondent; the few letters on business and similar subjects show that he wrote when it was necessary and then only briefly. His friend George Schweitzer writing from Brighton complained of his 'very short and business-like letter'. He would have preferred news of London's scientific and artistic life but 'you, a great man, an influential man ... are stingy not even to give me some crumbs from your superfluity'.[14] Perhaps Morson's brevity led to the destruction of his letters.

Soon after the Society was formed, several periodicals started to attack it. Their reasons were a mixture of conservatism, fear of competition, jealousy of Bell's success with the *Journal* and competition for readers; and, in one case, disappointment at rejection of a proposal to manage the *Journal* for the Society. In some cases, the attacks were personal and scurrilous.

The Chemist[15] went to great lengths to denigrate the Society and its officers, especially Bell, Morson and Squire. Bell and Morson were attacked jointly for running the Society for their own benefit in attracting attention to their products, so much so that they were accused of 'being the Society'. Charles and John Watt had started this journal a year before Bell began publishing the *Pharmaceutical Transactions*. They approached the Society in order to propose that the *Transactions* should be published by them in *The Chemist*. When the proposal was turned down, they commenced a vituperative attack which lasted for nearly ten years. Rejection was a disappointment and much affected their circulation. Bell was a pioneer in technical journalism and had the advantage of reporting and commenting upon the Society's proceedings. The Watts were dependent on repeating the material published in other journals, however good their translations from European publications were.

Their attacks on Bell concentrated on his editorship and accused him of financial irregularity; those on Morson, 'with one of the most lucrative businesses in London', of overcharging the Society for chemicals, of using the Society to promote his business and of hypocrisy in his support of the School of Pharmacy; Squire's technical achievements were denigrated and a very personal attack was made including remarks about his appearance and even his smile.

The Medical Times,[16] a very conservative journal, accused the Pharmaceutical Society in December 1841 of 'disturbing the whole arrangement of society'. With little real argument on their side, they continued the next month by referring to pharmacists as a mixture of 'tradesman and scholar, the trafficker and the gentleman', which says more for their snobbishness than for their ability to argue a case. They attacked the College of Physicians for 'an old intrigue' with chemists and druggists and said they were taking 'the field in conjunction with a trading class of the community'. It is extraordinary that those claiming an intellectual superiority conducted the argument at so low a level.

Other journals joined in, among them *The Forceps*[17] which carried an article praising Morson for his achievements but regretting that he had anything to do with the Society whose demise they predicted, saying that it was destined to become as offensive and useless as the Worshipful Society of Apothecaries. The Society survived, most of these journals did not.

Some of this opposition reflected the opinions of important sections of the community; the determination of pharmacists certainly exhibited the 'unwearied perseverance' that Bell knew would be needed. It is a tribute to Bell's leadership and the support he had that their professional institution survived and created the means of educating and training men worthy of it. They were not diverted by the internal arguments which developed into dissension in the 1850s although there must have been times when their resolve weakened and they wondered why they worked long hours in the interests of what Morson called 'their profession and trade' instead of attending to their businesses.

By September 1841 Morson, Squire and Bell, were visiting the lecturers selected by the Scientific Committee. They included Brande, Faraday, Pereira and Thomson, Faraday being the only one to refuse as he was so wedded to the Royal Institution and his work there.

In October, after their meetings had been held in Bell's, Pigeon's[18] and other houses, the question of permanent premises was discussed by Council.[19] Morson gave details of the accommodation available at the R.S.A. Eventually the R.S.A. agreed to help the Scientific Committee but would not offer any other facilities to the Society. By 15 November the Bloomsbury Square premises were being talked about and the rent of £100 was considered acceptable, so on 13 December a number of councillors went to inspect No. 17. They were sufficiently impressed that the whole Council agreed on 17 December that it was suitable.

The Society organised events very quickly, a move designed to maintain members' interest as well as give evidence of the Society's ability to attract senior scientists as lecturers. By early 1842, Dr A. T. Thomson had given the first lecture and within a year of the inaugural meeting courses of study and examinations of candidates had started. In October, a course of four chemical lectures by Fownes was given.

At the second anniversary meeting William Allen was in the chair, although he did not live much longer. He became ill in October and died at the end of 1843. D. B. Hanbury recorded the progress of his uncle's illness, writing that 'his recovery was very doubtful' on 28 October and ' W A will not last many days longer' on 22 December. These events are interspersed among entries that indicate the speed with which every aspect of the Society was organised. There were meetings to consider and finalise a draft of the Charter, which were followed in March 1843 by the very laborious job of the committee on the by-laws, which were eventually adopted in December 1844, the year that Savory became President and Morson Vice-President.

In February 1844, Hanbury joined the Finance Committee, not long after his son Daniel had entered his firm. Daniel Bell spent many hours on Society business and in September 1852 he succeeded Richard Hotham Pigeon junior who had followed his father in the Treasurer's job, and died after only three years. Hanbury remained Treasurer until his retirement from business in 1867.

It is a measure of the effort made by councillors that in 1846 Hanbury, who was no exception, recorded his attendance at 11 meetings and deputations for the Society; in 1855 it was 13. In 1852, he writes that 'the state of matters [is] far from satisfactory to me in various particulars'. He was, as with his business and work for the Friends, punctilious in his attendance at meetings. These sometimes lasted four hours, occasionally more, when he found them long and tedious. The most intensive discussions were about the additional by-laws and the circumstances of Acts of Parliament. Opposition by the 'Dickinson party' made the meetings very trying and on 6 September 1853 the meeting was stormy; Dickinson's conduct was hostile.

This hostility had been taken to extreme lengths. Dickinson and Bastick published an article which Pereira referred to in a letter to Bell on 5 January 1852: 'I have positively ascertained that the article on Pharmacy in the opposition journal, ascribed to Liebig, was written by Prof. Geiger and published by him more than 22 years ago! From the first moment of the advertisement I suspected some trick; but I had not time to compare the translation with the original until this afternoon at the Pharmaceutical Society, where I saw Morson and satisfied him of the fact.'[20]

Dickinson, with Bastick's support, was very critical of Bell both at meetings and in his editorials for the *Annals of Pharmacy and Practical Chemistry* which they published for about three years. Dickinson 'seized any opportunity to belittle' Bell's efforts,[21] even shifting his ground to maintain his attack[22] when the Pharmacy Bill (enacted in 1852) was under consideration.

Earlier the attack had been more personal. An article which they wrote in *The Chemical Record* of 6 December 1851, included: 'In vain may Dr Pereira bluster; in vain may Mr Bell think to set himself right with the world by assuming airs of bold defiance; in vain may the comfortable family circle of Morson, Redwood & Co think by redoubled blandishments offered to the pupils that the Pharmaceutical Society will maintain its present basis- deceiving still.' They finished with a firm prediction that 'the career of Mr Bell and his clique is at an end' – a classic example of speaking too soon.

It was Bullock who had been the centre of opposition to Bell and his friends, at an earlier stage, and he resigned in 1844. His experience in Germany and France led him to believe that British pharmacy should copy the Continentals, stressing chemistry. He openly criticised his colleagues for their ignorance of this science. He ignored the fact that British pharmacy had developed in an entirely different manner and totally free of government help or intervention. The councillors of the Pharmaceutical Society were men who ran successful businesses for which, increasingly, scientific knowledge and manipulative skills were required. It was unrealistic of Bullock to believe that another branch of his profession could be created which would exist without the trade of pharmacy to provide its funds. The councillors recognised that it was not possible to start afresh, even if they had thought this desirable. Because Bullock tried hard to persuade the Royal Institution and then the Pharmaceutical Society to concentrate on a school of chemistry with him at its head, one is left to ponder whether his ambition was really to be an academic.

Successively the opposition was slowly overcome and the Society started to become secure. This coincided with increasing business activity and the introduction of many new substances. Morson, in addition to all the alkaloids, contributed creosote, pepsine and an increasing range of inorganic substances to this trend. Feeling secure in their business and progress with their Society, its members continued to give Bell their support, certainly not uncritically but they recognised that the achievement of the main aims might mean the subordination of other matters. Additionally it is certain that they admired Bell's flair – no one else had it.

That they relied upon him meant that he made great efforts on their behalf, even entering Parliament to promote the Pharmacy Bill. It has not perhaps been sufficiently stressed in the writing about Bell's life that he was under considerable strain and worked extraordinarily long hours. As early as 1847, Fownes wrote to sympathise with him 'in his affliction', also referring to his own health which was 'in a very bad state – rapidly declining'.[23] The previous November Bell wrote to a Mrs White thanking her for the gift of some meat, saying that 'engagements during the day are so numerous and pressing that breakfast is the only meal I can rely upon with any certainty. It is, therefore, a good plan to start the day with a solid foundation.'[24]

This was six years after an attack of quinsy had detained him in Geneva while on holiday with Edwin Landseer, and several years before the full development of the laryngeal phthisis which caused his death. The 1850s saw increasing signs of the disease but he made no reduction in his enormous workload, although he had great help in his business from Thomas Hyde Hills[25] whom he made a partner in 1849. To those who worked closely with him, it was clear that he was getting worse.

Daniel Hanbury,[26] who had made such an impact even though very young, assisted in editing the *Journal* and referred to his 'very great sufferings'. After Bell's death, he wrote to de Vrij in Holland saying that Bell could not swallow and it was lack of nourishment that had contributed to his early death.[27]

Bell was as active as ever in editing the *Journal.* This was his means of promulgating his views and keeping in touch with his constituency. The question of the editorship was discussed at intervals from the start of the Society, a Council meeting on 4 December 1850 doing so 'at some length' but no change was made.

All these years, Morson was reviewing his draft leaders. Bell wrote on Christmas Day 1858, sending two for the next month's issue. It is as well to quote it in full:

My Dear Morson,

I enclose two of my leaders for the next month's Journal. The one on Juvenile Associations is intended rather to encourage that kind of thing and if possible to suggest a kind of nil desperandum idea. I hope I have not trodden on anybody's toes. In the other article I think I have placed Homeopathy in its true light. I believe the entire question of the honesty of the system is correctly stated in the sentence, against which I have placed nine [*sic*] marks.

Mr Roberts wrote to me to ask the price of the horse. I have been shut up all day here by very ungenial [*sic*] weather, wind rather blustering more or less rain. The extent of my walk was 3 hours. Off to Blackmore's to dinner where I found him in bed with a kind of rheumatic attack and swelled face – and after dinner I had the amusement of applying some leeches.

Yours Sincerely

Jacob Bell.

The article entitled 'Homeopathy in its true light' appeared on 1 January 1859. The sub-title was: The battle of the -opathics.

Even though he was working as hard as ever, he owned to being unwell and depressed. He called himself 'weak and incapable' in a letter of 8 January 1859 from Tunbridge Wells, where he had gone in the hope that his health would improve. His letter omits words, revealing that his concentration was affected. If he had been better he would have 'carried into more detail the suggestions about the Journal'. He was working on the arrangements for its transfer to the Society and needed Morson's views, so 'after a dose of sedative ... I have been favoured with a lucid interval and in great haste have written the enclosed .... The Library and Museum Committee meet tomorrow morning – some part of the enclosed might be worth consulting about but I leave it to you to do as you please. There will be a few more suggestions if I revive and live long enough to write them. The question about money is a delicate one. I think the proposal is fair at all events for a beginning and with the understanding that it is open to revision.'

By this time his writing had deteriorated, making some words difficult to decipher; and there is an almost complete lack of punctuation.

The letter confirms that Bell and Morson spent considerable time discussing the details of how the *Journal* should be transferred and the means to be employed for its future editing and management. Bell relied entirely on Morson to discuss any matter he thought fit with the councillors on the Library Committee. The only alternative open to Bell would have been to write formally to the committee. He chose to rely on the man whose counsel he had used for nearly eighteen years.

At the end of the month, Bell was no better. Among Morson's collection of Bell's letters is one written to Hills from Hastings on 27 January. It is typical of Bell that it is embellished with sketches. When he refers to their cook and her drinking habits, she is shown draining a glass – doubtless of Bell's port!

He was taking cod liver oil and 'quinine, two grains'. 'The enemy has not come forward yet – as soon as he indicates I shall take the opiate.' At a quarter to six, the enemy appeared and the opiate was taken. With the pain gone his wry sense of humour returned and he drew the devil of pain on his paper. He was trying

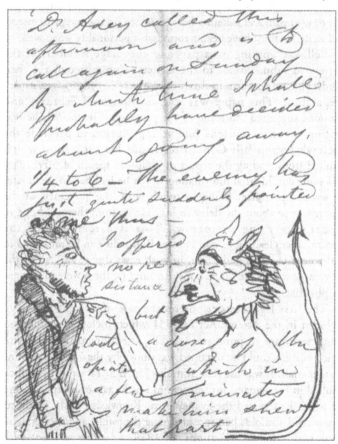

Figure 11: Letter, Bell to Hills, 27th January 1859

acetate of morphine in an ointment placed on lint 'on a raw surface, the skin being removed by a blister' which was about an inch across. Dr Williams had suggested this would be absorbed and avoid his having to swallow. He had taken 'Chloridine for a week. In some respects it is a very nice medicine but my throat is so tender that the stimulating effect seems rather too much for it.'

On the 28th he wrote again from Hastings to Morson: 'My hopes are in perilous condition unless I hear from you in the morning.' He wanted Morson to stay, together with Hills – 'that would be jolly. I want to talk to you about a few things if I can a day or two before the Council.'

The courage he displays in his determination to complete his few remaining tasks, especially the journal transfer, is extraordinary. If at this time of pain and suffering he summoned up the energy to discuss and write, he must have been a formidable personality when well.

Bell was working on a paper to encourage members of the Society to submit items to the General Committee of the then Medical Council for inclusion in the *Pharmacopoeia* under preparation. This paper was read for him on 3 February and revisions suggested to some of the processes. On the 9th he was writing about the Poisons Bill, asking Morson to persuade the Society's Poison Bill Committee about his suggestion which resulted from reading the report of Walpole's speech of 3 February and some confidential information which he had had. A week later he wrote again after being in touch with 'the Secretary' at the Home Office about the delay in his hearing from them. 'I hope to report something tomorrow.' This is a reminder of the circumstances leading to two Poisons Bills failing to be presented to Parliament in 1858 and 1859, in both cases due to the fall of the Government, but the discussions surrounding them were important for pharmacists.

The first legal restrictions on the sale of poisons had been included in the Arsenic Act of 1851 which included stipulations about warnings to purchasers. Public attention to the ease with which poisons could be obtained was drawn by the 1856 strychnine murder trials. It was the final stimulus for A. S. Taylor's work which resulted in his demand for restrictions on the sale of morphine, and for which he received the Swiney Prize. Knowledge of the ill-effects of powerful alkaloids had spread among the public and inevitably to those with criminal intentions. In 1858, a terrible accident with arsenic killed twenty people and ensured that a bill dealing with storage, labelling and control was drafted.

The discussions in Parliament were used by Bell to promote the interest of pharmacists and to oppose the old medical establishment, which had contrived to have included in a bill, in 1858 before the arsenic tragedy, a clause setting up a board of physicians and apothecaries to license sellers of poisons. Bell organised a petition and the bill was withdrawn. After the arsenic accident, the Pharmaceutical Society did not think they could oppose another bill and one resulting from such circumstances.[28] In February 1859, however, they decided to reaffirm their opposition to any bill which did not make proper provision for their professional interest. No legislation was presented because of the fall of Derby's government over the Reform Bill.

This is an amazing level of activity for a very sick man. If he consulted so much with Morson in writing under these conditions, their discussions when he had been well must have been virtually continuous.

Bell's brain continued to be clear and active. Writing again from Hastings on 23 March, he told Morson: 'I fear the Poison Bill will fail to do even the modicum of good that we hoped it might-as it is to be cut down in every distinction of rank or class ... I think so far as I can judge now the less we stir in it the better – what I am now afraid of is a rising of the Chemists and Druggists (on the Chartist principle). The enclosed is a specimen – I have seen several like it. This came from the Manchester Guardian. I don't know whether there is any need for me to come to the Poison Committee on Thursday, is there?' From Hastings to London in 1859 would have been a long journey for a sick man, even one obviously feeling stronger. He was, however, very concerned that his influence should be exercised to prevent what he suspected might become a serious disagreement about poisons legislation, a point made by a deputation led by Morson which had been to see the Home Secretary whom they believed was ill-informed.

On Thursday 20 April, he 'had nothing to boast of in the way of strength or sanitary reform – day by day I exist'. Nevertheless he asks if Morson had received a proof of a leader about Evidence of Soundness of Mind. 'I sent it to you before showing it to anyone else wishing to know if you see any objections to it. To me the case appears clear and a true parallel but I sometimes find that an idea may strike others differently.' He was working on other articles including one on the demise of the Poisons Bill, being entitled 'a false way of stating the truth'.

He wished to answer those who maintained that the Pharmaceutical Society was insignificant compared with 12,000 chemists and druggists. His article was published on 2 May 1859; it pointed out that included in the Registrar-General's definitions of druggists were 'grocers, oilmen, some apothecaries who keep open shops, keepers of drug stalls in markets etc.' It was only the members of the Pharmaceutical Society who worked to raise the standards of their profession.

The letter tells Morson that he was advised to go to Tunbridge Wells. There was another rare moment of depression: 'it matters not to me where I am I may as well go'. He intended moving on Easter Saturday, two days later.

All the humour had left him and he needed what strength remained to complete the few tasks outstanding. He still needed the support of his old friend, confidant and working partner, so was 'anxious to show you what I have written as my address to the members for Wednesday'. Morson read this address to the Society's 18th Anniversary meeting, Bell being too ill to give his Presidential address himself. It must have been a poignant occasion.

Bell's letter points out that 'very few of the members know the undercurrent which has had a material influence in making the Society and keeping it together in harmony'. This is the key to many of their actions and the answer to Bullock and Dickinson for their failure; in this respect, due in part to their ambition for themselves and not for the Society.

On 30 May, Bell was still in Tunbridge Wells asking to meet Morson to discuss the arrangements about the *Journal*. He wanted a little consultation 'to make the arrangement final and satisfactory', asking Waugh and Sandford[29] to join them at Langham Place so as to have allies to settle the matter with the Council on 1 June, two days later. Its importance was considerable since without a transfer, the *Journal* would have belonged to Bell's estate; the complications arising from that would have taken years to solve.

Bell had travelled from Tunbridge Wells to Bloomsbury and while they were at the council meeting he asked Morson to call on him. He then sent a note round to Southampton Row telling Morson 'there is no occasion to trouble yourself to call on purpose, that is for the regular meeting of the *Journal* Committee, of which you will in future be a member'. There was little that Bell had written on which Morson had not been asked to comment. Bell wished to ensure that Morson would continue to be, as Ince put it years later, the Editorial Committee's standing counsel.

The details of the Transfer of the *Journal* to the Society were published later in it. The final part differs little from the pencilled draft which Morson kept all his life in a small envelope marked 'J. Bell's last writing'. There is a note from Bell saying: 'the foregoing is adopted by Council – you approve this and I sign the whole leaving you in case of need to complete any details wanted'. Bell and Morson signed the transfer with Hills, witnessing their signatures.

Bell wrote three documents: one concerning the *Journal's* price, one on receipts and expenditure and the third with suggestions for future management. He had been working on these for weeks, consulting lawyers and even the publisher John Churchill. The difficulties under which all this was achieved are indicated by an undated note he sent to Morson, but it is near to his death; he says he has tried 'twenty times or more' to write. 'The one I sent by post I had only $^3/_4$ hr to scribble – I may have another lucid interval but very likely not.'

The sadness attendant upon reviewing a dying man's last actions is more than offset by admiration for his courage and strength of purpose. He adds a personal note to Morson: 'What I particularly desire is not to have lugubrious rumours spread about. The facts will be out soon enough and it puts me in a flurry [illegible] about it. I am also afraid of alarming my sisters.' Morson was at Bell's side until an hour before his death on 12 June 1859.

Morson and Hills saw to it that the facts were made known and kept to themselves these details of the circumstances. They, like other colleagues, remained loyal to his wishes.

The Council decided to commemorate Bell's death by establishing a scholarship in his name. Subscriptions were invited and, since the Council wanted a portrait of Bell, they felt that an engraving of it could be sold to augment the Scholarship Fund.

On 2 August 1859 Hills, who had been asked to see what could be done, wrote[30] to Morson to tell him that Bell's friend Sir Edwin Landseer had agreed to paint a posthumous portrait. Morson drafted his reply in pencil on Hills' letter, a not infrequent practice. He states that the Council were pleased to have a portrait from 'so highly distinguished a person and also from a personal friend of our late lamented President'. He thought that a publisher might purchase the copyright and 'a noble addition might be made to our Bell Testimonial Fund'. He concludes by asking Hills to 'act in such manner as may be most agreeable to the distinguished artist who so generously records his friendship for a lost friend'.

The Scholarship Fund was successfully established and benefited a number of students whose names and portraits are entered into a special album.

Bell's declining health had been obvious for some years and probably in anticipation of his death he was, in 1856, elected President of the Society with Morson as his Vice-President from 1859, a decision ensuring continuity. No one apart from Bell had contributed more than Morson to the creation of the Society, had a greater effect on the formulation of policy nor had greater knowledge of the 'undercurrents'. Morson had huge support in the Society. As early as 1843, he received the fourth greatest number of votes for Council after Bell, Allen and Pigeon. Later he was second only to Bell, although in 1855 he received the highest number of votes of all candidates. His work for the Board of Examiners had been unremitting, requiring not only the ability to examine candidates but the necessity to keep abreast of new pharmaceutical and chemical developments. Others, like Alsop, had admitted they could not do this and had resigned. Morson described it as 'an onerous and time-consuming duty; but it exerts a very important influence on the character of the Society'. He clearly had similar motives for carrying out another important duty – the Pharmacopoeia Committee that he joined from its first meeting in August 1854.

Morson assumed the Presidency for the second time on 13 June 1859 and remained in the office for two important years. Deane,[31] Waugh, Squire, Sandford and Morson's old friend Savory together with D. B. Hanbury had been part of the inner circle supporting Bell. It was D. B. Hanbury's son, Daniel, who perhaps summed up their attitude and support for Morson when he wrote to de Vrij,[32] the well-known Dutch quinologist: 'From his reputation as a scientific man and the other qualifications he possesses, the post, it is thought, is well filled up.'

That Bell's death left a void of leadership cannot be doubted but Morson quickly took over the reins and addressed the practical problems facing the Society. Also he changed the manner in which decisions were taken. The Council as a whole would run the Society in future. No one would again achieve the dominance that Bell had. A new phase of the Society's development was started.

The first matter was the *Journal.* Morson and Daniel Hanbury (who had been on the Journal Committee for some years) ensured that it was properly managed while Redwood, Bentley and Barnard were the paid editors in each of their spheres: Chemistry/Pharmacy, Materia Medica and the affairs relating to the shop. When he left the office of President, Deane ran the Journal Committee with Morson, Edwards, Hazelden and Waugh. By the end of 1861 new arrangements had been completed with the publisher Churchill for management and publication. His work completed in keeping the *Journal* well organised and in accordance with Bell's terms of transfer, Morson left the committee in 1863.

The day-to-day administration of the Society was in the competent hands of Elias Bremridge, who had joined the Society as Secretary in 1857 so had two years' experience by the time of Bell's death. He was a capable man, dealing with all the bureaucratic functions of the Society until 1884.

All those in the forefront of the Society were pharmacists and businessmen of success and importance in London, Edinburgh, Liverpool, Exeter and other cities. They had all recognised Bell's exceptional talent. He had the political skills, the determination and the time to give to the creation of the Society. His burning ambition to create a professional body was the result of his conviction about the need; and the suspicion that he had a limited time to achieve it. He was always careful to ensure that he had the support he needed, otherwise he could not have withstood the attacks from within the Society nor have fought the determined opposition from without.

Morson was no politician, he relied on his extensive knowledge of his profession and a wide – on occasion probably rather detached – view of the debate swirling round the Society. He knew they were taking part in a revolution in medicine and, consequently, in the structure of its organisation. He was highly intelligent and had considerable charm and had to rely upon these characteristics to retain the respect of such widely differing people as Squire and Hills, for example. He remained on good terms with people because he understood the reasons for their differences. He was more cautious, perhaps less emotional, than Bell – a factor in making their partnership so successful.

Two days after Bell's death, Morson held an informal meeting of councillors. This was prior to his first Council[33] meeting on Thursday 16 June. His attitude was clear. The Society was a unified body and had, at long last, been recognised as the professional institution of pharmacists. He was convinced, as he said in his annual report in May 1863, of the 'extent to which the value of these objects (protection, education and benevolence) has been recognised by the Medical Profession as a whole'.

The third matter, and in some ways the most difficult, concerned the School of Pharmacy. In one of the most important acts of his Presidency, Morson set up a committee to look into its finance and management. While the main aims of the Society were being achieved, the attention given to the running of the School was less than needed. This 'ladder by which we may hope to ascend to our proper place in the medical profession', as Bell put it, was not successful. It was costing more than had been anticipated and the number of students was declining. All this was against the background of the extraordinary decision to halve the subscription, thus reducing the Society's income very significantly.

A laboratory for the students was set up in 1844 and a year later one designed by Redwood was opened when Morson, as Vice-President standing in for Savory, invited members at the October meeting to inspect it. Andrew Ure had praised the new laboratory for its design.

It was not long before the manner in which the laboratory expenses were handled was criticised. As early as January 1846 there was the criticism that Redwood was not providing vouchers for the items he purchased. Morson must have been aware of this not only because he took a close interest in the educational aspects of the Society but because he was frequently taking council meetings in place of Savory. In April 1850, there were further comments but no action was taken.

The arrangement was that Redwood accepted the students' fees, taking half for himself; the other half he used for laboratory expenses, handing over any surplus to the Secretary. The auditors forced a change to this 'very unsatisfactory arrangement' in September 1850, the fees being paid to the Secretary and controls being introduced on Redwood's expenditure. In 1853, another change made Redwood the sole participator in the profit or loss connected with the laboratory. The only justification for such a measure might be that the Professor was thus encouraged to search for students and to keep the expenses low. In 1858, Redwood's balance from the 47 students was £196.

In 1860, the Council was persuaded to expand the laboratory favouring a plan to move it to the top floor of the Society's building and consolidating the School of Pharmacy there. Redwood describes the building surrounded by scaffold poles for this project to be effected.[34] It was to create accommodation for 60 students.

By early 1861, the expense of the project was running well ahead of that anticipated. So much so that Morson and Squire took over supervision of the building work, which Council had decided could be financed from Bell's legacy of £2,000.

The question of the running expenses was also within the remit of Morson's Special Financial Committee. Morson, Squire and six other councillors looked into 'the large expenditure lately incurred and the income and expenditure of the laboratory and lectures'. Perhaps in anticipation of what was to come, the Professors were formally requested to cooperate. The report was produced in less than two months with Morson, Squire and D. B. Hanbury playing a major part.

On 14 March 1861, Redwood submitted a memorandum, proposing minimal changes, and countered the expected criticism by asking for cooperation from the members. He also complained that he had had very little return for eight years of effort. However lax the Council had been, this challenge to their authority must have caused a sensation. When they published their committee's report it showed that Morson and his colleagues were dissatisfied with the 'industry, order and neatness' which were lacking and they entirely disagreed with Redwood. They also accused the Library Museum and Laboratory Committee of a failure to supervise, thus leavening the criticism of Redwood, for the Committee was composed of councillors. They also hoped that Redwood would cooperate in better management of the laboratory. He said he would give increased personal attention to the students after the Committee had, at D. B. Hanbury's suggestion, discussed the report with him.

It seems likely that the Library Committee had been lax, but their defence would certainly have included the closeness of Redwood with Bell. This must have been the reason why earlier attempts at control had not been pursued. With Bell's death, Redwood was left without his patron. It is inconceivable that Bell had been ignorant of the criticisms of Redwood, but he chose not to support any action. Whether this was due to his illness, his heavy involvement in parliamentary matters, or a desire to avoid unpleasantness or even scandal about his protégé cannot be known. Morson grasped the first opportunity to act. This and his initiation of the review of finance and of the policy towards the School of Pharmacy ensured that the Society made further progress towards its stated objectives. In respect of the School of Pharmacy it was a belated return to a situation similar to that when Fownes was appointed, although it could not recover the ground lost: the chance of creating the national school of chemistry. Fownes had made no secret of his desire in an address to the Pharmaceutical Society[35] that its school should become a College of Chemistry.

In spite of Redwood's promise to improve, the cleanliness of the laboratory deteriorated even though it had only ten pupils. The Council had had enough. They decided to appoint a Director, leaving Redwood doing his lecturing on pharmacy only. In March 1862 Attfield[36] was appointed. He quickly restored order and reputation, although one incident suggests that relations with Redwood were difficult. Redwood was asked for an inventory of his equipment, stocks etc., identifying what was his and what he would like the Society to take off his hands. Clearly the laboratory had become a personal fief and he had failed to respond to the changes following Bell's death.

The relationships between Bell, Morson and the Professors were one of the complicating factors which made Morson's position difficult. It is to his credit that matters were resolved in a straightforward and honourable way, even though it inevitably upset Redwood.

In the first years of the Society four professors were appointed. Pereira was Professor of Materia Medica, Thomson of Botany, Redwood of Pharmacy and Fownes of Chemistry.

George Fownes had worked as assistant to Morson's friend Graham, and had studied at Giessen. It was Morson's knowledge of Fownes, and his influence in the Society, which had obtained the professorship for this brilliant young man. It cannot be doubted that the presence on their staff of eminent men, especially Pereira and Fownes, would enhance the prestige of the fledgling Society. Morson had a scientific liaison with Fownes over Furfurol, which had caused great interest in January 1840 when exhibited at the Royal Institution. It was the first production of a vegeto-alkali; Fownes was later to describe it as 'in many particulars resembling substances occurring in cinchona bark'.[37] He received a Gold Medal from the Royal Society for this work. Morson exhibited a sample he made at the Great Exhibition of 1851. It was included in the firm's sales catalogues until 1899.

Unfortunately Fownes' health was poor, he contracted tuberculosis and his health forced him to leave England for Barbados in the hope of getting better. He wrote[38] to Morson from Government House where he was staying with the Governor who provided him with 'a little cottage in the garden for a laboratory'. He wrote that 'he cannot express to you my sense of obligation to Mr Graham for his kindness in taking charge of the pupils', an arrangement obviously made by the three friends, but also an example of Morson's frequent role as a facilitator whose influence was important. In this case, Fownes' pupils at University College were temporarily in the charge of the Professor of Chemistry at London University.

The letter includes an account of Fownes' discovering that the bitter Camara contained hydrocyanic acid but 'Dr Davy tells me that my discovery is old so we must say nothing about it. I have no books to refer to.' A few months later in 1848 he returned to England and died the year after, aged only 34. His health had forced him to resign his Pharmaceutical Society appointment in 1846. He was not replaced, the Society feeling it had to economise so they appointed Redwood as Professor of both Chemistry and Pharmacy. If Morson tried to have Fownes replaced with someone of equal reputation, he failed.

The same policy of retrenchment had resulted in the Scientific Committee, suggested by Pereira in 1844, being a short-lived affair. When setting it up, Morson's influence had been paramount, most of those invited to serve were his scientific friends. Two measures reducing the Society's scientific reputation were a blow to one who believed that this was an important part of its work. Morson, however, had to bow to the members' wishes, short-sighted as he knew they were.

This was not the only item debated for hours in Council in the middle of the 1840s; the editorship of the *Journal* and the School of Pharmacy would have been casualties if they had not had Bell's powerful support. The former was run at very small cost to the Society, Bell bearing virtually all the costs and subsidising it from his own pocket, but it was the means of communication and publicity. The latter was central to raising the educational qualifications of members and thereby of a profession in need of greater expertise. The strong personalities on the Council made sure these subjects were debated, Daniel Bell Hanbury recording the fact that several council meetings took four hours or more to complete their business. This was not a rubber stamp for what John and Charles Watts in *The Chemist* described as the 'ruling clique' in 1850 when referring to Bell and Morson.

Redwood's appointment as Professor of Pharmacy was due to Bell. Apprenticed to a Cardiff apothecary, he had experience of the wide range of duties of a country practice from compounding medicines to minor surgery. In 1823 he went to complete his training with John Bell's pharmacy, a move initiated by a Quaker friend of his father. Here he met Jacob Bell with whom he formed a lifelong friendship. He made a worthwhile contribution to the business both in running the dispensing counter and in re-designing the shop. He left to run his own business in 1832 but sold it to a Thomas Bigg in 1834 from whom Curtis, of Baker Street, bought it. Redwood went into the manufacture of chemicals and pharmaceutical preparations but does not seem to have been any more successful than with his retail business. He joined Bell late in 1841, as sub-editor of the *Pharmaceutical Journal* and *Transactions*.

A second link with Bell was that they had both been brought up in Quaker households. While Bell's family had been in the Society of Friends for several generations, Redwood's parents were converts. His father married twice; one of Theophilus' half-brothers was Isaac Redwood who made a large fortune as a coalmaster and property-owner in South Wales, where Theophilus had a property after his father's death.

Thus, there were close personal and professional links between Bell and Redwood.

Another of Bell's appointments was that of Robert Bentley as Professor of Botany (following Thomson's death) and later of Materia Medica. He was Professor of Botany at King's College from 1859–1887. He had been an assistant at Bell's pharmacy.

Among the accusations and misrepresentations levelled against Bell and Morson was one of nepotism and of using place-men. In Bell's case, there was some validity, for neither Redwood nor Bentley had the kind of reputation that Fownes had earned, and no one had dared to impugn wrong motives for that appointment. The fact that Redwood became Morson's son-in-law after his appointment at the Society did not prevent the Watts from making snide remarks but they were invalid except in so far as the addition of Chemistry to Redwood's duties was concerned; but that could be said to have been caused by the members.

Redwood was the longest-serving of the Professors at the time Morson was President. His close understanding with and support from Bell allowed him greater freedom of action than would otherwise have occurred. He was a first-rate pharmacist and was dedicated to improving the education of pharmacists, an attitude which may have been a factor in his approach to Council. Perhaps he suspected that they were less dedicated to the School than was Bell. Redwood also made a successful contribution to pharmaceutical literature and was appointed to edit the British *Pharmacopoeias* of 1865, 1874 and 1885; he also wrote the supplement to the 1867 edition.

It is interesting to attempt to explain Redwood's attitude. His challenge to Council was a mistake that so clever a man should have avoided. It may be that he had become so central a figure in the Society that he had grown careless. Fownes' death and his liaison with Bell resulted in his running the Museum and Library in addition to his duties as a professor which included the Laboratory. He was sub-editor of the *Journal*. With the formation of the Cavendish Society he became its Secretary. *The Chemical Record*, the short-lived predecessor of the *Annals of Pharmacy*, both owned and edited by Dickinson and Bastick, the enemies of Bell and the Society, pointed out that too much was expected of Redwood but also that he received nearly £900 a year in fees for the posts that he held. They omitted that a small part was in turn used to employ an assistant in the laboratory. Redwood himself wrote[39] that more and more duties were piled upon him, but he did not restrict his involvement in outside activities, among them societies like the Cavendish and Chemical, nor his attempts to enter the chemical industry.

He made the mistake of delegating teaching to his assistant and, according to Morson's committee, only passing through the laboratory during the day, thus avoiding what they called euphemistically 'all interference'. It is not surprising that they concluded that the decline in numbers of students was due to 'defective arrangements in the laboratory itself'.

In this connection, the evidence of one of the first two Bell scholars is very apposite. William Tilden was apprenticed in September 1857 to Alfred Allchin, once an assistant in the School of Pharmacy. He attended lectures in 1858 and again in 1860. In an article[40] written by invitation of the editor of the *Pharmaceutical Journal* in 1923, he points out that a condition of his apprenticeship was attendance at the School's lectures and spending his last year in its laboratory. He so impressed Dr John Stenhouse, who had a private research laboratory in Islington, with his chemical ability that he was offered a post as a chemical assistant. He worked at 17 Bloomsbury Square for nine years, thus he experienced supervision from both Redwood and Attfield. Tilden left London in 1872 for a permanent appointment at Clifton College, Bristol, having decided to give up pharmacy. He became Professor of Chemistry at Birmingham and then the Royal College of Science; he became an F.R.S. and was knighted.

In his article, he hopes that he does not upset his pharmaceutical friends but nonetheless points out that, while enjoying the first lectures at the School in 1858, after which he did a great deal of private study, he was bored by the second year's lectures and escaped to attend Hoffmann's 'exciting' ones. These were in a 'new world of scientific chemistry'. He refers to Redwood's lectures as 'utter rubbish, entirely behind the knowledge and experience of the time'.

It is surprising that Redwood felt able to spend so much time on activities other than those of his main function and the source of his reputation and most of his income.

He omitted any reference to the incidents with Council in his section of the *Progress of Pharmacy*. His excuse that many duties had been heaped upon his shoulders, if meant to explain his failures, is weak. He was the most senior of the Society's staff, and the longest-serving. He had ample opportunity to suggest alterations to his duties.

With the efforts to hold members together and to persuade Parliament to legislate in their favour consuming so much of the available time, there is some reason to excuse members of Council, who were part-time, for their reliance on Redwood. We are forced to the conclusion that he failed the Society in so far as the School of Pharmacy was concerned. There is a difference between a failure to control expenditure and a failure to implement, being in a pivotal position, one of the main aims of the Society: the creation of a new generation of scientifically trained pharmacists.

The French had Professors of Chemistry and Pharmacy in Paris but Redwood's attempt to combine the two was unsuccessful. Student numbers dwindled and their standards of chemical knowledge cannot have been high if their Professor's lectures were 'rubbish'. Had the examiners noticed any effects and did they, including Morson, call the Council's attention to the problem?

There are also two longer-term questions which Redwood's performance raised. The failure of the School of Pharmacy to attract students disappointed the reformers and led many students to go to the College of Chemistry.[41] A smaller number of poor- quality students left the School to go into practice. If their technical standards were no higher than that of the older generation, there is little likelihood that the general standard in the profession was rising. It may be that standards were not even being maintained. The possibility arises that the failures in innovation and pharmaceutical chemical production later in the century were due to the earlier absence of an adequate supply of more highly trained pharmacists. Since standards were not rising, the objections to the inclusion of chemists and druggists qualified only by apprenticeship or experience in the Pharmaceutical Society's membership may not have been felt valid.

The information from the Council minutes and references elsewhere to the important work of particularly Morson, Squire,

T. H. Hills, Webb Sandford and others reveal more of the history of the Society at this time than Redwood wrote in his part of the *Progress of Pharmacy*. Reviewing some parts of his writing in this light reveals them to be a somewhat egocentric account of events. This is disappointing as there was no one working for the Society who had a greater knowledge of its early days. Also it seems that Redwood has had an effect on subsequent accounts of the Pharmaceutical Society's history. The emphasis on parliamentary activities is to the detriment of a more balanced record of the professional, scientific, industrial and commercial activities of pharmacists and also of an assessment of the success the Society has had in achieving its aims.

In 1854, in his evidence to a Parliamentary Committee, Redwood stated that he was 'engaged in chemical manufacturing operations'. There are no extant records of these, but he signed a lease on 25 March 1859 for the rental of 168 High Street, Homerton. His occupation of these premises continued for years; entries in rate books provide confirmation that he was operating at Homerton throughout the 1860s, and 'Redwood and Co.' appear as occupants in 1872.[42]

There is oblique confirmation of Redwood's chemical activity by Morson's younger son Robert, who was writing to his brother from Spain, in May 1868, where he worked as a construction engineer. He states that: 'I wrote to Redwood last night but forgot to ask him the price of alkali per ton.'

The extent of Redwood's business cannot be gauged, but his trade with Morson's chemical plant at Hornsey was substantial. The ledgers of Morson's account at the Bank of England record regular payments of varying amounts starting in 1856. By 1859, they had reached £1,000 and continued through the 1860s, slowly declining from £728 to £196. The last year of entries is 1868 and coincides with the last rate book entry apart from the 1872 one, which appears to be a repeat after Redwood had left the site.

This date matches the statement in the obituary of Morson in Boase which says he set up his factory at Homerton in 1869.

By this time, Redwood's business was failing, if not bankrupt. Morson took over the factory which was described as a gelatine works; gelatine appearing in Morson's sales lists and advertisements at this time. In his Will, which left his son his business, he also leaves him the 'works at Homerton, transferred to me for money advanced to Theophilus Redwood'.

Financial failure carried a stigma in Victorian times, so both of Redwood's failed attempts in business would only have been referred to in private. That Morson knew of Redwood's business activities in 1861 is proved by the bank ledgers, nor was Morson his only customer. He may have supplied Bell. It is surprising that he continued with a business whose activity was unrelated to any research or invention which he was able to exploit. Williamson[43] licensed his scammony process, Pelletier and Guibourt, professors in similar institutions to Redwood, ran factories using their discoveries and process developments. Redwood did not have such techniques to exploit. His business was a quite separate venture. There is, however, a clue to his reason – he needed more money than his academic activities provided.

Redwood married Morson's daughter, Charlotte Elizabeth in 1845 at St George's, Bloomsbury. Thus he automatically renounced his Quaker upbringing. Bell was a witness. It is curious that Redwood described himself as 'Gentleman' as he did his father, Thomas. It seems pretentious to have used the term, when 'Professor of Pharmacy' would have done better, and it implies a financial independence which he did not possess.

The Redwoods had children at speed in the mid-Victorian manner, Charlotte having live births at intervals averaging 16 months. She became ill with tuberculosis and died, aged 46, in Boverton, Redwood's home, where she had gone to avoid London's smoke.

Morson was generous to the newly-weds. From the receipts signed after her death by her children for their share of their mother's dowry, it appears that Morson settled about £3,000 on Theophilus and Charlotte; this would have provided Charlotte with £90 a year in interest, a better- than- average income. In addition, they had £500 as a present and in subsequent years between £60 and £125 was given in each year. With a much above average income from professional activities, the couple could have lived quite well at 19 Montagu Street, on the east side of the British Museum and not 200 yards from the Society's house. The Census of 1851 reveals that they had three servants and that of 1861, four servants; there were then six adults and seven children in the house.

According to a leading article of 1852 in *The Chemical Record*[44] they felt it would be fair to ask 'of the Professor of Chemistry what he had done and where the fruits of his labour are recorded'. Although this publication was critical to a venomous degree, one point is factually made: Redwood not only had a wider range of duties in the Society than might be expected, he received fees and payments separately as Lecturer, Librarian and Director of the Laboratory amounting to £645 in 1851. In addition, he received

£75 as Secretary to the Cavendish Society. There was also rumoured a fee of £150 as sub-editor of the *Pharmaceutical Journal*. Thus his income exceeded £750 a year when a labourer's wage reached barely £30. He was able to live in Montagu Street with, according to the 1851 Census, a nurse, cook and housemaid in addition to the five in the family at that time. He had, as well, a generous father-in-law.

While their income was considerably less than Morson's and a fraction of Bell's, whose lavish entertainment scandalised his fellow Quakers, they were comfortably situated. Possibly Redwood tried to keep pace with his father-in-law and his sponsor; he certainly was never happy with his income. Even when his grandchildren were adults, Morson's cash book shows regular sums paid to the two elder ones. These were in addition to the regular payment of £50 per quarter to Redwood which was agreed at the time of Morson taking over the Homerton lease. Morson also paid 100 guineas a year for a life assurance policy, which was part of the marriage settlement. The life policy apart, payments at this time varied between £400 and £600 a year. In today's money, this is worth about £10,000. Such a father-in-law must be exceptional.

From all sources, Redwood's income was more than sufficient for anyone not either extravagant or imprudent. Redwood, however, caused Morson considerable irritation as is shown by a letter of 30 April 1872, which he addressed simply to 'Dr Redwood':

I have received your letter. It did not astonish me as according to custom no sooner was I absent for a few days than a demand for money was addressed to my son. You state truly that it is over three months since you had a cheque but you are not ignorant that this was given you in advance. I doubt not you are in want of money but have I ever known you otherwise? and it is quite evident that you will do nothing to assist us with the least good will – but the contrary. The accounts for the last quarter have not been delivered although half an hour's work is all the time required.

He requested that the ledger be sent to him so that the accounts could be compiled. If that was done, another £50 would be advanced. Whatever his irritation with Redwood, he asked after his grandsons, finishing with the hope that the eldest was not leading an 'idle life'. One can assume that this was not the case, at least for very long, as he became a successful oil chemist, advising Lord Fisher as Chief of Naval Staff on the conversion of the Navy's ships from coal to oil before the First World War, besides inventing the Redwood viscometer and receiving a baronetcy.

Redwood's reply may be imagined from Morson's second note:

38 Queen Square
9 May, 1872

Dear Redwood,
I enclose you a cheque for £50, the further advance I promised you,
receipt of which you will acknowledge to me. Had you devoted to
the sending out the 3rd and 4th [quarter's] accounts, half the time
occupied in writing me a faithless, unkind and I may say insulting
letter I should have been spared the necessity of writing what you
consider a sharp letter. Every day brings with it some painful
discovery and I think we have suffered enough from you not to be
subjected to the addition of insult to injury.
Yours truly,

TNR Morson

Relations could hardly have been worse. A more complete
judgement of the situation would be possible if we knew what the
painful discoveries were. A ledger needed to be kept because Morson
took over not only the site but also the firm of Redwood & Co., for
whose taxes he became responsible. He appears to have been paying
Redwood £200 a year, providing he accounted properly for
expenditure the details of which are unknown. Two years later when
Morson's son took over, the arrangement was changed. A nominal
rental of £200 was paid to Thomas junior so that the commitment
to Redwood could be continued.

The fact that stands out is that money was a long-standing
difficulty for Redwood. Knowing what he was, perhaps it was
Morson who proposed to the 1861 Committee that, after all
outstanding bills for the laboratory at 17 Bloomsbury Square had
been paid, a limit of £2 should be placed on individuals before
reference for approval had to be made. Such a low limit speaks
volumes for the Committee's views about both their previous
controls and the financial reliability of Redwood.

In his 1861 address to the 20th Anniversary meeting of the
Society, Morson started by paying tribute to his friend, Jacob Bell,
who 'devoted not only the greater part of his time, but also no small
share of his wealth' to the Society. It would appear that the Professor
of Pharmacy was subsidised to the extent that his income was half as
large again as the fees and payments he received from the Society!
Redwood was content that this should remain so since he accepted
this situation, undignified as it would have been to a man with self-

respect. It is not surprising that this state of affairs was concealed; it is a complete mystery why Morson allowed it to happen. An explanation might be that he was concerned for his daughter and grandchildren and that what started as generosity became, under whatever circumstances, an unavoidable commitment.

However upset Morson was with Redwood, he did not allow this to affect his attitude towards his grandchildren. He was generous to the sons and, in his Will, left £100 to Mary Ann who had been born in 1848.

The question of what would have happened if Redwood had become insolvent is also relevant. It is possible that his career with the Society would have ended amid embarrassing stories about his finances. There could also have been an adverse effect on Morson's business.

Morson included a reference in his address to Bell's achievement in uniting the 'in many instances, unkindred spirits of our trade'.[45] Surely a suitable comment on Bell's difficulties.

The first point that Morson made was that progress from the satisfactory position they had reached, depended upon providing facilities for the best possible education of students. To this end he was to set up a committee of councillors, with wide terms of reference, to consider the future objectives and the means of realising them. In all this he had the support of Deane, Squire and MacFarlan,[46] even if the latter did not live many more months, for the next year Morson had to report the death of his much-respected friend from Edinburgh.

One of the most important subjects for this committee was consideration of the means of increasing the Society's income and putting its finances on a better footing. As the report in the *Pharmaceutical Journal* put it: 'some new adjustment of the means of providing an income adequate to the requirements of the Institution will be necessary'.[47] It was Morson's opinion that fees should be paid annually by all members and that the practice of composition fees giving life membership should end.

With solid achievement behind them, the Society turned its attention to two internal matters. Morson wanted the Society to maintain its stability by better financial arrangements. One means of achieving these was to persuade members that they should open their doors to those 'whose age, respectability and long connexion with the trade ought to have ensured' their membership. There can be little doubt that Morson was referring to chemists and druggists. The debate about their membership had been going on for a long time and may explain why there was no proposal to apply any tests to these proposed new members.

Morson's experience obviously led him to the conclusion that a School of Pharmacy needed to be continued. As no provision existed for scientific pharmaceutical education, the Society had included in its original aims that of setting up an 'efficient means for supplying the scientific knowledge required by Pharmaceutical Chemists'. The need was confirmed during Morson's Presidency even if a few members expressed the view that the Society should not sink into a 'mere Academy'. The achievement at this stage had fallen short of the scientific status at which the Society aimed. It was also lower than that reached in Germany and France. In his Presidential review in 1861 Morson expressed his disappointment thus: 'In what respects are we not progressing? I should answer in the advancement of the science of pharmacy.'[48.]

Thus Morson guided the Society out of difficulties to some extent created by the need to balance the academic and trade requirements of the members and to place it upon a sounder financial footing. The man Hills described as Bell's right-hand man since the inception of the Society was true to the original aims.

Morson continued to serve the Society as a councillor for more than ten years, taking part in the discussions and joining his colleagues in deputations to Government departments, at the same time supplying the knowledge that only long service can. His interest in education resulted in his being an examiner for 28 years, quite apart from his many visits to the School with eminent scientists, especially men like Liebig, Cap, Dorvault and, in earlier times, Rose and his fellow student Mitscherlich, Guibourt and equally prominent French pharmacists – occasions which appear to have excited the interest of the pupils as well as the staff. It was a similar attitude to his interest in his own employees, some of whom became well known in their own right and served the Society in senior posts. One of these was John Williams who spent ten years at Southampton Row, leaving to start a firm with William Hopkin, who was an assistant to Morson in the 1840s. Their reputation in the manufacture of pure chemicals became as high as Morson's. John Williams was serving on Council at the time of Morson's death and later became President of the Society.

Morson's close interest in the Society's affairs is apparent from a letter he wrote to H. B. Brady in 1869.[49] He objected strongly to the proposal to allow reporters to be present at council meetings. 'Heaven help the Councillors' was his comment. While he regretted the action being taken, he did not allow his views to cause him to forget sending his respects to Brady's family.

Morson's technical contributions, both formal and informal, cover a period of over thirty years; the first being on 9 June 1841: 'A sketch of the rise and progress of pharmacy'. The greatest number of papers is on opium and morphine, which is not surprising in view of his pre-eminent position as both scientist and manufacturer. It is significant that he never presented a paper on quinine. As we have seen, his interest waned in the 1860s in the face of competition from Howard's and others, especially those in Europe. It is our loss that he never sought to describe the history of this first modern medicine and his part in its manufacture and sale.

Additionally, he took the chair at meetings, addressed by old friends like Richard Phillips on subjects as varied as potassium iodide, the action of lead in distilled and river waters- both in 1844- and Thomson's review of 'new combinations of iodine;' there was also a paper by Pereira on rhubarb which included the display of samples from Siberia and 'Buchara'.

Samples were an important source of information and were also used for reference purposes, so the Society formed a Museum to which Morson contributed especially opium specimens, the countries of origin being all those in the Middle East, India and China as well as England and Australia. It would be very interesting to have compared these samples, many being complete cakes in their original wrapping, but in ignorance of their importance and probably a false assumption that they still contained some alkaloid, they were destroyed when transferred to the Royal Botanic Gardens at Kew. No photographic record was made to help us assess what it was like to handle this substance, so valuable and important over a very long time.

The chemical museum contained many interesting samples of nineteenth-century products. It is to be hoped that, with modern analytical techniques requiring very small samples, they can be tested as well as catalogued at Kew. Comparisons of the purity achieved then with modern products might provide useful information.

The contributions to this museum include some of the first Furfurol that Morson made. It was this material Fownes used to prepare Furfurine, a sample of which Morson also presented. Phosphoric acid, gallic acid, coniine hydrobromate and a substance named menthyl hydrate were presented as well as Meconin (opianyl) which was described in the Society's list as a magnificent specimen crystallised in a glass basin. There was also a sample of uric acid extracted from the excrement of a boa constrictor at London Zoo. When this fact was related by Sir John Hanbury from a story he had been told by Thomas D. Morson, a great-grandson of T. N. R. Morson, it seemed unbelievable but the records of the chemical museum are clear. Besides, Tilden recalled that he operated such a process at Bloomsbury Square. Final confirmation is provided by the firm's 1899 catalogue which includes the item: 'Ammonium urate (from Boa's excrement), 1/= per ounce'.

Presidents held conversazioni and there exhibited personal possessions as well as products to advertise their wide interests. At his, Morson exhibited[50] piperine and red prussiate of potash, so recently discovered by his friend Playfair. Tennant was persuaded to display a case of minerals. Morson brought two flower pictures by Mrs Augusta Withers, who specialised in flower painting.

The pictures are still in the family so it is possible to comment that the *Journal's* reporter does not seem to have been a gardener, since he described a gloxinia as a foxglove!

Morson attended all the British Pharmaceutical Conferences. The *Yearbook* for 1874 records that a few months after his death, his son displayed alkaloids, rare chemicals and opiums; also the W. J. Muller picture, *The Laboratory*, of Morson's alkaloid manufacture at Hornsey. Interestingly there was also exhibited a Chinese opium-smoking apparatus. If this was the carefully made brass device, with its containers for opium powder and cleaning probes, which was preserved until recently, it was a good example of design and workmanship. The other exhibits were no doubt ones which Morson himself would have shown. The opium apparatus, however acceptable earlier in the century, may have raised an eyebrow in 1874.

The conversazioni were opportunities to invite friends. In May 1866, Morson's interest in art resulted in his inviting George Cruikshank who brought his picture of *Shakespeare's Birth*. Since his youthful visits to art galleries in London and Paris, he was interested in painting. Once his income rose to allow him to start a collection, he showed his knowledge and good taste in the quality of the pictures he bought. He would have been influenced by Cornelius Varley who sat on the Chemical Committee of the Society of Arts because of his interest in optical instruments and in the City Philosophical Society. Several pictures by John Varley, Cornelius' brother, were in his collection. When he became well-off Morson was part of the intellectual support and friendship for artists and writers. His collection included pictures by Constable, Morland, Thomas

Danby and the pupil of his friend Muller, Harry J. Johnson. Morson was friendly with John Henderson, who lived in the same street as the Redwoods; he had many Muller pictures, which he left to the British Museum. The habit of collecting was shared by Morson's son who had a number by Whistler which were lost in a fire at Southampton Row in 1873; in all more than thirty paintings were destroyed.

Their greatest interest, however, was in Cruikshank's works. The collection started when Morson was less than 40 and resulted in Thomas junior becoming very friendly with Cruikshank. We can speculate that in addition to their artistic and literary interest in his work, they enjoyed laughing with Cruikshank at many aspects of nineteenth-century life as well as looking askance at the cruelty to boy chimney sweeps, drunkenness and other features of Victorian life, which he depicted in his drawings.

The collection was used to assemble a catalogue[51] of Cruikshank's works by the Keeper of Prints and Drawings at the British Museum, who referred to the fact that the Morsons were probably the first to collect Cruikshank's works and possessed 'many varieties and proof states of the artist's finest work, forming the best series in existence'.

The collection was sold at Sotheby's in 1871. There were 182 lots, a large proportion of which included six or more drawings; the sale lasted two days.

The Shakespeare drawing, described as his first appearance on the stage of the Globe in 1564 with some of the members of his company, showed him in his cradle with friends round him and creations of his after-life. It took a long time to complete. Cruikshank wrote in February 1866 that he was still working at it. He had talked to a Mr Graves, a publisher in Pall Mall, who wanted it exhibited at the Royal Academy in April 1867. He had suggested it was worth £250. In October 1868 Cruikshank acknowledged Morson junior's second £50, completing payment for the Shakespeare drawing, with the admonition: 'don't tell Mr Graves what my friend gave me for it'.

At the end of the letter Cruikshank commiserates with his friend on the deaths of Charlotte, Mrs Redwood, and of Robert, his brother. This is a reminder that the 1860s were a sad time and, while Morson continued to manage his successful business with his son's help and also to pursue his scientific interests, death removed both relatives and friends from Morson's life. His wife Charlotte Elizabeth died, after many months of suffering from a circulatory complaint, in 1863. She was buried in Highgate Cemetery in the part reserved for scientists, proof that a decision was taken that Morson himself would be buried there, not far from the graves of other eminent men, like Faraday who died in 1867 after many years of decline, including loss of memory. Antoine Claudet and William Brande died the year before. In the same year as his two children died, his very old friend Thomas Lott was buried, as also was, John Elliotson. In 1869 Thomas Graham and John Barlow died and this was the same year that John Edward Gray had one of the more serious of a series of strokes.

A friend with whom he had close technical and business ties, MacFarlan, died in 1861. In a decade many of Morson's closest relations and friends, whom he had known throughout his career, had left him. One of these was Richard Solly who had died in 1858. In view of his influence in Morson's career, his death would have been particularly poignant.

He had helped a number of men and organisations, using his scientific knowledge and his wealth, and must have been mourned by them also.

This was also a decade of increasing difficulty in business, with a decline in trade and serious competition from Germany. The Franco-German war saw the siege of Paris in 1871, an event which caused great sadness and which Morson would have viewed as he did the events of 1848, when he commented in his Presidential address that attention had been directed more to the manufacture of bullets than to science for the benefit of mankind. This is a reference to the Revolution in France in February 1848 after which Louis Napoleon, who had been living in England, went to Paris to offer himself for election firstly to the Constituent Assembly and then for the Presidency. There were riots in Paris in February, with the Tuileries Palace pillaged. In Sicily there was violent revolution, as also in Vienna. In March Charles Albert of Savoy, Sardinia and Piedmont declared war on Austria. Even as he spoke in June 1848 there were serious riots in Paris and Lyons. There was, however, good news that the US-Mexican war had ended in February.

His last visit to Paris was in 1872, when he was photographed by the famous Frenchman, Nadar, the portrait revealing how very much older he looked.

He did not stand again for election to the Pharmaceutical Society's Council and retired from all activities outside his business.

Notes

1 *The Forceps*, 2 (1844–5), 13. A journal of dental surgery and the collateral arts and sciences, published fortnightly, 1844–6.

2. Royal College of Physicians; Minutes of Carey Street and Bishops' Court Dispensaries; also Lesch, 'Dispensary Movement', *Bull. Hist.Med.* 55 (1981) 322–42.

3. Worshipful Society of Apothecaries of London; 'Laboratory Stock Audit Book', 1803–57.

4. Loudon, Irving, *Medical Care and the General Practitioner, 1750–1850*, London, Clarendon Press 1986.

5. Hanbury, Daniel Bell (1794–1882); 1808 apprenticed at Plough Court pharmacy; Partner 1824. Treasurer, Pharmaceutical Society 1852-67. Father of Daniel Hanbury, F.R.S.

6. *Pharmaceutical Journal,* 1841–2, 23.

7. Bell, J. and Redwood, T., *Historical Sketch of the Progress of Pharmacy in Great Britain,* London: Pharmaceutical Society, 1880, 97.

8. May, John; 33 Chapel Street, Stonehouse. Secretary, Plymouth and Devonport Branch; original member of the Pharmaceutical Society (no other details discovered).

9. Russell-Gebbett, Jean, *Henslow of Hitcham,* Lavenham, Suffolk: Terence Dalton, 1977, 13.

10. Private archive; letters, Bell to Morson, between 1841 and 1859; quotations from these letters are made throughout the chapter.

11. *Pharmaceutical Journal,* 4 (1844–5), 293–6.

12. Ince, Joseph (1826–1907). M.P.S., F.C.S., F.L.S. Son of William, President Pharmaceutical Society 1850–1, whom he succeeded in 1853 as Director of Godfrey's Laboratory which Robert Bøyle had founded in the seventeenth century. Successful teacher of pharmacy and contributor to the *Pharmaceutical Journal* from 1853 when he joined Jacob Bell on the Editorial committee. Attended Professor Daniell's lectures on chemistry at King's College, London 1843–4, while apprenticed to William Hotham Pigeon 1841–5. Paris Schools of Pharmacy and of Medicine 1845–7. School of Pharmacy, London 1847–50. Assistant at Godfrey and Cooke's pharmacy 1850–3. Pharmaceutical Society Council Member 1866–9 and Examiner 1867–73.

13. Cloughly, Burnby and Earles (eds), *'My dear Mr. Bell',* American Institute of and British Society for, the History of Pharmacy, 1988.

14. Personal archive; letter, G. Schweitzer to T. N. R. Morson, undated.

15. *The Chemist:* a monthly journal of chemistry, chemical manufacture and pharmacy, 1840–1858. This journal was extremely quarrelsome

and 'served as a weapon of propaganda more than as serious pharmaceutical, chemical or medical information'. See Brock, W. H., 'The Chemical News 1859–1933', *Bulletin of the History of Chemistry*, 12 (1992) 30.

16. *The Medical Times*, 4 December 1841, 114; 8 January 1842, 17; and 22 Jan 1842, 199.

17. *Op. cit., note* 1 above.

18. Pigeon, Richard Hotham (1789–1851). Wholesale druggist 1841–50. Treasurer of the Pharmaceutical Society. Also Treasurer of Christ's Hospital where he was very successful in both obtaining funds, improving the facilities and helping pupils to go to university. During the periods of argument in the Pharmaceutical Society, he was conciliatory.

19. Royal Pharmaceutical Society of Great Britain Archives; *Minutes of Council.*

20. *Op. cit.,* note 13 above, 95.

21. Holloway, S.W. F., *Royal Pharmaceutical Society of Great Britain1841–1991*,London:Pharmaceutical Press, 1991.

22. *Op. cit.,* note 7 above, 229.

23. Pharmaceutical Society Archives; letter G. Fownes to J. Bell, 27 January 1847.

24. Wellcome Institute Library; letter, J. Bell to Mrs White, November 1846.

25. *Pharmaceutical Journal,* 22, 3rd series, 1891–2, 445–6.

26. Hanbury, Daniel (1825–1875). Son of Daniel Bell Hanbury. Entered the family firm 1841; studied at the Pharmaceutical Society's Laboratory 1844, pupil of Pereira. An accurate and careful researcher, his papers appeared frequently in the *Pharmaceutical Journal* from 1850. With Flückiger he completed his greatest work, the *Pharmacographia* in 1874, a storehouse of reliable information (*Pharmaceutical Journal,* 5, 3rd series, 1874–5,. 798). F.L.S. 1855; Treasurer at his death. F.R.S. 1867; Councillor 1873. Member of the Juries of the 1862 and 1867 International Exhibitions. Pharmaceutical Society's Examiner, 1860–72. Like Morson, was fluent in French; read German. A practising Quaker all his life.

27. Pharmaceutical Society Archives; 12318 (1–59). Letters of Daniel Hanbury to John de Vrij.

28. For a description of the circumstances surrounding the attempted bill, see Earles, M.P., Ph.D., 'Jacob Bell and Poisons Legislation in Britain', *Farmacia & Industrializacion*, Madrid, 1985, 137–55.

29. Waugh, George (1802–1873); M.P.S., Oxford Street, W.1; neighbour and friend of Jacob Bell. Original member of Pharmaceutical Society,

Vice-President 1850. Reliable and steadying influence on the
Council during the difficult years with Dickinson. Refused the
Presidency and later resigned as a councillor when members of
Council decided that 'new blood' from the provinces was needed.
Sandford, George Webb (1813–1892), M.P.S. After his
apprenticeship in Norfolk, joined Herring's in London in 1832 and
remained there all his life. 1857 Council member. Vice-President
during Morson's presidency. President 1863 and for many years
after. His achievement was to hold such influence with the Medical
Council that it withdrew its proposals for regulating pharmacy and
proposed to the Home Secretary that a bill should be enacted to
make the Pharmaceutical Society responsible for the education,
examination and registration of pharmacists. Sandford's diplomatic
skills ensured that the Pharmaceutical Society and the United
Society of Chemists and Druggists eventually agreed to the
enactment of the 1868 Pharmacy Bill. This achieved direct
recognition of the Society by Parliament, an original aim of the
founders of the Pharmaceutical Society.

30. Private archive; letter, T. H. Hills to T. N. R. Morson, 2 August
    1859.
31. Deane, Henry (1807–1874). M.P.S., F.L.S. A Quaker until his
    marriage in 1843. 1825, apprenticed to John Fardon in Reading;
    then worked for J. Bell & Co. before starting his own business in
    1837 with a loan from Richard H. Pigeon. His important
    improvements to the processes for making tinctures established his
    reputation. Joined Pharmaceutical Society 1841. Examiner in 1844.
    Councillor 1851, Vice-President 1851–3, President 1853–5.
    Member of the Pharmacopoeia Committee 1854.
32. *Op. cit.*, note 27 above.
33. *Op. cit.*, note 19 above.
34. *Op. cit.*, note 7 above, 294.
35. *Pharmaceutical Journal*, 4 (1844–5), 202.
36. Attfield, John (1835–1911). Ph.D., F.I.C., F.R.S. Director then
    Professor of Practical Pharmacy, P.S.G.B. 1862–96.
37. *Pharmaceutical Journal*, 5 (1845–6), 414
38. Letter, George Fownes to T. N. R. Morson dated Barbados, 25
    January 1848. University College Library Ms. Misc 2F. Morson has
    written on the envelope: 'Fownes 1848. Interesting letter from
    Barbados in which most honorable [*sic*] mention is made of Mr
    Graham'.
39. *Op. cit.*, note 7 above, 306.
40. *Pharmaceutical Journal*, 110, 4th series, Vol. 56, 1923, 286.

41. Roberts, G. K., 'Chemistry by profession', *Historical Studies in the Physical Sciences*, 7 (1976), 437–45.

42. City of London Record Office, Land tax and rates records, 6017 R&B; Post Office Directory 1807–1905, address given 168 Homerton High Street.

43. *Pharmaceutical Journal*, 18 (1858–9), 447. The extraction process was licensed to McAndrew & Sons, King William Street.

44. *The Chemical Record*, 28 February 1852, 146.

45. *Pharmaceutical Journal*, 1, 2nd series, 1859–60., 591.

46. MacFarlan, John F. (1790–1861). M.P.S. Head of J. F. MacFarlan & Co., Edinburgh. Trained as a surgeon but practised only for a short time before starting the firm of chemists and druggists. Joined the Royal Medical Society of Edinburgh in 1818; Treasurer, 1830 and Honorary Member in 1850. City Councillor and magistrate.

47. *Pharmaceutical Journal*, 2, 2nd series, 1860–1, 538.

48. *Ibid.*, 536.

49. Private archive; T. Morson letter book, 1866–73.

50. *Pharmaceutical Journal*, 9 (1849–50), 551–2.

51. Reid, George William, Keeper of Prints & Drawings, British Museum, *A descriptive catalogue of the works of George Cruikshank*, London: Bell & Dalby, 1871.

8

Conclusion

Late in January 1874, Morson had a stroke, perhaps not the first if the marked deterioration in his handwriting a few years earlier, and then an improvement, is assumed to have been the result. It may also have been the reason he spoke of being aware that he was unlikely to reach a very old age at the time he gave up all activity outside his business.

On this occasion he was paralysed and after five weeks, he died at his house in Queen Square on 4 March. His grandson, Thomas Pierre, and his daughter, Isabelle, who had looked after him for eleven years, were present.

The burial was at Highgate Cemetery, the coffin being placed in the same chamber as his wife, Charlotte, and his younger son, Robert. It is covered by a slab of pink Aberdonian granite on which their names are carved. When Isabelle died in 1905, her coffin was placed in this grave, but sadly, her name was not added to those of her parents and brother.

The obituaries of Morson give some impression of the esteem in which he was held by his contemporaries. It was to be expected that the *Pharmaceutical Journal* and the *Chemist and Druggist*, which had published a biographical article in 1870, would publish lengthy ones, the former repeated in the *Transactions of the Linnean Society*. His wide reputation, however, caused the *Illustrated London News* to accord him half a page and a reproduction of Claudet's portrait. Up to that time no other pharmacist had been given such treatment. Bell had had a short obituary only and his death was merely recorded in *The Lancet*. This would have been because he had no reputation as a scientist and was not, therefore, viewed in the same light as Morson. The editor of *The Lancet* made an

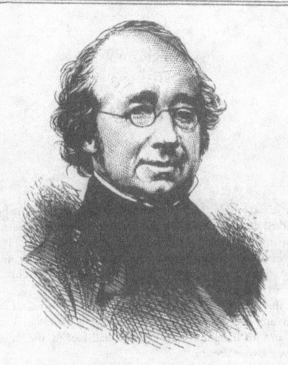

THE LATE MR. THOMAS MORSON, CHEMIST.

An eminent scientific and practical chemist, the late Mr.
Thomas Newborn Robert Morson, died the other day at his
house in Queen-square, Bloomsbury, aged seventy-five. He
was born at Stratford-le-Bow, and was apprenticed to an apothecary in Fleet Market ; but the study of chemical science, in
which he had the companionship of Faraday to assist and to
improve his early efforts, proved more attractive to Morson than
the medical profession. In the establishment of M. Planche, a
pharmacien at Paris, he acquired a high degree of knowledge
and skill. On his return to London he succeeded to a business
as chemist and druggist in Farringdon-street, where he carried
on, with his ordinary trade, experimental researches and inventions of different useful kinds. The first sulphate of quinine
made in England and the first morphia were produced in Mr.
Morson's laboratory. He was also the inventor of a medicine
called "pepsine," designed to aid the nutritive processes for
the assimilation of food in cases of diseased spleen and other
disorders of the digestive organs. From Farringdon-street he
removed, after his marriage, to Southampton-row, Bloomsbury,
and some time later established a manufactory in Hornsey-

Figure 13: Obituary picture from
The Illustrated News, 11 April 1874

210

'exception to the general rule in going beyond the limits of the profession in obituary notices'. Morson's European reputation ensured that there was an obituary in the *Repertoire des Pharmaciens* as well as notices in such as the *Journal de Pharmacie*. His friend Chevallier repeated the obituary from the *Repertoire* in the *Journal de Chimie Médicale*.

An obituary also appeared in the *Annual Register,* another indication of Morson's fame reaching beyond the pharmaceutical world.

The Council of the Society sent a letter of condolence to Morson's son on the day he died; Bottle, the Vice-President, John Williams, the Treasurer, and Morson's friend G. Webb Sandford who had been President for six years, longer than anyone else, drafting it for the President, T. H. Hills, to sign.

Thomas wrote[1] saying that he was presenting a portrait of his father to the Society, hoping they would 'recognise the likeness of an old friend'. Hills' reply[2] assured him that 'the gift of the portrait of your excellent father will be appreciated by every member of the Society with which he was so intimately connected from its foundation'. As an old friend of the family, he ends by asking Thomas to accept his personal thanks 'for your kind present', and sending his 'kind regards to Mrs Morson, yourself, sisters and family'.

Hills' letter is dated 2 April so Thomas had acted swiftly to ask his artist friend, Francis Wyburd, to paint the posthumous portrait using the Maull photograph which had been taken about twenty years previously. Wyburd's technique produced a very smooth finish and the portrait suffers from showing Morson without a line in his face; it therefore lacks character. Wyburd had met Morson so could have used his memory as well as the photograph.

Wyburd wrote in August 1868 to commiserate with Thomas on the death of his brother, Robert, in Spain. Thomas' interest and support for artists were shared with Hills. They both knew the Swedish artist Lundgren. There is a humorous photograph showing Hills and Lundgren with another artist friend ,Alfred Elnore, and Sir Henry Thompson, a surgeon, with the title, 'The Four Pilgrims'.

Lundgren wrote to Thomas to dissuade him from going to Spain in 1868 to collect his brother's body. The country was in a very disagreeable state and the heat in the south would be very fatiguing and 'is not to play with'. Lundgren had met Robert in Spain in the previous spring.

Morson's life had spanned an extraordinary period in the history of science. Its start coincided with the final abandonment of the fruitless search for the philosopher's stone and the elixir of life, making way for the acceptance of Lavoisier's conception of chemistry which was raised to its leading position among the sciences. It was Antoine Laurent Lavoisier[4] who realised that Joseph Priestley[5] and Karl Wilhelm Scheele[6] had discovered a separate element and that it was essential to combustion. Lavoisier called it oxygen. Joseph Black[7] discovered 'fixed air' or carbon dioxide in 1756 and Henry Cavendish[8] was the first to recognise hydrogen as a distinct substance. This work led to a belief in the compound nature of, for instance, water. Lavoisier demonstrated that water was composed of two gases, thus exploding the phlogiston theory, that all flammable material was expelled on burning. Lavoisier's concepts enabled chemists to address questions of the nature of chemical composition and of combination. Acceptance of the idea that chemical compounds had fixed compositions was explained by John Dalton's theory of atomic weights announced in 1807.[9] Humphry Davy reasoned that electrolysis offered the most likely means of decomposing substances into their elements.

With Joseph Louis Gay-Lussac[10] showing in 1811 that equivalent amounts of different elements could combine together and Jöns Jakob Berzelius[11] drawing up a table of accurate atomic weights, the behaviour of inorganic substances began to be better understood.

These were also the steps necessary for analytical chemistry to make progress. The initial failure to understand and use molecular weights in devising formulae resulted in different formulae for the same compound. It helps to explain confusion about analytical results in the first half of the nineteenth century. The chemical techniques in use were all new and some barely developed when Morson went to Paris.

Organic compounds created further difficulties until it was realised that groups of atoms acting as one, radicals, could combine with others and that carbon atoms had the ability to link into chains. Final resolution of this problem had to wait for work by Liebig on benzoic acid, and Williamson's on etherification showing that ether and alcohol had molecular structures like water, and then Edward Frankland[12] introduced the concept of valency in 1852 followed by Kekulé[13] in 1857, whose researches led to a better understanding of the structures of organic compounds. During the greater part of Morson's life, therefore, the manipulation of chemicals and an understanding of the theory were developing side by side.

It was the development of phyto-chemical methods begun by Scheele and extended by the chemist/pharmacists in Paris which led to exciting new possibilities.

The discovery of the alkaloids was one of the most brilliant chapters in the chemistry with which the imaginative French had enriched the world. It supplied a scientific basis for the practice of medicine. The replacement of vegetable medicines by chemical preparations started at the end of Morson's apprenticeship. Chemistry came to the aid of the management of disease to an ever-increasing extent during his life; it was also used to begin the study of body fluids, contributing to an understanding of their function and of the associated organs.

Morson's manufacture of quinine, morphine, strychnine and other alkaloids, his introduction of substances like creosote and pepsine and his large-scale output of a range of pure inorganic chemicals was the beginning of the fine chemical industry. He was, therefore, one of the greatest contributors to the first scientific advance in medicine and to the creation of a new industry. He lived long enough to see the second in Perkins' search for a synthesis of quinine in 1856 which led to the discovery of synthetic dyes which, in its turn, led to the discovery of aspirin. During his adult life, science had become a part of everyday life and he probably felt some satisfaction in the contribution he had been able to make.

Morson was a man of medium height with small but regular features. He had 'a remarkably keen eye and an intellectual countenance'.[14] He was affable, Hills describing him as an interesting and genial companion.[15] He loved discussions and used his sense of humour to lighten them. An example was his sending to Sandford, President of the Society, a parcel just before a small dinner party which followed the passing of the 1868 Pharmacy Bill, due largely to Sandford's efforts. The parcel contained a toy white elephant with the message: 'Pharmacy Act 1868 by G.W. Sandford. What will he do with it? Absit omen.' Morson showed a sympathy for his fellow man but this compassion was of an intellectual rather than sentimental kind, in keeping with the attitudes of his time.

It is far from impossible that there was a connection between this and a desire to use medical chemistry so that medicine progressed beyond the crude stage of his early life. He knew what surgery was like, just as Edward Osler did in 1816 at Guy's when Mr Travers, the surgeon, 'castrated an Irishman who roared most lustily'; not even whisky could guarantee that no pain would be felt. The Irishman's cries frightened a tailor who was waiting to have an operation for hydrocele. 'He gesticulated at Mr Travers who was persuading him; and the whole theatre was kept in a roar of laughter. The tailor trembled and slunk downstairs to his ward amidst the laughter of the pupils and the hootings of the patients who collected at the doors of the wards to see him pass.'[16]

There were more serious effects of studying surgery. Edward relates how a student cut his finger while examining a patient who died of 'inflammation of the vein following bleeding'. The student's axillary glands were swollen the next morning and he died later. Guy's 'lost' four students, with a fifth not expected to recover, between October and July.

Turning away from surgery was the first stage leading Morson away from medicine. His attitude was further altered by the chemical lectures at Guy's and then those of Brande at the Royal Institution. Brande, as an important link[17] between chemistry and medicine, was a formative influence. Finally, Faraday, with other members of the City Philosophical Society, convinced him that his most rewarding course would be the study of chemistry.

Morson's ambition, moulded by these influences, was to become an operative chemist, although why a man whose family had no background in science or medicine chose a scientific career in medical chemistry, cannot be fully explained. The choice of his apprenticeship was perhaps his mother's shrewd decision at a time when such a career was popular and would lead to a step up in the world. Once he was orphaned, his pleasant personality seems to have attracted the help of older men. He was not shy in approaching them, as is shown by his seeking to speak to Berzelius at Thénard's lecture in Paris. He drew on his resources of character, particularly his self-reliance and determination, to ensure that he obtained the training he needed. Hence his refusal to go into business in Paris, 'not wanting to be so much my own master'. He persuaded Planche to provide what was needed; 'he stipulated for and undertook the superintendence of the pharmaceutical preparations in Planche's laboratory', was the way *The Forceps*[18] put it.

His early successes with alkaloids followed. The recognition of his talents came early from Copeland and other medical men. He was able to exploit a period of intensive interest in and increasing demand for medicines. By 1830, he had made a considerable reputation as scientist and manufacturer. It grew in the next decade, such that he took his place among eminent scientists in France and England with his membership of the Société de Chimie Médicale and his fellowship of the Linnean Society. He had become one of the successful middle class whose ideas and aspirations enhanced the prestige of institutions like the Society of Arts and the Royal Institution. Groves,[19] a 'real chemist' according to Sir William Tilden, said that 'no man was listened to with more respect in scientific discussions. He was not only the first manufacturer in this country of many of the rarer chemicals but reputedly the best.'[20]

His reputation for supplying such items led to Dan Hanbury[21] seeking information from him when de Vrij asked for supplies of rare chemicals. An example was Churra. On 6 October 1855 Hanbury wrote that Morson was the only chemist in London who had any of this preparation of Indian hemp. It was made from 'Ganja, the herb form of hemp with long stalks'. A year later in October 1856, de Vrij asked for codeine for which Morson was charging 8/- per dram. MacFarlan charged 10/- per ounce. 'Macfarlan's codeine is in powder form but its purity may be relied upon.' A difference of nearly eight times in the price is not explained by the Scottish advantage in spirit costs.

In the introduction to his 1825 catalogue, Morson drew attention to a parallel activity by writing: 'To the preparation of the chemical reagents included in this catalogue I have devoted much attention, and trust they will be found pure and to be relied upon by those engaged in chemical pursuits'. He was nothing if not consistent in his desire to raise the standards of chemistry, in this instance by supplying a comprehensive range of analytical reagent chemicals. By the 1860s these were available to the increasingly large number of industrial laboratories, dye works and analytical consultancies, not only in England but in many other lands. Later, a large business was established in A.R. chemicals, as they became known later in the nineteenth century, when universal standards started to be drawn up; most of this was in bulk for the laboratory-furnishing suppliers to sell under their own labels.

Advice and supply to those whose hobby was chemistry resulted in them visiting Southampton Row. One such was Lord Salisbury in the 1860s, who needed supplies for his experiments in the laboratory he had created at Hatfield House.[22]

Morson's own skills at analytical work brought him a countrywide practice. This increased markedly when attention was directed in the 1850s to the quality of water supplies. Records exist of tests on samples from as far away as Jersey, as well as Swansea, Hastings and several parts of London including the New River. The earliest reference to his service is a letter from Lord Palmerston, out of office at this date (September 1843), asking for a soil analysis of two samples from his Broadlands estate in Hampshire. One was from 'Marks Field mown this year' but the second was not identified. Palmerston asks if they are suitable for agricultural purposes and whether they have any deficiencies. Morson's opinion was that they were good absorbent soils but any recommendation he may have made for special attention to them has been lost.

Morson was always quick to exploit new discoveries which appeared to offer commercial success. This trait was recognised by Professor Armstrong in his remarks when inaugurating the 1928 session of the School of Pharmacy.[23] He remembered Morson, Daniel Hanbury and David Howard, to all of whom 'science was knowledge but there was not the slightest value in it unless one knew how to apply it'.

His decision to manufacture medicinal creosote is a good example. Nor was this success spoilt by a tendency, evident at times, to move on to a new venture when one had been mastered, preventing him, for instance, from exploiting his achievements with quinine. Creosote was an example of complete success.

Charles, Baron de Reichenbach, had used his time while imprisoned by Napoleon I in the fortress of Hohenasperg to study science. Once released, he established a factory for carbonising wood which provided the funds for purchasing land on which his raw material grew. In late 1832 he published a paper[24] announcing his discovery of a distillation product of wood tar which he called Kreosot, literally flesh preserver, because of its ability to preserve meat. It was one of five new chemicals he found in wood tar: creosote, paraffine, eupione, picamar and pittacal. Creosote was the only useful one and beechwood tar contained up to 25%. In 1833, Morson had purchased some in France and set about its manufacture straightaway. A brief description of the process was published in the *Journal de Chimie Médicale*;[25] it involved six successive distillations of tar obtained from beechwood, although work was done in Munich on pine tar which was said to be a simpler process and to produce a product of equal quality.

Reichenbach sent Pélouze a sample of colourless creosote in 1833, a year before Morson presented one to the R.I. He had already sold some to Allen & Hanbury – 32 ounces at 6/- an ounce, the price in France having been £1 an ounce.

The demand increased rapidly, creosote being used for seasickness, deafness, toothache, ring worm, birthmarks and especially as an expectorant; in cases of pulmonary tuberculosis it was hoped it would act as a cure but this was not to be. Elliotson's paper for the Medico-Chirurgical Society[26] in 1835 states that he used it in July 1834, so there had been little delay in its manufacture. He found it beneficial in the early stages of tuberculosis, for diabetes and some skin conditions but was cautious about its use for other complaints.

It was quickly placed in the *Pharmacopoeia* of 1836 by Pereira and remained in successive editions for many years. It was not until 1968 that it was deleted from the Codex. Savory's early prescription books show that both Elliotson and Thomson were prescribing it regularly.

The Lancet[27] reported that the addition of creosote to a calomel and opium pill had made it successful in treating cholera. In a paper[28] read to the Medical Society of London, Morson's friend Snow outlined the principles on which the treatment of cholera should be based. After discussing symptoms, including the analysis of blood carried out by some colleagues, he recommended the use of creosote, pills of which had been in use since 1841, the famous physician Sir James Clark prescribing them in October that year.

In these early times, there was confusion between the phenols derived from coal tar and the similar substances obtained from wood tar. Morson's creosote was a genuine wood tar product. The confusion lasted many years. The adoption of the description phenol or carbolic acid for the coal tar derivative removed some of the difficulty. Morson developed a test for medicinal creosote to check that it was free from carbolic acid. His last contribution on this subject was a comment in the *Pharmaceutical Journal* in 1872.[29] It would have been doubly satisfying for him to have known that an American doctor would report in the 1930s that Morson's Creosote was the only one answering to the glycerine test.

Morson's labels and advertisements always stated 'Beechwood Creosote' in an attempt to stress its authenticity and distinguish it from ordinary medicinal creosote. For the product he had always made from beechwood tar he used a pink label; Kreosote 'Morson' differed from the substance specified in the 1898 *Pharmacopoeia*. The firm made creosote from pine tar conforming with the specification of later pharmacopoeias and labelled this with a white label. It was continuously manufactured for 106 years until the 1939 war prevented the raw material from entering the country. Until then it was exported all over the world.

Generations of patients in the earlier years of this century became familiar with the taste of creosote not only in proprietary expectorants like Famel syrup, but also as a result of visits to dentists, with whom it was popular. This applied particularly to those in the United States where eminent men did a great deal to maintain interest in Morson's product. It had been in the U.S. *Pharmacopoeia* since 1842 where it was named creosotum, although reference to its use in dentistry was first made in 1834 in the *London Medical and Surgical Journal*,[30] which stated that 'one drop applied to a carious tooth is considered to be a certain cure'.

As recently as 1926, in New Orleans, Dr Edward Kells[31] confirmed that he had used a paste of zinc oxide and Morson's creosote to fill dental cavities, which was removed after a year when a 'perfectly satisfactory condition will be found beneath'. The cavity was then 'filled with zinc oxychloride (with or without creosote, as may be advisable) and a thin veneer of gold or amalgam completes the operation'. Such fillings had been perfect after fifteen years' use. He had used creosote in a variety of other circumstances, commenting 'Morson's Beechwood Kreosote has been my religion from the beginning.' He asked Morson via the agent if there was any information on a comparison of germicidal activity with phenol. He did not get any help so asked a bacteriologist to make some tests. He was surprised to find that it was 'just one and a half times as potent as phenol'.

With constantly increasing demand, larger facilities were required for a process using quite large equipment, the last expansion being made in 1932. What was needed in 1834 occupied 400 square feet involving six stills with dual receivers to enable distillates to be separated at succeeding stages of the process and to enable vacuum to be maintained on the still itself. In addition, stirred tanks for treatment of the wood tar with sodium sulphate and then potassium carbonate were of at least several hundred gallons' capacity. The technology was not complicated, although Morson may have needed to consult his distiller friend Bowerbank, regarding the design of the distillation equipment.

At the time of Reichenbach's paper, Morson had decided to buy a country cottage and decided on a property in Hornsey. The contract was signed in July 1834. There was a cottage, semi-detached, with about an acre of land which cost £302 10s.-0d. The site sloped gently to the south-west from the ridge along which Hornsey Rise runs. The cottage had three living rooms and six bed and dressing rooms, a kitchen and scullery; the lavatory was outside. There was an attached conservatory on the south side and it was filled with plants, both foliage and flowering. A greenhouse was situated half-way down the garden, which was over 200 feet long.

On the land at the bottom of the garden Morson built the factory, part of which is depicted in Muller's picture. The buildings covered about 5,000 square feet and had open yards for storage. Maps of the period and other documents reveal that the ink factory was already in production next door, having been started about 1828. The area was rural, not exclusively residential, with nurseries and a few small businesses. It could be reached easily, with horse buses leaving Holborn several times a day; in 1847, the Post Office Directory said that 'omnibuses leave every twenty minutes'. In 1840, Pigot's Directory wrote that 'Hornsey – a village about six miles from the 'Standard' in Cornhill – is agreeably situated in a vale with hills commanding prospects as beautiful as they are extensive, including various views of the metropolis. This neighbourhood is considered one of the most agreeable round London.'

In 1842, Morson had the opportunity to buy the house next door, so making it possible for his factory foreman to live on site and have his own garden. Morson paid £600 for the cottage and a further £100 for the 12' 6" wide roadway on the south-east side providing good access to the factory. His final purchase, on 7 September 1844, costing £410, was for two strips of land between the roadway and his own garden. He now had a rectangular piece of land, on which the two cottages stood, of about two acres in area and this had cost him £1,412 10s.0d. for which some of his wife's money acted as surety. There were now two greenhouses, a poultry house and chicken run. Some 6,000 square feet were used to grow medicinal herbs and vegetables.

The 1869 Ordnance map shows a surprising amount of detail including the layout of Morson's flowerbeds. It is the same as in an

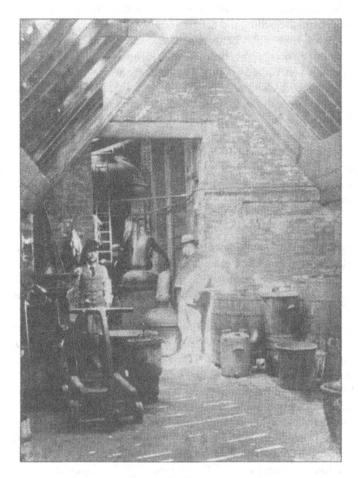

Figure 13: Photograph of Hornsey Factory, 1870,
by Henri Claudet

1870 photograph, by Henri Claudet, which shows some of the
family and a stone grotto, a rustic wooden table, a planter and a
statue on a plinth at the top of the garden.

All the chemical-processing operations were moved to Hornsey,
some of them like those for chloroform on a scale not only
impossible at Southampton Row but larger than that for creosote. It
became a very busy factory with its manufacture of the complete

range of Morson's chemicals, many hundreds even in the 1850s and being added to as new substances, like aniline dyes, were developed.

In 1854, Morson created a partnership with his son, but this excluded the Hornsey factory which he continued to run himself, keeping a separate account at the Bank of England and arranging for the retail business to pay for their materials and the bulk pharmaceuticals sold by the wholesale business. This change towards fine chemical manufacture with the retail and wholesale businesses run from Southampton Row was a reflection of Morson's interest and his conviction that the chemical manufacturing activity was more than able to exist independently. He was to be proved right. His was one of the earliest changes in a trend to manufacturing in the 1850s; new products, greater demand and the need to increase the scale of production caused the first moves towards factory operations and away from the laboratory bench. The change in organisation may also have had tax advantages as well as providing a definite position for Thomas junior who ran the wholesale and retail business.

The sale of bulk medicines included chlorodyne, whose invention in 1848 by Dr Collis Browne when he was in India, provided another opportunity for Morson to supply wholesalers who could use their own labels. There are indications, but no more, that Davenport's, who had obtained the sole rights to manufacture and market Collis Browne's formulation in 1856, sub-contracted the product's manufacture to Morson. This sort of arrangement has always been a feature of pharmaceutical manufacture and Morson had had experience of this type of product since before 1840.

In the early 1850s Morson started a programme of work on 'digestive ferments'. Liebig had initiated such studies in Germany, where the earliest references to pepsin are to be found. During the 1840s work started by Schwann, then Wassmann and continued by Vogel, who became Professor of Chemistry in Munich in 1846, resulted in a product from pigs' stomachs. It was unpalatable but not as bad as a similar extract which the French made from the rennet bags of sheep, whose taste was described as repulsive.

Morson marketed a palatable product which he named 'Pepsine Porci', a formulation of pepsin, extracted by his newly developed process which produced a pure product, and sago starch. It became famous and continued in production until the 1920s. It was sold pure, in lozenges and globules 'so that they may be carried in the pocket', and also as Pepsine Wine. There was extensive advertising in books (for instance in Cassell's *National Library* reprints of good literature which – even bound – cost only threepence), in periodicals like *Punch* and in the daily and weekly papers. On one occasion at least eleven London morning papers, all except *The Times*, carried advertisements pointing out the advantages to digestion of this product made by the original manufacturer, and warning against imitations.

These latter came onto the market first from France about 1856. Boudault developed a process making pepsine from sheep not

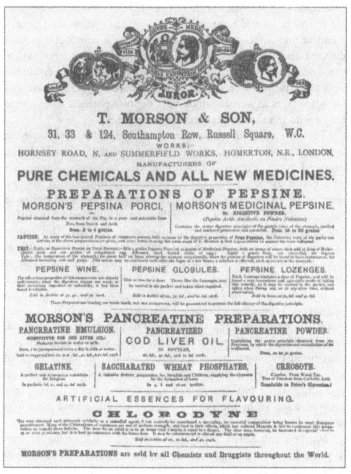

Figure 14: Advertisement for Pepsine products, circa 1870.

merely palatable but good enough to persuade a Dr Chambers to write in *The Lancet* that it was an 'elegant and agreeable' product. He called it 'poudre nutrimentive' and soon exported it to compete with Morson, appointing Squire as his agent. Bullock, using pigs' stomachs as raw material, was another competitor. By the late 1850s these three, particularly, competed strongly with one another, Morson extending his range to include his own 'poudre nutritive' which he also called 'Medicinal Pepsine' but made from calves' stomachs, the only one to use this source. Visits to Smithfield Market to buy his raw materials were frequent. It must have been a surprise to the traders to find someone buying what had previously been wasted.

Packaging was used as a means of helping the user. A hollow stopper was made so that it could measure out the doses. Morson sent his product to a firm in Dijon called Theomot, as well as his chlorodyne, to be made into lozenges which were a popular formulation.

The competition had not improved the products sufficiently to prevent Hazelden in 1859 from complaining in the *Pharmaceutical Journal* that 'uniformity of strength and preservation' had yet to be achieved. Morson's product, however, was odourless and non-hygroscopic, thus making it suitable for use in the tropics where the competition product rapidly deteriorated.

Trade fairs were another opportunity for promotion and the large exhibitions of the 1860s saw all three firms showing off their products. Morson's success was resented by the French, especially when they discovered that pepsine was being imported in bulk and sold by French firms under their own labels. Morson was the largest supplier to the Paris firm of Grimault, who decided to promote his product by using Morson's name on his labels and in his advertisements, in spite of an agreement that he should not do this. Morson probably realised the effect this might have on the French with their sensitivity to matters of digestion and their pride in matters gastronomic.

Unfortunately Grimault also criticised the non-digestible properties of competing products. There were, naturally, varying opinions about the action of pepsin as a medicine. The French authorities did not like Grimault's mode of advertising, one which they determined to stop by making him the first to be prosecuted. Immediately after this case, Thomas went to Paris and consulted with Grimault and their lawyers. After seeing the presiding magistrate, he no longer considered giving evidence on appeal, realising that an example was being made of Grimault and that there was no chance of the judgment being reversed, only the risk of further bad publicity, even though Morson's had not caused the trouble.

What effect this had on Morson's sales is not recorded. He continued to export and extended his market to Germany, also making a similar arrangement with another firm in France as he had done with Grimault. The formula he sent them used one part of pure pepsine, three parts of starch, specially prepared from sago flour, and 1/16 part of tartaric acid. After mixing and drying (a point stressed in the instructions) a little caramel was added 'to render it darker'.

Morson had no difficulty in meeting the French specification when they introduced one into their Codex. This followed the work of a committee which included Boudault and his friend Dr Corvisart whose early recommendation of Boudault's product had benefited his sales. Pepsine continued to be a major item in the firm's sales line, gaining a prize, as did their creosote preparations, at the London Exhibition in 1909. Pepsine sales continued at substantial levels until the 1930s.

Bismuth salts were another item in Morson's lists throughout the century. It was sales of the sub-nitrate and the carbonate which steadily increased from his earliest time in business. As a result he became a substantial purchaser of the pure metal by the 1860s, when the price started to rise, finishing four times as expensive as the price, only 2/6d. a pound, with which it started the decade. This price rise caused him to search for supplies of ore through his friend Hood in Australia. Provided it contained not less than 10% of pure metallic bismuth and cost no more than £10 per ton, he was prepared to import half a ton. He suggested a trial at £8 a ton but nothing came of it. He was using about 15 tons a year so a cheaper source of metal was worth some effort.

Iodides and iodoform, a popular antiseptic, were also a major concern. Morson probably used in his later years up to 10 tons of iodine a year since records show such quantities being purchased at the turn of the century when iodide business was at about the same level, although it increased considerably in the 1920s when up to 30 tons a year were used.

One benefit of Thomas junior's experience at Béral's pharmacy in Paris was the knowledge he brought of the process for producing water-soluble products in the form of scales, introduced by Béral in

1831. A solution whose concentration is high enough can be painted onto glass, dried and scraped off as shiny scales. At a time when most preparations were made up in the dispensary, a quickly soluble form was a great advantage. Large quantities of scale preparations like iron ammonium citrate, iron quinine citrate and iron citrate with strychnine were produced for inclusion in tonics of varying formulation.

The range of products produced at Hornsey and Southampton Row was large. There were over 500 chemical substances manufactured in the 1860s. These were made in all grades of purity up to that for analytical reagents. There were also over 250 essences, extracts and tinctures; the proprietary preparations and gelatine completed the range. Requests to manufacture little-used substances made in small quantities for a particular customer were almost always met.

Less pure chloroform was made as an antispasmodic years before its use as an anaesthetic. It was certainly in Morson's list, so like many of his competitors he was quick to supply anaesthetic-quality product as soon as demand increased, following the publication of Sir James Y. Simpson's famous pamphlet in November 1847. There is an invoice of February 1848 for a supply to Allen & Hanbury's of 2lbs at 14/- per pound and another for 3lbs three days later. As was always the case, Morson was interested in maintaining quality and sharing his knowledge with others. Chloroform provides an example of this. In July 1848, he drew attention to the 'spontaneous decomposition of chloroform' in a letter to Bell which was published in the *Pharmaceutical Journal*.[32] Dr Christison wrote to him from Edinburgh stating that decomposition did not occur in chloroform made in Scotland. Pereira[33] picked up the point and wrote to Guibourt on 3 October 1848. He mentions that 'our friend Mr Morson' had passed on the news of his daughter's marriage and goes on to ask if the French also found that light and air caused decomposition of pure chloroform. He might have added that the decomposition also occurred when light and air were excluded. At the Pharmaceutical meeting[34] on Wednesday 7 November when Morson was in the chair, he used the opportunity to raise the problem, pointing out that he had obtained samples from 'all the principal makers in England and Scotland before writing his letter and therefore what he wrote applied to all of them'.

His results showed a wide variation in the rate and speed of decomposition. The cure was said to be washing with sulphuric acid although no one had investigated what was removed. One of the students at Bloomsbury Square had obtained a very similar substance when making chloral but it did not darken with sulphuric acid. Morson suggested that better control over the distillation might produce a purer product which would not require the acid wash; alternatively the initial processing might be the cause.

The following March, Dr Gregory read a paper[35] to the Royal Society in Edinburgh. He had attributed the headache and nausea sometimes experienced by patients to the presence of oils. In a piece of curious logic he said that the oils in the best Edinburgh manufacturers' material were so small that it caused adverse symptoms in only a 'few peculiarly sensitive persons'. He said a test was needed because chloroform made in Edinburgh was better than that made elsewhere. He ignored Morson's paper and went on to discuss Simpson's experience that the 'purest chloroform he had used not unfrequently causes vomiting'. When Simpson used less pure chloroform, the symptoms did not appear. Gregory was at pains to point out that this chloroform was not made in Edinburgh!

In the absence of a standard, it was surely a matter for physicians to arrange a test of the material they purchased, the demand for chloroform being so great, with many firms making it, that some variation in quality could be assumed.

Morson's manufacture continued for many years. Not until the 1930s after the equipment had been transferred first to Homerton and then to Ponders End in 1902, did production cease.

Chloral, which is a fairly powerful hypnotic, became very popular in the 1860s; it was also used as a sedative in cases of whooping cough, convulsions and delirium tremens. One agent imported almost ten tons in 1870[36] and the *Pharmaceutical Journal*[37] estimated a consumption of 30 tons over an eighteen-month period.

Complaints of differences in quality caused Alfred H. Mason to test several samples and review the test method. He criticised Morson and German makers, and finished his discussion with a recommendation that pharmacists had a 'decided obligation' to dispense only Liebreich's product. This blatant promotion angered Morson who wrote to point out that this was a departure from the rule from the foundation of the Society that 'no article injurious to members should be printed'. In any case Mason's results were faulty, a fact he admitted and apologised for.[38]

The Council instructed the editor to avoid any such incident in future and the President called on Morson to apologise to him and to ask in what way they could make amends. Even though he was

72 and retired from Council, his reputation in the Society ensured that the man Hills described as 'one of the brightest ornaments that ever adorned our ranks' was not tarnished by the editor's failure.

The Great Exhibition of 1851, followed by those in Europe and America, were grasped as opportunities by fine and pharmaceutical chemical manufacturers to display the best examples of their production. Morson's exhibited at eleven in 60 years and gained prizes at all including Philadelphia in 1876, a part of the celebrations of the United States Centennial. At the 1851 Exhibition Morson gained his prize medal among a total of 21 awarded; they were given on the assessment of the Jurors and not on any arbitrary rule devised before the Exhibition started. Firms from many countries were among the prize-winners; more than half from the UK, including Hopkin & Williams who had only joined forces a year before, but Sardinia, Tuscany, Germany and France were represented, along with one from the U.S.A, Powers & Weightman, whose exhibits were presented to the Pharmaceutical Society's Chemical Museum.

The Paris exhibitions of 1855 and 1867 were also successes for Morson, the latter earning him the only silver medal awarded in his class. At the 1862 London Exhibition, he was a Juror sitting with Daniel Hanbury and Theophilus Redwood among a very international group of people. They awarded medals to MacFarlan for 'a large basin of crystals of opiates'; to Ménier of Paris whose opiate alkaloid crystals were among 'the finest we ever saw', but their size was exceeded by Merck. Morson earned a medal for his narceine and aconitine, which was 'well-known for its superiority in virulence, a fact which enables it to command a very high price', an accolade earning a reference in *The Lancet*[39] to Flückiger's comment that Morson's product was identical with the one obtainable from 'Napaul aconite root'. Flückiger and Hanbury refer to this product in the *Pharmacographia*. Morson, 'the well-known manufacturing chemist' had long had a great reputation for his aconitine which he produced in large well-defined crystals for the exhibition. Previously it had been known only in the form of an amorphous mass. This achievement in chemical manipulation was recognised as a remarkable one by his peers.

Thomas Groves had stated that Morson's preparation of aconitine was the only one which was pure. At the 1862 Exhibition 'every Pharmacist must have noticed with surprise and pleasure the magnificent specimen in perfectly defined large crystals made by Morson'.

Aconitine was discovered in 1833 by Geiger and Werse. It is very

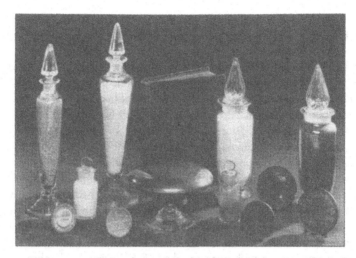

Figure 15: Prize medals, exhibits and hand catalogue of the 1851
Exhibition. The medals are, left to right: Paris 1855; Gold medal
Paris, 1867, London 1908; Great Exhibition 1851;
London 1862 (juror).

poisonous but important in alkaloid chemistry and in providing an
opportunity to improve techniques both of extraction and of
purification. Groves referred again to Morson's achievement in 1873
in a paper to the Pharmaceutical Conference.[40]

The demonstration of these skills in extracting and purifying this
substance was recognised as a *tour de force* by his contemporaries.
Taking account of the state of chemical knowledge and the equipment
and apparatus available to Morson, his achievement was remarkable.

The Jury's report provides a sidelight on the competition for
pepsine, with exhibits from Squire, Morson and Bullock whose
product 'was of superior strength'.

The Jury awarded a prize to one of Morson's oldest friends in
France and whom he entertained in London. Cap[41] was given a
medal for his bismuth tannate, proposed but not much used at that
time for treating diarrhoea. Morson included it in his list.

Great pains were taken to present specimens attractively, Morson
using stoppered glass display bottles, a few quite elaborately cut and
in a great variety of shapes, some more like cut-glass vases.
Resublimed iodine was in a flat, wide bottle with a narrow neck and
a stopper which formed the base.

Trade was difficult during the last five years or so of Morson's life
due to the trade depression throughout Europe. He had made his

firm dependent mainly upon the sales of bulk fine chemicals, speciality products and proprietaries as varied as pepsine and potassium iodide, of which he was the leading manufacturer. The interest in the pharmacy was less, though it remained profitable. Even the interest in opiates was less, with manufacture no longer continuous. This change may have been due partly to age and partly to his son being less technically competent than he was, for they did not introduce any new products. Thomas junior's contribution, however, to the general running of the business was done with skill and commercial flair.

Trade depression and German competition were the main causes of difficulty. Germany had already succeeded France as the country producing able chemists. Following their political unification, state backing was given to their industries. The chemical industry used inexpensive loans to create excellent research facilities from which soon flowed a succession of new products and techniques. By the 1870s, they led Europe's chemical industry. A small result of this was the presence on Morson's warehouse shelves of many bottles of Merck's alkaloids and of Böhringer's quinine, with rather less of Morson's products on theirs.

Even so, Morson had organised a continuous expansion of the range and volume of his production. During his life factories had replaced the bench at the back of the shop, although these had seen little change in the technology used.

Some of the continuing success of his firm was due to the reputation established throughout the medical profession when Morson's new products were being prescribed for the famous by the most eminent physicians in London and dispensed by the leading pharmacists like John Savory, whose prescription books[42] in 1836 and 1837 include entries for Princess Victoria. The Princess's family kept the dispensers fairly busy with a prescription almost every week. These included alterative pills (ipecacuana and hyoscamine), aperient pills of senna and 'dinner pills' of aloes. Whether they achieved their purpose is doubtful as many pills were gilded or silvered. If this meant coating with silver foil, it is probable that they passed through the alimentary canal without releasing their contents.

The Princess must have had a cough after Christmas 1836 for she was prescribed hydrocyanic acid with potassium carbonate and nitrate flavoured with lemon syrup; a tablespoonful was to be taken every morning. The following March, she developed a fever, a prescription being dispensed for quinine sulphate with dilute sulphuric acid and distilled water, a tablespoonful of this mixture in as much distilled water being taken twice a day. On 21 March she was given camphorated oil and alterative pills. The quinine was repeated on 14 April with a gargle and again on 14 August by which time she was Queen. In between these dates, she had a 'simple camphor liniment' exactly a week after her accession. It is likely, therefore, that in the two months prior to her becoming Queen, her symptoms were alleviated by two of Morson's important products.

It was a wide reputation for innovation, quality and reliability which resulted in Morson being invited to join those who were trying to organise their profession. After some hesitation to become involved in pharmaceutical politics following their resurgence in the late 1830s, he took his place among those who realised that full recognition of pharmacy by Parliament and the medical professions was only obtainable if they rejected any moves towards forming merely a trade association or an academic institution. Neither would have been awarded a Royal Charter. Bell, Morson and their colleagues correctly assessed the value to the public of their new science-based skills and that it was essential to form a professional body.

Morson's enjoyment of scientific discussion and application of science to industry ensured that he was an active member of the Society of Arts, the Royal Institution and the Société de Chimie Médicale. Nor should the Zoological Society be overlooked; his friend Gray and doubtless Owen enjoying his company there. He was a member in 1834.

He was never invited to become a Fellow of the Royal Society possibly because he had no academic background and was known mainly as a manufacturer. It is not surprising that he joined the Cavendish Society, started just two months before the Pharmaceutical. He took an active part because it provided an opportunity both to learn what progress science was making on the Continent as well as to further his interest in education. The Society's object was to promote chemical science by providing English translations of foreign papers and works on chemistry.[43] Morson arranged for the use of facilities at Bloomsbury Square by the Society whose Secretary Redwood became. The Cavendish published *Chemical Reports and Memoirs* in 1848 when the scientific circle, of which Brande, Fownes, Odling, Schweitzer, Playfair, Phillips, Prout and Brodie were members, included Morson's friend Alfred White. Its President was Thomas Graham, in whose house at 4 Gordon Square the annual meeting was held. Morson was an auditor and proposed the resolutions accepting the annual report and thanking the officers for their services. In 1862, Williamson, who had succeeded Graham as professor at University College, was a Vice-President and so this circle of friends maintained contact with one another and with men like Owen whose interest was not primarily in chemistry.

Morson's friendliness worked as a catalyst in bringing scientists together. Due to his reputation, they were the most important men in European chemical science. His friend Bennett wrote that Cap, Liebig, Rose and Mitscherlich were all guests at his house. 'He formed acquaintances which ripened into friendship with the greatest chemists and philosophers of the age.' The list is a long one: Pereira, Bell, Williamson, Playfair, Graham, Brown, Bennett, Bowerbank, Gray, Daniell, Forbes and Faraday in England; in France there were Pélouze, Boudet, Robiquet, Guibourt and Robinet. The *Repertoire des Pharmaciens* said that 'all these were received with cordial hospitality, and among them not one will forget the pleasant face and happy smile of the excellent Mr Morson'.

Many different occupations are represented in these friendships, physicians, lawyers, biologists, architects and zoologists as well as other disciplines close to his own. There was a wide range of age and background among his friends, a catholicity consonant with liberal views.

The famous Robert Brown was a whole generation older, and almost as great a difference separated Morson from Richard Phillips and R. H. Solly. In France, Robiquet and Guibourt were more senior while Pélouze was seven years his junior. Dan Hanbury was a generation younger and from a Quaker family with a long lineage. *The Forceps*, in its perceptive article, commented that Morson was a member of many of the scientific societies, 'where you may frequently observe him ensconced in some retired corner discussing knotty points with some young Sir Humphry'. Irrespective of age or background, the common interest was in science and it kept them in touch with an intelligent and pleasant companion.

His associations with the older members of this group started in Fleet Market when he joined the City Philosophical Society, whose members wanted to improve their understanding of science and shared a desire for self-improvement.

The latter helped some of the members and could be accepted as worthy by anyone. The understanding and use of science was a new trend and evoked the whole gamut of reactions.

Taking account of what they did, it seems that Faraday and the group he had gathered in the Society of Arts' Chemical Committee wanted to demonstrate the advantages of science, in the first instance by showing how it could be exploited for improving everyday life and not merely as an adjunct to the old empiricism. Morson helped to guide the committee jointly with Faraday and then Hennell over a period of seven years. The record of their many and diverse 'encouragements' was substantial.

At this period, science was not the accepted tool for the solution of practical problems, in medicine least of all. Suspicions and resentments to its encroachment abounded. Chemistry in particular – and this is where men like Faraday, Brande, Phillips and Morson are so relevant – had only recently emerged from its 'secretive, deliberately obscure' alchemical origins.[44] The whole development of chemical technique had been concentrated on the hopeless pursuit for the transmutation of metals. The eighteenth century saw the first important changes, Lavoisier being the one whose work initiated the move away from earlier thinking. The French in the early nineteenth century took the necessary steps to utilise chemistry for discoveries which were to transform attitudes to medicine. Though there were outstanding discoveries made by English and Scottish scientists in the later years of the eighteenth and early ones of the nineteenth century, chemistry in England was seen as a pastime to be indulged in by those with money and leisure. It had now to have its advantages demonstrated so that it became a catalyst for change.

Whereas the French, excelling in the application of the new chemical ideas, and Germans accepted the change, the English were cautious, some even resenting an intrusion into their cosy world of a new way of thinking as well as of inconvenient new facts. Morson's Continental friendships, especially those with Rose, Pélouze and Robiquet, all with international reputations, marked him out as strongly influenced by foreign conceptions. It is far from unlikely that he, and others who had taken the opportunity to visit Paris and Berlin to learn of the latest ideas, suffered from unspoken post-Napoleonic Wars xenophobia. From early in his life he was part of an international network of scientists. In Robiquet's company he learned of the disciplined approach to chemistry that his colleague had been taught as a pupil at Vauquelin's school of analytical chemistry[45]

Battley's apparent refusal to accept new methods and Hennell's inexplicable disregard for some published work are specific examples among those who failed to open their minds to the possibility that change would be beneficial and to progress in analytical chemistry. Others like Dickson and Elliotson saw it all as an opportunity to improve their expertise and so their patients' lives. Thomas Hodgkin

(1798-1866), who was later to have a disease (actually a cancer) named after him, sought out new concepts and new ways to view disease. He knew that after the 'cessation of hostilities in 1815, British and American physicians collected in Paris to learn' from the French[46]. He arrived there within weeks of Morson leaving in 1821.*

The belated acceptance of new knowledge about opium has a pattern which illustrates the range of attitudes. Robiquet and Magendie had removed the confusion about opium by using chemistry to prove the presence of a sedative (morphine) and a stimulant (narcotine), and physiology to demonstrate the implications. A scientific explanation of an age-old treatment which had caused problems was available, but was far from being widely accepted. However, it was not 'Magendie's work alone that evoked hostility but the whole contemporary trend to bring the sciences to bear on medicine'.[47]

Magendie enunciated the advantages of pure substances, thus dismissing the idea that the extracts previously used, with their varied processing and effects, were superior. He stressed that 'only a precise knowledge of the active principle classifies the pharmaceutical preparation of medicines, makes known rational formulae and distinguishes them from those that are empirical, absurd and often dangerous'.[48] Such ideas were resisted by interests, commercial, technical and institutional, which wanted only to

---

*   American doctors went to Paris in the 1820's in considerable numbers; as many as 105 having been identified as having travelled from Boston. Philadelphia, New Orleans, Baltimore and New York. (cf Jones, Russell M., *Bulletin of the History of Medicine*, 1973, Vol XLVII, p.40.) These visits varied from several years of serious study to a few weeks of "medical tourism" (cf Warner, John Harley, 'Remembering Paris; Memory and the American disciples of French medicine in the nineteenth century', *ibid.*, Vol 65, 1991, p.303.)

The English were particularly interested in the new phyto-chemical discoveries and the associated physiology. They also took great interest in the organisation of French scientific institutions.

Parisian science was at the forefront of both medical and chemical discovery. This reputation attracted a steady stream of Englishmen wishing to find out for themselves what these achievements were as well as those, like Morson, who went to study. He was one of the first to do this. Other visitors were Pereira, Fownes, John Savory, Bullock, Squire, Ince, Playfair and Williamson. Among medical men were Copeland, A.S.Taylor and Samuel Solly, who trained in Paris.

perpetuate established ways.

Morson was a member of the Medico-Chirurgical Society, alone among pharmacists, so that he had an unrivalled opportunity to hear the reactions of physicians to the new scientific approach. Elliotson, Roots and Copeland could let him know of their clinical work and conclusions as well as the opinions of others, including those who found too difficult the acceptance of a new concept.

He also took an interest in the medical politics of his earliest times in Southampton Row. The evidence for this is in Filkin's letters. The two young men enjoyed the latest gossip about Johnson and Wakley, who began editing the new journal, *The Lancet*, in 1823. The two friends knew the wide differences in opinions, the result of varying degrees of medical competence, among medical men. They knew, too, of the social status reserved for those who had graduated from one of the two ancient universities and had become members of one of the Royal Colleges as well as, to a lesser extent, the general practitioners of the Society of Apothecaries.

This status, however, concealed serious short comings. During the cholera epidemic of 1831/2, the section of the population most affected was the less well-off. They suffered from a failure by medical men to use remedies known to be effective at least in treating the symptoms. In addition, there was much rivalry to obtain appointments to the new local Boards of Health, followed by dissension within them. The 'collective image of medicine was one of inter-professional squabbling and weakness'.[49] The challenge to competence provided by the epidemic revealed the low standard of the profession and the state of medical education.

As the decade of the 1830s progressed, Parliamentary inquiries and debates in the B.M.A. revealed the 'derisory state of medical education in the older universities'.[50] The opinion in which medicine was held could not have been lower but the Government did not think it right to interfere. This permitted a continuation of the 'complacent acceptance of this implied hierarchy and the laxity of standards of performance that often accompanies the substitution of status for achievement'.[51]

The establishment of University College and then London University was a beginning of reform, although it provided a focus for argument among medical men. For the first few years it was 'racked with dissension and its scientific direction was a heated issue.'[52] One of the reasons for this was the introduction of new ideas by 'Paris-trained medical graduates [who] were flocking to London to staff the new university'.[53] By 1834 five medical professors had resigned. One student, who was the son of the Professor of Materia Medica, A.T. Thomson, later a Professor at the Pharmaceutical Society, was expelled for his views and for organising riots during an unpopular professor's classes.[54]

The agitation was general and not confined to the University. Pereira's reputation at the Aldersgate Street medical school, a private one closed in 1848, was that of a radical and he was seen by some to have been influenced by Parisian materialism. The school became a centre of debate. Pereira had adopted Grant's anatomical classification as well as French teaching methods in an attempt to raise the level of expertise. The same applied to Samuel Solly, also trained in Paris and a cousin of the Solly who wrote the memoir of the artist Müller.

Medicine was far from alone in this reform process. The 'demands for democracy to end privilege' which was 'as endemic in medicine as in other sections of British society'[55] were part of a widespread trend. The 1830s saw the famous Reform Act which began to widen the parliamentary franchise, satisfying the less politically aware. It was inherited and conferred privilege which reformers wanted to see at least reduced, while the most radical preferred to see it all swept away – an attitude creating fears of Continental-style revolution. An intense debate was hardly surprising when viewed in retrospect as it combined arguments about technical, social and religious matters.

In the later 1830s at the Zoological Society, the voices being heard calling for a change were 'those of the new professional and trading classes'.[56] Morson became a member in 1834 just in time to hear the criticisms made of the Council. Ballots for councillors and public access to the gardens were issues hotly debated. Owen played a considerable part by being in favour of change but restraining the radicals, among whom was Gray who was known for the forthright expression of his opinions. Darwin became alarmed by the 'snarling',[57] so the debate was at the least a vigorous one. Slowly, however, the Society introduced some restraints to the power of the executive and introduced moves to make the Council representative.

Such changes were introduced into other scientific institutions, many men being members of more than one.

Morson became a member of the Royal Institution in 1831 and his contribution to its affairs steadily increased, reaching a peak in the 1840s, by which time the influence of the aristocratic and landed proprietors was already on the wane. Changes sought by industrialists and other middle-class men successful in a variety of fields were initiated, and as a consequence, the R.I. played a central role in confirming a new social image of science and a model for its support. The R.I. had also been identified with the 'Benthamite teaching empire which included the S.D.U.K..'.[58] The Benthamites worked for the greatest happiness for the greatest number and their technical education schemes were devised primarily to provide expertise to those who were entering government. They were supported by the medical radicals.

By 1850 most scientific institutions had been reorganised because technical advances were being made; and also the popularity of Faraday's lectures were playing a part in this process. A new younger, largely self-educated group without inherited wealth had grasped the power previously wielded by the traditionally minded aristocrats. The new professional middle class had, over twenty years or so, established their position. The social composition of scientific societies had changed from 'the oligarchs of the old science to the mandarins of the new'.[59]

There were casualties among those whose views became extreme in either an organisational or technical context. Grant[60] led such open and severe criticism of the Royal College of Physicians that his unpopularity caused his practice to shrink and his income was reduced to a small fraction of that of his successful colleagues. Elliotson ruined his career by his fascination with mesmerism, which led to his resignation in 1838 from all his official appointments. It seems likely, however, that some of his colleagues' motives may have been incited by his reputation as 'the strongest materialist' of his day.[61]

The importance of religious orthodoxy at this time has to be stressed. The place of religion in British life was important and was expressed in a social as well as religious context. The Catholic Emancipation Act had been passed in 1829, but this did not reduce religious bars at once. Few non-Anglicans joined the Royal Colleges,nor were they accepted in the teaching hospitals. Feelings ran high about all the changes after such a long period when questioning of entrenched attitudes had little effect. Tyrrell[62] was denied the opportunity of lecturing at St Thomas' and so started one of the private medical schools, most of them set up because religious reasons had been put forward as the basis for refusing appointments.

Such extreme attitudes were incompatible with Morson's character. He was cautious in these as in business affairs, a trait probably reinforced by the knowledge of what had happened to

Elliotson and Grant.

Morson's close professional association and, in many cases, social contact with so many eminent academics, physicians and surgeons is not only a reflection of his attitudes, but also evidence that far from all Victorian medical men tried to elevate themselves by pretending that 'in some mysterious way trade was denigrating'.[63]

While favouring change in order to provide opportunity and to raise levels of competence, Morson knew that his relations with other medical men generally were vital to his business. He may be best described as a conservative radical; nevertheless one who contributed to the introduction of chemistry to medicine.

The Royal Society was not insulated from the processes of change taking place elsewhere. The late 1830s found it adjusting under the general pressure. It had been possible for nominations for Fellowships to be made at any time and the scientific credentials of a candidate were less important than the reputation of his proposers. In the late 1840s, a committee was set up to review candidacy and it sat only once a year to consider nominations. The Society had become aware that its scientific standing was at stake. In future, scientific achievement would be the criterion for a Fellowship.[64]

The 1840s were an extraordinary decade. The Industrial Revolution was in full spate. Railways were shattering the peace of the countryside, much of which had not changed for centuries. The speed and convenience of travel, if not the comfort, changed beyond recognition. The topography of London with new bridges over the Thames, public and private developments, railway stations, theatres, even the road surfaces altered the appearance of the greatest metropolis in the world to an extent that made parts of it unrecognisable. Abroad, continuing expansion of Empire coincided with political reform at home, egged on by movements like the Chartists'. Even attitudes to religion were changing; no longer was the hand of an overruling Providence seen in every turn of events.

The publication of Darwin's *Origin of Species* in 1859 brought to a head the debate about man's origins. However, there were scientists who were not unduly bothered about Darwinism. Morson may have been one of these; he could not take the problem into his laboratory and verify it by experiment. At this time he had much to occupy his mind and so it is likely that he was content that the problem belonged to others.

This was a period when he was extraordinarily active even if he was over 60 at its end. He ran his expanding business for which he developed new processes and products, organising a change in scale of operations from a few gallons to hundreds. He was active in scientific societies in London and Paris. In the 1840s he was a Vestryman. He took part in London's artistic and literary life. He continued his interest in music and organised his Sunday scientific meetings. Without neglecting his family or friends, he took an even more demanding role in the establishment of the Pharmaceutical Society.

The social foundations of science were being transformed[65] and Morson and his friends were part of the new scientific culture which grew as a result of its increasing acceptance.

The evolution of more scientific treatments had begun and there was some insight by 1850 into the chemistry of the body. *The Lancet* had come to the conclusion that there was far more chemistry in medicine than physicians were inclined to believe. Golding Bird was referred to as a chemical physician because of his work on medical botany and urinary pathology in 1843 when he was lecturer in Natural Philosophy at Guy's Hospital. Medicine was slower, however, to recognise the benefits of chemistry than agriculture, which was persuaded of its advantages by the publication in 1840 of the *Chemistry of Agriculture* by Liebig,[66] the most famous of European chemists. Playfair, who arranged the printing of the English edition, commented, in a letter of 5 October 1840 to Liebig, that his work 'must change the whole face of agriculture'.

An event which marked the sea change in attitudes was the Great Exhibition of 1851. Playfair had a vital role in its planning, especially with his scheme of classification of the exhibits. Among those who contributed to its scientific success were Owen, Edward Forbes, Barlow and J. E. Gray, all of whom took part in the selection and preparation of the papers published in the comprehensive *Official Catalogue*, which consisted of four large volumes.

Although there had been such exhibitions in France, they had not been much supported nor attracted other than local interest.[67] The Crystal Palace was on a scale altogether different. It covered nineteen acres, a supreme feat of technology on which the organisers decided to place their emphasis. It was universal and 'the world responded enthusiastically'. It set the seal on the achievements of middle-class entrepreneurs and demonstrated the possibilities of science.

The secular spirit of the radical dissenters spread and strengthened professional power. This power had reformed scientific institutions, democratised them and, especially in medicine, greatly reduced privilege.

Science had been demonstrated as successful and medical institutions accepted that the new concepts and disciplines it brought were needed as an integral part of medical thinking.

The application of these concepts, whether in the professional and scientific spheres or in his laboratory, business and home, is a consistent theme in Morson's life. Henry Roots once wrote to him that he knew 'your love for the advancement of science'.

Notes

1. *Pharmaceutical Journal,* 4 (1874), 726.
2. Private archive; letter, T. H. Hills to T. Morson, junior, April 1874.
3. Wyburd, Francis (1826–1893); exhibited 1846–89.
4. Lavoisier, Antoine Laurent (1743–1794). After studying law began in 1770 his studies on combustion. 1777 made the full report of his oxygen theory. 1783 announced water was composed of hydrogen and oxygen. 1789 reclassification of the elements with Berthollet.
5. Priestley, Joseph (1733–1804). A dissenting clergyman. Discoverer of oxygen. 1766 F.R.S. for his *History of Electricity.* 1773 Copley Medal for his work on dissolving carbon dioxide in water.
6. Scheele, Karl Wilhelm (1742–1786).Discovered chlorine, 1774. Discovered oxygen in 1774; he remained a believer in the phlogiston theory.
7. Black, Joseph, M.D. (1728–1799). His experiments on magnesia and other alkaline substances opened the door to 'pneumatic chemistry' (1756). Lavoisier, Priestley and Cavendish followed his lead from his discovery of fixed air or carbon dioxide.
8. Cavendish, Henry (1731–1810). F.R.S. 1760. The first man to recognise hydrogen as a distinct substance (inflammable air) and carbon dioxide (fixed air). Carried out in 1783 experiments to determine if air is of fixed composition which led to his discovery of the compound nature of water and the composition of nitric acid.
9. Dalton, John (1766–1844). F.R.S. 1822. Developed modern atomic theory. He gave an account of it in his *New System of Chemical Philosophy* in 1807.
10. Gay-Lussac, Joseph Louis (1778–1850). Professor of Chemistry, Ecole Polytechnique. 1832 Professor of Chemistry, Jardin des Plantes. 1805 discovered, with Humboldt, that water was composed of two parts hydrogen and one of oxygen.
11. Berzelius, Jöns Jakob (1779–1848). M.D. Uppsala 1802, Professor of Chemistry, Caroline Medico-Chirurgical Institute, 1815–22. Discoverer of selenium, thorium.

12. Frankland, Edward (1829–1899). Advanced the theory of chemical equivalents. Worked with Playfair in London and Bunsen at Marburg. 1851 Professor of Chemistry, Queen's College, Manchester. 1863 Professor of Chemistry, Royal Institutio ;1865–85 succeeded Hofmann at Royal School of Mines.

13. Kekulé, Friedrick August (1829–1896). University of Giessen at which he attended Liebig's lectures in 1848. 1851 went to Paris and then London in 1853 at St. Bartholomew's Hospital. Returned to Germany in 1858 after which he was appointed a Professor in Ghent. In 1867 he became Professor of Chemistry in Bonn.

14. *The Forceps*, No. 2, 1844.

15. *Pharmaceutical Journal* 4 (1874), 938.

16. Wilkinson, Anne, *Lions in the Way*, London: Macmillan, 1957.

17. Royal Institution, *Managers' Minutes* ;Introduction to Vol. VI.

18. *Op. cit*. note 14 above.

19. Groves, Thomas Bennett (1829–1902). M.P.S., F.C.S., distinguished pharmacist. Well known for his scientific investigations, especially his researches into alkaloidal chemistry including work on aconitine, aloin and opiate alkaloids. He was, therefore, in an excellent position to judge the value of Morson's work. The gift of Fownes' *Chemistry* from his father stimulated his interest in pharmaceutical chemistry. Attended the School of Pharmacy in 1850, a fellow student of William Squire. His first publication was in 1854 on the alkaloids present in English poppy capsules.1856 succeeded to his father's business in Weymouth but continued with his research.1870–1 Councillor of the Pharmaceutical Society and a corresponding Member of the Philadelphia College of Pharmacy. President British Pharmaceutical Conference, 1874 and 1875.

20. Presidential Address, British Pharmaceutical Conference, 1874.

21. Pharmaceutical Society Archives; P.12318 (1–59).

22. Cecil, Lady Gwendolin, *Life of Robert Marquess of Salisbury*, Vol. 1, 1921, 174–6.

23. *Pharmaceutical Journal*, 121, 4th series, Vol. 67, 1928, 329.

24. Schweigger-Seidel's *Journal fur Physik und Chemie*, Vol. 65, 1832, 461.

25. *Journal de Chimie Médicale*, Vol. 9, 1833, 617–20.

26. *Medico-Chirurgical Transactions*, February 1835, 'The Medical properties of Creosote', John Elliotson, M.D., F.R.S.

27. *The Lancet*, 2 (1848), 194.

28. Medical Society of London, 21 January 1854.

29. *Pharmaceutical Journal*, 2 (1871–2), 921.

30. *London Medical and Surgical Journal*, 1834.

31. Kells, Dr. C. Edmund, D.D.S., *Three score years and nine*, New
    Orleans, 1926; Kells, 'The conservation of Natural teeth', *Dental
    Cosmos*, August 1923.
32. *Pharmaceutical Journal*, 8 (1848-9), 69.
33. Pharmaceutical Society Archives; Pereira, letters to Guibourt,
    1831–42.
34. *Pharmaceutical Journal*, 8 (1848-9) 278.
35. Gregory, William (1803–1858), M.D., F.C.S.; Assistant to Professor
    of Chemistry, London University 1829. Studied with Liebig at
    Giessen before being appointed in 1837 Professor of Chemistry,
    Andersonian College, Glasgow. 1839, Professor of Medicine and
    Chemistry, King's College Aberdeen. 1842-8, Professor of
    Chemistry, Aberdeen.
36. *Pharmaceutical Journal*, 20 (1871), 457.
37. *Ibid..*, 11, 3rd series, (1871-2), 369.
38. *Ibid..*, 1, 3rd series, 1870-1, 691.
39. *The Lancet*, 1 (1882), 235.
40. See *Transactions of the British Pharmaceutical Conference;*, Groves,
    T. B., 'Further Experiments on Napaul Aconite'.
41. Cap, Paul Antoine (1788–1877); pharmacist in Lyon, then Paris,
    where he died. Worked with Henry. Published a *Treatise
    on Pharmacy*, 1838 and a *History of Pharmacy*, 1851.
42. Savory & Moore archive at Macarthys Ltd. Savory, John,
    (1800–1871), L.S.A. 1825, nephew of Thomas Field Savory, founder
    of the firm. Took over his uncle's share of the business in 1831 and
    bought out Moore in 1846. He had several well-situated pharmacies
    and a large manufacturing business. His firm was an official supplier to
    the War Office, the supplies covering medicines, field dressings, even
    ambulances fully equipped. In 1855 sales to the Government reached
    £50,000. Their medicine chests were first issued in 1836 and were sold
    for domestic use as well as Army use complete with a copy of *Savory's
    Compendium*. Some indication of the size and profitability of the firm
    is provided by Savory's ownership of three houses, one in London,
    needing ten servants in 1851. He was the inventor of the ribbed
    poison bottle.Savory was President of the Pharmaceutical Society,
    1844-8. He visited Paris in 1819. He purchased a book entitled
    Oeuvres de Madame la Marquise de Lambert, published by Libraries
    chez Ganeau, Bauche fils and D'Loury, Paris, 1751. It now belongs to
    Mrs S. Savory whose husband, the late Mr D. Savory, was a director
    of Savory & Moore from 1951 until he retired in 1980. John Savory
    wrote on the flyleaf of the book: 'John Savory, 1 November 1819, 19
    Rue Vivienne, Paris'. He was nearly two years younger than Morson

and was therefore eighteen when he went to Paris.

43. *Pharmaceutical Journal,* 6 (1846-7), 340.

44. Sherwood Taylor, F., *The Alchemists,* London, Heinemann, 1951 3.

45. Lesch, John E., *Science and Medicine in France, 1790–1855,* Cambridge, Mass: Harvard University Press 1984, 143.

46. Kass, Amalie M. and Kass, Edward H., *Perfecting the World,* Boston: Harcourt Brace Jovanovich 1988, 64.

47. *Op. cit.,* note 45 above, 159.

48. *Ibid.,* 143.

49. Inkster and Morell (eds), *Metropolis & Province, Science in British culture, 1780–1850,* London: Hutchinson, 1983, 27.

50. Loudon, Irvine, *Medical Care and the General Practitioner 1750–1850,* Oxford: Clarendon Press, 1986 297.

51. Desmond, Adrian, *The Politics of Evolution,* University of Chicago, 1989, 297.

52. *Ibid.,* 92.

53. Desmond, Adrian, *Archetypes and Ancestors,* London: Bland and Briggs, 1982, 375.

54. *Op. cit.,* note 51 above, 96.

55. *Ibid.,* 14.

56. *Ibid.,* 135.

57. *Ibid.,* 144.

58. *Ibid.,* 30.

59. *Ibid.,* 92.

60. *Ibid.,* 87.

61. *Ibid.,* 165.

62. *Ibid.,*155.

63. Burnby, Juanita G.L., 'A study of the English Apothecary from 1660 to 1760', *Medical History,* Supplement No. 3, Wellcome Institute for the History of Medicine, London, 1983, 111.

64. *Op.cit.,* note 49 above, 125.

65. *Op.cit.,* note 53 above, 83.

66. Briggs, Asa, *Victorian Things,* London: B.T. Batsford, 1988, 21.

67. Greenhalgh, Paul, *Ephemeral Vistas,* Manchester University Press, 1988, 10.

9

Thomas Morson & Son Ltd.

Under his father's Will, Thomas Morson junior inherited the business together with the premises at Hornsey and Homerton; the pharmacy and warehouse in Southampton Row were rented under contracts made by their partnership. The pharmacy was re-numbered as 124 in 1864 and was continuously occupied from 1824 to 1900 when the London County Council took over the premises before demolishing them to widen Southampton Row. The first warehouse was at 46, being used for eight years when it became too small, and 31 & 33 were rented from 1865, until 1904 when the warehouse was transferred to Elm Street, just off Gray's Inn Road.

The house in Queen Square with its contents were left to Isabelle who inherited Morson's shares in the Gas, Light Company, a reminder of the link with Faraday and Winsor in the 1820s. The research laboratory continued to be operated at Queen Square by the business.

Three of Morson's most treasured possessions were mentioned specifically: a 'silver waiter', a present from Dr Roots whose friendship dated from the move to Bloomsbury, the small but beautiful equestrian statue of Wellington by Count d'Orsay, a present from Jacob Bell, and the Muller watercolour of the alkaloid factory at Hornsey. The statue was passed in 1908 to Thomas' second son who left it to the Thames Yacht Club, when he died in 1940. What interest the Club had in a statue of Wellington is doubtful; they have no knowledge of its whereabouts.

At the age of 49, Thomas became the sole owner of a famous pharmacy and a world-wide business in fine chemicals and pharmaceutical specialities. He had been educated at University College School before going to Paris to study chemistry at the

Institut Mathé, after which he served an apprenticeship in the Rue de la Paix with Monsieur Béral whose reputation was second to none. Like the rest of the family he was bilingual at an early age. He married a French pharmacist's daughter, having two sons and two daughters, all born in Southampton Row. The sons were 22 and 18 when their grandfather died.

Thomas had been helping the development of the business since he qualified. For a time, he lived at 46 Southampton Row supervising the wholesale business while the pharmacy was run by Robert Taubman, who later became a partner, after joining the firm in 1858 as an assistant. Taubman was very competent and soon ran the wholesale business while keeping an eye on the pharmacy.

In 1865 Thomas moved back to live in the apartment over the pharmacy and continued to do so until he moved to Gordon Square in 1881. He was widowed in 1878. He recorded all his children's births and those of his grandchildren until 1880 in the bible which his godfather, Thomas Lott, had given to his wife 'on her wedding day with my young friend'. It is an Anglican bible; under his wife's influence he became a Roman Catholic though his sons did not follow his example; their two sisters did.

Thomas continued the practice his father had started of support for close relatives. His cash book[1] shows some regular and many occasional payments, especially the dowry to his daughter of £37 10s.0d. per quarter. It was only right that his sister Isabelle had an income from the firm. Isabelle continued to live at Queen Square until she died on 15 July 1905. Hers was a life typical of Victorian times. Born during the Regency, she was brought up in Bloomsbury and was 11 when Victoria became Queen. She was a well-educated, cultured woman with literary and musical interests. She was a skilled needlewoman. She was 36 when her mother died and dutifully ran her father's house with skill and charm for eleven years. She was small, always beautifully dressed and had her father's sense of humour. Spending over 30 years alone at Queen Square enjoying her private life and interests, the frequent visits of great-nephews and nieces were a particular pleasure. She saw London develop to reflect the circumstances and riches of Empire, enjoying the opportunity provided by being the daughter of a famous father.

Isabelle's sister Mary helped to run the house at Queen Square until she and their elder sister Charlotte went to live at Boverton in 1863 in order to avoid London's smoke. In Wales, she met Isaac Redwood, half-brother of Theophilus. He was a very wealthy coalmaster and property owner who had been widowed some years earlier. His wife, Lydia Price, was the daughter of an ironmaster who, as a Quaker, was also a pacifist. Isaac's half-sister Margaret married Charles Vachell, a chemist and druggist and an apothecary of Cardiff to whom Theophilus Redwood was apprenticed in 1821. Mary Morson married Isaac in 1864, Charlotte and Theophilus being witnesses. No details of their life together are extant. Mary continued to live in South Wales after her husband's death in 1874. His Will left all his property to his niece who inherited practically the whole of a fortune of £60,000. Mary died in 1895.

Thomas junior inherited a business whose sales of chemicals and proprietaries were worth at least £30,000 a year. It is not possible to be precise because such account books as have survived cover only a part of the business. It is clear that substantial sales were made to the Apothecaries' Company, who recorded their outstanding debts to suppliers and Morson's name appears regularly for a long period of years. The only entry in Morson's books shows sales of £1,330 in 1870. The famous London hospitals including Guy's and Thomas's were also regular customers, as were all the larger wholesalers and some retailers throughout the British Isles. Australia was an important market, but was overshadowed by Canada and the United States. Firms from Montreal to St Louis were good customers and warranted Morson taking part in the Philadelphia Centennial Exhibition of 1876, at which the Prize Medal was won. Business was conducted with such firms as Schwartz and Haslett in Pittsburgh, Paine Bros. in New York and Avery and Co. in Boston. The firms in Canada were all offshoots of English ones such as Evans, Lescher. Contacts continued until the Second World War, when the business interruption was complete and restarted only with such specialist substances as Osmo-Kaolin, a specially prepared form of kaolin used extensively for face powders and other cosmetics besides being used in morphine and kaolin mixtures.

A gold medal was awarded to Morson's exhibit of alkaloids at the 1904 Louisiana Exhibition at which an extensive range of products was shown. The Exhibition was attended by Thomas junior's grandson, T. D. Morson, who took the opportunity to visit Finlay's in New Orleans; they had been important customers for a long time. Creosote continued to be a substantial export until 1940. During the years of the war, the Americans developed alternative supplies and in 1945 the Hayden Chemical Company in New York was in a position to export both beechwood creosote and the U.S.P. quality. They offered to supply Morson's, a confirmation, if one were needed, of the continuing demand for creosote.

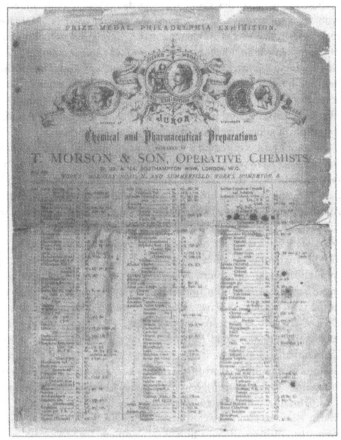

Figure 16: The front page of the 1878 price list.

France, Germany and China were sending orders quite frequently and India was fast becoming the major export market during the last quarter of the nineteenth century.

By the time of Morson's death, the profitability of the retail side had declined. Southampton Row continued to dispense and sell the usual range of a chemist's shop. Interest, however, had switched away from this part of the business. There were fewer residents in Bloomsbury, its houses being used as offices and some of the larger ones as hotels. Some of these, together with the big purpose-built ones, were very popular with American tourists; a steady stream of these, recently landed from the transatlantic voyage, called in for remedies to cure their sufferings! One which was popular was based on delphinine, which Morson had started isolating in 1821.

The years following Morson's death were used as an opportunity to make some necessary changes. Up to this time, profits had been continuous and sufficiently large for accurate accounting to be unnecessary. Under his son's influence, Thomas decided to sell the Hornsey property. They certainly did not need two factories. In July 1875, Hornsey was first mortgaged for £1,500 and then sold to Edward's, the ink manufacturer, for £2,500.

All the manufacturing equipment was transferred to Homerton, even some domestic items being transferred; a photograph shows some of the garden ornaments which had previously been at Hornsey.

For some years it must have been clear that retail profits were shrinking. In January 1869, the Bank of England lent the firm £700. This was repaid in six months together with 2% interest. It was, however, the first time a loan had been negotiated. One of the causes was the very extended credit given to customers. With expansion of the manufacturing side, with larger individual transactions, cash-flow problems must have been anticipated. It was not unusual for a year's credit to be given, a practice which had grown up much earlier in the century; a book entry of Isaiah Deck, a well-known Cambridge pharmacist and scientist, shows that he paid Morson in March 1847 for goods supplied in April and May 1846. In 1870, Morson complained of extensive credit shrinking margins further 'so that a microscope is needed to see them'. Profits had come more easily in former times.

The only surviving account book reveals that the factory at Homerton continued to be run separately but all wages were paid from the Bank of England account. Not all transactions appear to have been recorded. The business had grown to a size that required better bookkeeping and comprehensive accounts but the attempts made before Thomas junior's death do not appear to have been wholly successful.

If profits were more difficult to achieve, the business was still one of the largest in its field in London. Their licence[2] to store 'spirit' under the new Petroleum regulations in 1869 was the fourth largest of the 177 issued in London, and larger than their rivals Howard's and May & Baker. Other comparisons are also revealing. In December 1868, the York Glass Co. was paid £150, some twelve times as large a payment as was made by Ransom's whose national business was at Hitchin. Large payments were made for raw materials, nearly £800 for bromine and one payment out of several for citric acid was nearly £200. This was all in addition to the payments for alkaloids and other materials purchased from Europe; Schering, Böhringer and several French firms like Menier in Paris, being sent up to £100 at a time. Sales of Morson's narceine and codeine would be discussed in letters requesting despatch of his supplies from these companies.

The business had already been steered towards manufacture and trading in pharmaceutical chemicals, the retail side making an increasingly minor contribution until it was abandoned following losses in the last years of the century and the decision by the London County Council to take over the Duke of Bedford's properties and widen Southampton Row in 1899.

By the 1880s, sales had reached £35,000 a year with profits of 25% of turnover, so the partners, Thomas and his son T. P., were sharing a net profit in excess of £2,000; exceptionally in 1882 this rose to £4,000 which was a very substantial income for the time, when a manager's salary did not exceed £300 even in the more profitable businesses. The Homerton wages book[3] reveals that experienced process workers had a wage of 25/- a week, the juniors 18/-. Laboratory staff varied from 13/- to 25/- and 'girls' from 7/- to 13/-, although 'Grace' had a pound. The entry for one of the laboratory 'boys' is a reflection of the times. He asked for more wages and was immediately given a 10% rise.

About five years after his father's death, and although Thomas junior was taking an interest in the business, it was his son, Thomas Pierre, who was in charge. He was not inclined to assume that 'tomorrow would be like yesterday' and developed the business in new ways.

'T.P.' was born in 1852 and passed the minor examination of the Pharmaceutical Society in the year of his grandfather's death. He, too, went to University College School and then to Mannheim University for two years, returning in 1870 to study at the Royal College of Chemistry founded in 1845. The final part of his training was spent as an apprentice at Ferris[4] of Bristol. He was there from February 1871 for two years under an agreement drawn up between his father and the three Ferris partners. The deed stipulated that he was to see all invoices, to know rates and prices, both buying and selling. This commercial apprenticeship cost 150 guineas. He was well trained for the tasks he needed to perform in continuing to expand the fine chemical business and, as circumstances dictated, to relocate the factory and warehouse, besides introducing some orderly method into the office work. Many years later, staff who had

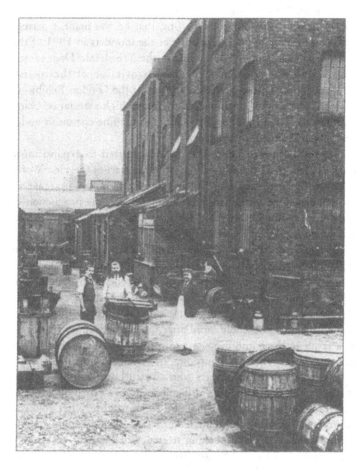

Figure 17: The Homerton factory, circa 1890.
Right to left are, Harpham, Works Chemist;
John Stevens, Manager and his son.

known him in the five years before he died in 1920 related how knowledgeable he was about every aspect of the business. These opinions were an echo of an article in the *British and Colonial Druggist* of 1910,[5] which described a charming, even debonair, man in morning coat and top hat attending the drug auctions in London, sometimes accompanied by Taubman. He was one of the most experienced buyers. He also had with him for these auctions a small notebook which was kept up to date by his staff and provided him with a record of his and others' transactions.

It is an indication both of his ability and of his father's confidence in his running of the firm that he was made a partner when only 27 in 1879. He was one of the founders in 1891 of the Drug Club, which in 1930 became the Wholesale Drug Trade Association and then in 1948, the Association of the British Pharmaceutical Industry. He was a Juror for the London Exhibition of 1909. The firm continued to maintain high standards, being awarded the Grand Prix at Turin in 1911 for fine chemicals and a Diplôme d'Honneur for reagents.

Under T.P.'s leadership, the business started to expand more quickly, the period immediately prior to the start of the First World War seeing a spectacular rise in turnover and an increase in profitability. One of the larger causes of this was the production of the double cyanide of mercury and zinc, the development of which was supervised by Taubman in the 1880s.

In 1865 the famous surgeon Joseph Lister began his work on antisepsis by using carbolic acid, one of the substances distilled from coal tar using a process invented by the Frenchman, Laurent, in 1831. During the 1840s Manchester had one of the two largest distillation plants in the country, the other being at Leith. Calvert's name became a household word after they started up in 1859, and as a result of their improvements to quality by 1864, the acid was pure enough for medicinal purposes.[6]

The work of manufacturers who assisted Lister and the dates of their contribution have been difficult to unravel, partly because of lost records and partly by an understandable wish to keep commercial details confidential. Lister was always careful to give credit where it was due, making reference to the help he received from manufacturers. The articles in the *Chemist and Druggist, Pharmaceutical* and *British Medical Journals* can be augmented by the Lister letters deposited by T.P.'s son, A. Clifford Morson, at the Royal College of Surgeons[7]. They were used for a paper given to the Royal Society of Medicine by Dr Basil C. Morson[8] in 1971. Lister wrote these letters to Robert Taubman and, later, to Thomas D. Morson, Clifford Morson's brother, who quite naturally did not think of giving him internal memos from the firm. These have now come to light. At MacFarlan's in Edinburgh, there are letters and notes concerning the work they did with Lister and these too record important details relevant to the development of antiseptic dressings and the preparation of catgut for ligatures.

Lister started his work while Professor of Surgery at Glasgow Royal Infirmary and used a carbolic acid spray in the operating theatre and gauze soaked in the acid for dressings. He was a great experimentalist and tried carbolic oil, putty and Lac plaster as well as ligatures of catgut treated with the acid so as to avoid the use of silk, which was not absorbed and its removal from wounds was difficult and painful.

At first, Lister worked with Apothecaries' Hall[9] in Glassford Street, Glasgow who later supplied MacFarlans with Lac plaster before they made their own dressings in Edinburgh. Lister visited the Hall as frequently as twice a week, leaving his wife in the carriage contentedly knitting!

At a Pharmaceutical Society meeting[10] under Morson's chairmanship in 1868, William Martindale described the dressings he was making at University College Hospital. He stressed they were made in accordance with Lister's antiseptic system. Lister's work had already spread throughout the country. After first using a carbolic acid putty (boiled linseed oil, whiting and carbolic acid), which was 'clumsy and inconvenient', they tried a plaster of olive oil, litharge, beeswax and crystallised carbolic acid spread on calico. This was followed by a mixture of shellac and carbolic acid which was spread on muslin; gutta percha being applied to prevent adhesion but allowing the carbolic acid solution to permeate.

If University College Hospital was experimenting in this way, there must have been other hospitals copying these developments.

In 1869, Lister went to Edinburgh as Professor of Surgery and continued his work, impregnating gauze with various antiseptic solutions. In 1870, he\approached MacFarlan[11] since they were the leading manufacturers in the city. Mr David Brown[12] developed a technique for carbolising gauze with which Lister was satisfied, the most important requirement being an even spread of the solution. MacFarlans soon received many orders for their dressings from surgeons and hospitals, and within a year or so were exporting them to Germany and the U.S.A.

Records at MacFarlans mention stocks held for this manufacture: a cask of paraffin, of rosin and a bale of muslin; there were stocks too of Nos 2, 3 & 4 antiseptic mixtures (not further identified) and also of antiseptic gauze. One of Mr Brown's letters, 10 January 1901, concludes that the experimental stage was passed and since these stocks were recorded in February 1871, it must have been 1870 when Lister started working with Macfarlan. There was some friction between MacFarlan and Milne, who had worked at the Edinburgh Royal Infirmary as a jobbing joiner until 1878, when he is said to have joined Lister in London. Milne issued a price list in April 1900 claiming precedence in the manufacture of Listerian dressings. Their rebuttal on 4 January 1901 was robust. In order to collect together the facts as MacFarlan saw them, they asked Brown and others for their views and, fortunately for us, these notes are extant except for Milne's reply. From the latter's point of view, his assistance to Lister constituted manufacture of a kind; even so, there can be no doubt that MacFarlan's were the first firm to develop, manufacture, and market Listerian dressings.

In July 1871, Lister reported his success in the *Edinburgh Medical Journal* and stated that it was MacFarlans who had supplied the dressings. This is confirmed by a reference in the *Pharmaceutical Journal*, 13 July 1872, by William Martindale[13] and by Dr Newman of Stamford Infirmary who was supplied by MacFarlan.

Iodoform and other substances were tried. A field dressing using iodoform was proposed in 1888 by Surgeon Major Bourke of the Army Medical Staff at Woolwich.[14] This was widely used as a first field dressing, the iodoform being dusted on from a small bag. MacFarlan's sales of this dressing and Morson's sales of iodoform, were quite significant.

In 1875 Lister published his so-called diffusion method for impregnating gauze, a development he introduced at the Infirmary, and hospitals were enabled to produce their own dressings. Not

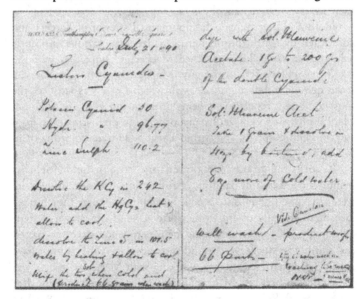

Figure 18: Formula for Double Cyanide, 21 July 1890.

surprisingly MacFarlan was disappointed that Lister appeared to ignore the efforts they had made to experiment and meet his requirements when he encouraged hospitals to prepare their own dressings.[15]

The efforts had included, for instance, staff[16] spending a whole day at a horse knacker's yard in Glasgow to collect five gallons of horse blood to make the serum with which the first 'Sero-sublimate' was made to impregnate gauze. It was so named as the serum was mixed with perchloride of mercury, the impregnated gauze being dried before use. It was not, however, sufficiently absorbent. One of MacFarlan's staff recorded that Lister wrote 'considerably later' asking the firm to destroy their stocks and stop production. He does not provide the reason.

Lister next tried Sal-alembroth, a double salt of bichloride of mercury and ammonium chloride. It was stained blue for identification purposes but had the disadvantage of irritating the skin.[17]

In 1877, Lister took up an appointment in London, always on the look-out for better antiseptic substances and experimenting with alternative dressings. In 1884, the *British Medical Journal* published his address on the use of corrosive sublimate as a surgical dressing.[18] By now, he was no longer using carbolic acid except sometimes for moistening a dressing with a weak solution immediately prior to use. The man on MacFarlan's staff who had collected the horse blood, Alex Macdonald, now living in London, maintained that corrosive sublimate gauze was not introduced by Lister but by a surgeon at one of the London hospitals, a Dr MacCormac. Lister wrote to MacFarlans at this time asking them to drop his name from their label which stated Lister's Corrosive Sublimate gauze. Perhaps his urgent letter was sent to prevent his name being associated with a development not initiated by him. By implication, he was authorising the use of his name in connection with Salalem broth and iodoform dressings.

William Martindale recalled that he worked with Lister in 1886 and that he had suggested the use of the cyanides of zinc and mercury.[19] He wrote that he had made some to supply 'one of the dressing manufacturers' but also that they worked for some time making experimental lots of dressings themselves. Alex Macdonald, writing in 1927, believed that the double cyanide most nearly approached Lister's conception of an ideal antiseptic and that it was first prepared by Morson's. Why Lister stopped working with Martindale and started with Morson's is not known. Lister may have believed that further progress could not be made without a specialist chemical firm to develop the chemistry of the double cyanide, leaving the impregnation of the material of the dressing to another specialist.

Lister decided to get in touch with Taubman almost certainly at Martindale's suggestion since the two chemists had worked together at Southampton Row for four years and remained friends. It is possible to speculate that Lister had discussed his problem with Playfair with whom a discussion of chemistry would have been likely and who would have remembered his work with T. N. R. Morson dating from the 1840s. It was Playfair, nine years after Lister's approach to Morsons, who introduced Lister into the House of Lords after he had been created a baron.[20] Whatever the background, Morsons worked to improve the purity and understanding of the chemistry of the substance and organised its production on a manufacturing scale. In their 1913 Catalogue they state that they first manufactured it in 1884. While this date differs from Martindale recalling he had suggested its use in 1886, there seems no doubt that Morsons were the first manufacturers, as Alex Macdonald confirmed.

Morsons believed they had originated the double cyanide because the Southampton Row laboratory developed the process,[21] Lister arriving (in his barouche and pair which was a familiar sight on the streets of London as the great man went to his appointments) to examine and discuss methods of manufacturing antiseptics. Morson's letter states that 'Lister's double cyanide was originated' in collaboration with the then Sir Joseph whose name they used on their labels until about 1930. During the Lister centenary of 1927, Morsons received a large Government order for double cyanide. The last batch was made in 1933, after which hydrocyanic acid was made only for internal medicinal purposes.

After the development work was completed at Southampton Row, the Homerton works started manufacture early in 1889. They were estimating the quantity of mercury left 'in liquor' and in the compounded powder on 10 May 1889. A costing[22] dated 8 August confirms they were then manufacturing at a cost of 10/4. per pound and waiting to recover mercury cyanide. A label records a batch quantity of 11³/₄ oz of product and an 'actual cost' of 8/- per pound. A note from the Works Manager provides the information that 14lb quantities would present no difficulty but that anything above that would require 'extra plant'. The latter was procured and the quantities made increased steadily. Over the following twenty years production continued to rise, with the period immediately before and during the 1914 war seeing a spectacular rise. In 1915, it was necessary to manufacture 500 lb lots of hydrocyanic acid to satisfy commitments. This increase in scale brought the product cost down to 2/- per pound, the sale price being maintained at 18/-, the same level as published in the 1899 catalogue.

An early problem was retention of the antiseptic on the gauze; 'dusting out' is how it was described. The Lister correspondence with Taubman indicates how this was overcome. Lister had tried paraffin added to a carbolic/resin mixture, but this had not proved satisfactory.[23] It was solved by the use of the comparatively new aniline dye and with the help of its discoverer, Perkin.[24] The affinity of double cyanide for mauveine (there is no chemical reaction) ensured that adhesiveness, as Lister called it, was achieved and at the same time, the distinctive colour of mauveine distinguished double cyanide dressings. Morson's 1899 catalogue confirms the use by referring to the double cyanide as 'dyed'.

Morsons accumulated considerable experience in the production of aniline dyes; 'aniline colours in crystals and solution' was an item in the July 1878 price list, with aniline included in two grades: 'pure' and 'commercial'. By 1899, they listed no less than thirty of these synthetic dyes.

One of Taubman's letters to Lister (23 September 1890) refers to John Milne[25] who opened a firm at Ladywell, Lewisham in 1878 for the manufacture of antiseptic dressings. Milne had helped with the introduction of the diffusion method between 1874 and the beginning of 1875, operating Lister's first apparatus for impregnating muslin with antiseptic at the Edinburgh Royal Infirmary. It seems that he decided to exploit this skill in London. If Lister was involving his firm in 1890, he may have done so from his earliest days in London.

Another link with Lister occurred in 1907 when he wrote to Morson's asking them for their process for the manufacture of chromium sulphate. The exchange of correspondence reveals some of the difficulties in using this substance for preparing catgut so that it could be used aseptically for ligatures. The draft of T. D. Morson's reply is among the surviving letters[26] and points out the intensely hygroscopic nature of this salt and the consequent problems in its use.

Lister wrote to MacFarlans in 1894 asking how they achieved consistent quality of chromium sulphate, as the commercial products were unsatisfactory. He also wanted to know if they immersed the catgut in the solution of chromium sulphate after it had been stretched out on a cylinder or frame.

The first catgut ligatures had been immersed in carbolic acid and were made by the Glasgow Apothecaries' Company when Lister was working at the Infirmary there. Alex Macdonald recalled what the method was at MacFarlan's. They immersed the lengths of catgut in a carbolic solution for two months; this was reduced to six weeks after some experience. This maturation was further hastened when Lister had the idea of using 'chromic carbolised catgut'.

Because there had been cases of anthrax in patients in Germany and it was traced to imperfectly sterilised gut, Lister laid great stress on the treatment the catgut be given before winding and drying. There was also a test introduced to check that the treated ligature bore a specified tensile strain depending on its thickness.

Lister wanted the ligatures to be absorbed by the living tissues only after twenty days and his methods were altered to achieve that result. When chromium sulphate in a solution of corrosive sublimate was used, the period of steeping was reduced to a day.[27] The chromium sulphate was used in order to prolong absorption time while the wound was healing.

Morsons had a letter from Lister dated 3 August 1907 stating that he gave instructions to a manufacturing chemist and a surgical instrument maker in 1894. The former must have been MacFarlans, the latter was a firm named Matthews who copied them out and Lister sent them to Morson's.

These instructions recognised the very hygroscopic nature of chromium sulphate and, as the concentration of the solution was so important, its preparation involved 'various important details'.[28]

Lister's purpose in reviewing these matters with the two manufacturers so closely involved in his work, was to prepare a paper[29] in which he pointed out that chromium sulphate treatment produced the best results, but it was not a germicide so the addition of corrosive sublimate was necessary. Lister usually gave credit to those who worked with him and, on this occasion, included a footnote mentioning Morsons who had 'devoted a good deal of attention to this salt'.

At this time, there was still some reluctance among surgeons to use catgut and though Morsons made chromium sulphate available, its sale was small. Eventually the London Hospital sold sterile catgut commercially in about 1912. There are records of Morson sales to this hospital as to most others but there is no specific reference to chromium sulphate. However, it may be significant that T. P. Morson was a life Governor of the London and from him they may have obtained the salt and Lister's method.

In the last years of Lister's life his letters seeking confirmation about both chromium sulphate and double cyanide seem to have been designed to enable him to record for posterity the details of his work. It is fascinating that what he first announced in 1865, he persisted with over such a long period constantly, improving his techniques.

The huge quantities of double cyanide made during the 1914 war, and continued afterwards until nearly 1930, are themselves a tribute to Lister's pioneering work.

Their contribution to the Morson company's sales was one of the reasons for turnover more than doubling between 1914 and 1916. It rose from £115,000 to £285,000, the first full year after incorporation. These are the first totally reliable figures and indicate that the earlier figures do not accurately reflect the size of the business conducted from Hornsey and then Homerton.

At the start of his period in business, there were four managers who assisted T. P. Morson. Robert Taubman was the most senior and was assisted by Thomas Trask, who won the prize for Materia Medica in 1849 after being examined by Pereira as a student at the School of Pharmacy. He became a curator of the Museum, in which T. N .R. Morson always took a great interest.

Bletsoe was the office manager and Taylor, the former apprentice, returned in 1871 to act as a salesman, travelling the country collecting orders and dealing with customers, the majority of whom were visited annually by T.P. who also paid quarterly visits to Scotland and the West Country.

In addition to these four, there were just over 30 employees at Homerton and in Southampton Row. Some had worked at Hornsey and many were to have quite extraordinary records of service, which was a feature of the times and particularly of process industry and of printing.

The most famous of these employees was Mary Ann Bowden. 'Polly' worked from 1876 until 1932, starting when she was 15. The earliest entry for her wage is January 1878 when she was earning 5/- a week. She was employed at Homerton, weighing out and packing alkaloids for many years, proof of her accuracy and reliability. She left in 1932 when earning 33/- a week on a pension of 25/-. Her peak earnings were in the early 1920s when her wage and bonus totalled 50/-.

Shortly before Polly started, a boy aged 11 was taken on at Southampton Row. On 28 March 1872, Robert William Courtenay joined the firm. He became a highly skilled operator under Taubman's supervision at first then under the foreman at Hornsey,

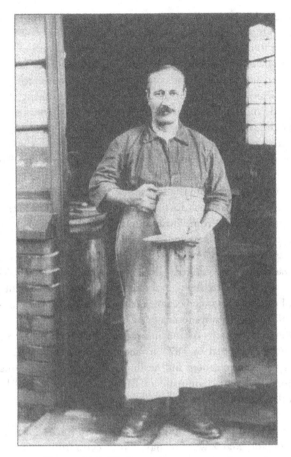

Figure 19: R.W. Courtenay, process worker,
worked from 1872 until his death in 1928.
Photograph taken about 1920.

William Semper. Courtenay moved to Homerton when the factory
was transferred there, working under the chemist Harpham and
the Works Manager Tipping, receiving a wage of 5/- at the
beginning and 32/- in 1896. In 1917 he had £3 2s. 6d. when he
was transferred to a salaried position and given 50 preference
shares in the company. In 1927 after 55 years' service he was
encouraged to start late and leave work as soon as he liked. The
habit of factory hours of working prevented him from taking full
advantage of this arrangement. He died in his son's arms at work
on 20 November 1928.[30]

He was one of those who passed his skills, through on-the-job training, to younger generations of process workers, helping to maintain the standards of operation which ensured that quality was always achieved.

In addition, they taught young men to handle dangerous substances long before there were Factories Acts and Regulations concerning chemicals. Due to their skill, bromine, iodine, inflammable solvents, dangerous acids and even explosive substances were handled without accidents over a very long period. In 50 years of using bromine, Ponders End suffered only one accident which caused a serious burn, but William Collier returned to work in a month.

Another notable record of service was by Arthur C. Burr. He was recruited in 1893 when he was 21 and had been working for MacFarlans at their London warehouse in Moor Lane. His wages doubled in the period of the First World War. He was salaried after the war and earned £230 a year, which was much above average for a man qualified by his extensive experience only. He completed 44 years' service, all as a warehouseman. After his death in 1937, his wife wrote to thank the Managing Director for a letter of sympathy. Her reply was most carefully composed and beautifully written.

The most incredible performance was that of John Stevens, who started work at Hornsey when 14 in 1858 and was pensioned in 1924 after 66 years' service! Such a record must be very nearly unique.

It was part of John's job to keep the wages book. There were so few people at Homerton in 1878 when he started his last book that he had no use for surnames, easily distinguishing between Charles on line 6 at 18/- and Charles on line 8 at £1 1s. 0d. The wages money was delivered to the site by one of the partners who brought it from the Bank of England. In 1880 John saved himself the trouble of writing out all the names every week. He noted the standard amount and any variations for absence or increases. These were few at a time of great stability in working hours and in the value of money.

No sooner had the new century been welcomed than the partners in Morsons were advised that their Homerton site was being taken over for expansion of the hospital next door. By this time Taubman was a partner, having joined Thomas junior and his son in 1891 and sharing in the satisfactory profits that were made, even though they steadily declined between 1900 and 1905. In 1892, the partners shared £5,243 and in 1905, £1,537. Taubman had been apprenticed to a Mr Bowman in the Isle of Man and had passed the major examination of the Pharmaceutical Society in June 1849, being one of the first to do so. He made an early impact on joining Morson's in 1858 and supervised the technical work once T. N. R. Morson had died, even though his managerial function was to run the warehousing and distribution. One of Robert Taubman's sons, F. H. Taubman, was also a pharmacist. His hobby of sculpture turned into a considerable success, his bust of William Martindale being placed in the hall at Bloomsbury Square.

The Hospital Guardians paid £6,750 for the lease, the site being cleared by a Mr Carey, who completed his task in November 1902.

Meantime, T. P. Morson was searching for a new site. After inspecting premises in West London, Stratford and other developing areas, the site at Ponders End was selected. In view of it being owned by Corbyn, Stacey, it is possible that business contacts with this famous wholesaler led to knowledge of the site. The first purchase was of 3 acres, the conveyance being completed on 8 May 1901 and the cost was £1,000.

The Lea Valley in which Ponders End is situated was traditionally a horticultural district. There were many nurseries round Stoke Newington when T. N. R. Morson was a schoolboy. As London expanded, the nurseries moved north along the valley, expanding the area, especially near Enfield, which had a long tradition of horticulture and market gardening. Residential property was built near the new factories, providing homes and creating a demand for shops.

Morson's site at Ponders End was next to the London-to-Cambridge railway, which made travel easy and provided a siding from which goods were delivered. The rural character of the area in 1900 is confirmed by the deeds which record that the land had been let as allotments; and there can be no doubt that they were very productive, being cultivated by experienced men who worked in the nurseries. The deeds gave the owners the right 'to pass and repass on foot and on horseback and with horses, cattle, sheep, carts, waggons and wains' along Wharf Road which was the only means of access. It is within living memory that cows strayed from their grazing on land which is now a large reservoir into the chemical factory-unwelcome visitors in the days when liquid raw materials were stored outside in 10-gallon glass carboys.

By December 1908, the opportunity was taken to purchase a second parcel of land, making the total area 6 acres, 2 roods and 28 perches in the old measure of area: now 6.68 acres valued at £300 per acre. Industrial land within outer London now commands a price of £300,000 an acre and more if official permissions for development have been granted.

The cost of the move and setting up the factory and facilities was £20,000. The site was mortgaged in December 1901 for £5,000 at 4%. A further mortgage was taken out in 1934, bringing the total borrowed to £8,000. All the equipment was transferred from Homerton including the 1,200-gallon chloroform still, but volumes were increasing and considerable amounts of plant and equipment were purchased.

The site was provided with a house for the manager, whose garden was planted with roses, shrubs and trees. It had three bedrooms and was built as solidly as the factory building. The first occupant was a man named A. J. Tipping who was Works Manager at Homerton for a short time before working at Ponders End. When he died in 1915 the house was used as offices, there being some pressure on space at the beginning of 1915 with the sudden expansion and increased business in export markets since the site was first operated in 1904. Besides, the need for a manager living on site had ended.

The house at the entrance to the Homerton site had served a similar purpose, but the occupiers were a factory foreman, William Harrison, and his wife, Emma. He had lived at 168 Homerton High Street for more than twenty years before he had to move. He spent most of his working life making potassium iodide, retiring after 50 years' service in 1930. He gave a party to celebrate the occasion, the invitations having a piece of appropriate doggerel:

> For fifty years I've led a life of 'iodised' enrapture,
> And crystal gazing is for me an Art I need not capture,
> A casual nod to Pot. Iod. does not grow crystals faster,
> The laws of Chemistry, I know, take years and years to master,
> If Iodine is in my spleen when I perforce depart,
> You'll find inside 'Pot. iodide' engraven on my heart.

The literary ability of William Harrison and of Mrs Burr contrasts with the illiteracy in 1915 of at least one employee who made his mark against his name on an address the staff gave to T. P. at the works summer party, which was held in the cricket field across the road from the factory. The land is now a colony of small factories.

After ten years of operation at Ponders End, Morson's range of products had extended beyond the pharmaceutical to include oleates, resinates and other substances used in the manufacture, as an example, of linoleum, which was manufactured in the area, although Kirkcaldy in Fife became a much larger centre of production. Lithium, strontium, cadmium, cobalt, zinc and aluminium salts in great variety were made in technical and pharmaceutical grades. With the establishment in the late nineteenth century of standards for analytical reagents, the range and volume of these were impressive. No attempt, however, was made to establish them as branded products. No less than 200 chemicals were sold direct and in bulk to laboratory furnishers.

Medicinal sodium sulphate, Glauber's salt, was made in various forms, with the acid sulphate made in ton lots for making tablets for treating drinking water for the troops in France.

It must not be assumed that the older products were ignored; valerianates, hydrocyanic acid, amyl nitrite* and some alkaloids were still manufactured, large spaces being needed for the storage and grinding of vegetable drugs for extraction of such as podophyllin, emetine, colchicin and aloin. An example of increased volumes is hydrocyanic acid of which 10,000 lb of 2% strength was made in 1930.

If all the substances made, even if only once a year, were counted, the total approached 2,000, although this was considerably less than the 3,000 items in the 1899 catalogue.

All of this was achieved with about 60 staff in addition to the few supervisors and a manager. This was nearly double the number, 35, employed in Southampton Row and Homerton when Morson's took over that site.

The management style at all firms, particularly those like Howards, Hanburys and Morsons, was paternalistic. T.P. saw himself as a father-figure but he was not unapproachable; anecdotal evidence exists for employees expressing their views to him about matters which were of concern. While there were no formal arrangements for sick pay, pensions or other 'benefits', it was normal to continue paying absentees, the period being judged by the circumstances, and the length of service. 'Staff', which meant those who were monthly paid, sometimes promoted to this category due to service, received their money for six months before a review was made. Pensions were entirely *ex gratia*. With such informal arrangements there were perhaps individuals who felt they had been treated less generously than others but the policy was hardly different from other firms and the pay was always as good as could be obtained from other employers and usually better.

---

* Amyl nitrate was discovered in 1844 and used as a medicine from 1870. It was in Morson's 1878 Sales List, the oldest one extant.

The remuneration of more senior staff also provides examples of competitive salary. After a period of working in the warehouse in Southampton Row in 1893 when he started at a salary of £32 a year, W. B. Fletcher was made office manager and, in 1915, became Secretary of the newly incorporated company. His salary that year was £600 with a bonus of £400. An income of £1,000 at such a time provided for a good standard of living, equivalent to about £35,000 today. Fletcher was an avid railway time-table reader and could quote train times and suggest routes as easily and accurately as anyone employed to do so by the railway company. He retired in 1944, so had been intimately connected with the company for 51 years. He lived to be a centenarian and, though very deaf, retained a clear mind. Soon after his 100th birthday, he made the comment that Taubman and he believed that 'Morsons were no good with money' in the context of a question about business affairs in the early twentieth century.

During the period between 1910 and 1930, large quantities of the main products were produced. The peak was reached before the Great Depression of 1931, when 350 tons of fine chemicals were made. Morson's share of some markets, while not dominant, was very substantial. The actual production of citrates reached 200,000 lbs, that of bismuths 70,000 and of iodides 83,000, of which 65,000 was potassium iodide, thus continuing an important place in a market entered in 1821. At one time the annual output of iodoform reached 7,365lb.

Under one of the cooperative arrangements of the 1930s all English manufacture of resublimed iodine was consolidated at Ponders End and sold through a company set up for the purpose, in which Whiffens had an interest. More than 10,000lb had been made in 1924 but this was to be many times increased by 1950. The method used was to place the crude granular iodine in a shallow unglazed ceramic dish whose cover was the same as the base, both being made with a wide flange which provided a perfect seal. They were made by Doultons. The dishes were set in rows in a sandbath supported by a steel plate, a gas or coke fire was lit at one end with a chimney at the other, the gentle heating warming the dishes and vaporising the iodine. Slow cooling caused the iodine vapour to crystallise on the inside surface of the upper dish. It was only on hot summer days that the operation had to be stopped because the iodine started to vaporise. It was a really low-technology but highly effective method which was operated by one man with occasional help for an output of up to two tons a week. The output of iodine products increased steadily until Morsons became the largest manufacturer in the UK in the inter-war years.

It is fascinating to see that the same method, even to the shape of the ceramic dishes, was used by Merck & Co. in their New Jersey plant. In their case it was probably the transfer from the Merck factory at Darmstadt that was the origin of the method. Perhaps German practice was copied by Morson's or, conceivably, the simple method had evolved independently to produce the same result.

In cool weather, the removal of the upper dish revealed iodine crystals up to three inches long clustered against the surface. The sight of the metallic lustre of scores of wafer-thin crystals was beautiful.

At this period, there was considerable standardisation of quality but not of physical form. Customers wanted their chosen size of iodide crystal, and as many as six densities of bismuth carbonate had to be produced for wholesalers and the larger chemists' shops who had established their own formulations for products containing these inorganics.

The operating technique to produce these variations was developed by the experienced foremen, who over the years needed little help from the chemists. In the case of bismuth carbonate a little phosphoric acid was used to adjust acidity before precipitating the product. The details of the technique were held eventually in one man's hands, a fact unknown to management until he became ill for some weeks, with production badly affected! Perhaps it gave him some wry satisfaction to demonstrate an aspect of his job security.

During the First World War very large quantities of bismuth bromphenal were made. Originally a German proprietary, ton quantities were shipped to Archangel for the Russian Red Cross.

In practice, Morson's had operated batch recording, reference sampling and both final-product and in-process quality control for many years, starting with simple recording and leading to successive increases in sophistication.

For many years, the firm successfully marketed its products to the India Office for shipment to Calcutta and Bombay for supplying the hospitals of the Indian Medical Service. The quantities were substantial even for such a large country. In 1888, 961lb of chloral hydrate and 750lb of quinine were included in orders which totalled £2,000. Morson's chlorodyne (100-2ounce vials), 66 ounces of cocaine, and 350lb of phenacetin were also among shipments made in the 1890s. By the early years of the current century, the business grew such that a ton of iodoform, 21/2 tons of potassium iodide, 400lb of chloral hydrate and 11/2 tons of chloroform were shipped in one order which included 53 pounds (*sic*) of strychnine – in all valued at £6,500. All the items were packed in small containers ready for distribution to pharmacies. The largest order ever received was for £12,787 in 1920.

This was not untypical of Britain's pharmaceutical exports, a business that had been increasing since the first days of Empire. A huge range of products and surgical supplies was manufactured by Allen & Hanbury, Corbyn and many smaller firms. These businesses made and marketed these goods including 'drugs which provided the commodity upon which the modern business of medicine is founded.'[31]

There were few exceptions to these products being made at Ponders End, though production of strychnine was supplemented by purchases from Whiffens who usually supplied all the quinine.

The introduction of aspirin in 1898 was an opportunity grasped by Bayer in Germany to such an extent that there was very little production in England, a fact worrying the Government before the 1914 war. Dr Pearson and Dr Morell, two London chemists, knew the process but needed help with finance and marketing. Morson's undertook to supply them with their materials and acted as selling agents, an arrangement that continued for more than twenty years, the last record of sales being in 1941. Royalties were paid to Morsons. Pearson and Morell were the first English aspirin makers but were overtaken by Howards by the 1920s.

An entirely different product was an offshoot of Morson's long experience with collodion, made since 1849 for surgical, photographic and, later, printing purposes. The pharmacist at the Great Ormond Street Hospital for Sick Children, J.W. Peck, developed a lightweight, non-inflammable celluloid solution to stiffen the material applied to limbs after surgery. The proposal had originally been made in *The Lancet* in July 1912 by D F. E. Battern and a few months later Peck had announced his celluloid splints which were limb casings made by painting the solution on successive layers of gauze or stockinette, wound on a plaster of paris cast of the patient's limb. It was used for many years, production of the solution reaching 1,500 lb a year. It was eventually marketed by Becket and Bird Ltd, Peck receiving a royalty over a period of 30 years until about 1950.

Soon after the new factory was in operation, production of Liquor Trinitrini BP, chemically glyceryl trinitrate or nitroglycerine, produced for emergency treatment of angina, reached 31/2 gallon batches two or three times a year and this continued into the 1950s with output three or four times greater. The process was conducted in the same small building as collodion. After so many years of operation, it was a surprise to find that registration was necessary with explosives inspectors from the Home Office. When they discovered what was done, they insisted on closing down the production. But even bureaucrats can be flexible when told that there was no other source for an essential medicine. They relented to allow stocks to be made while Imperial Chemical Industries Explosives Division were persuaded to take on the job.

During the 1920s it was evident that the business was increasingly dependent upon established products. In the absence of research work, expansion could only be achieved by joint ventures. T. D. Morson, the elder son of T. P., who had the responsibility of overseeing the construction, installation and production start-up at Ponders End, was a well-known figure in the industry. He published a paper[32] drawing attention to the circumstances of the industry at the beginning of the 1914 war and took an active part in the Society of Chemical Industry, a technical group covering every aspect of technical operations. He was an original member of the committee of the Association of British Chemical Manufacturers, a trade association, and became Treasurer of the Association of the British Pharmaceutical Industry. Most of the credit for the firm's progress between the wars is due to him.

When chocolate laxative tablets were introduced in the late 1920s, Morsons were in a position to exploit their process, which they developed in the 1870s, for making the aperient substance used. Phenolphthalein was included in the *Pharmacopoeia* 1867 and its production reached a peak of 80–100 tons per year.

When Menley and James, a subsidiary of Smith, Kline and French in the 1930s, needed their products manufactured in England to overcome the heavy import duties of the inter-war years, they turned to Morsons who started toll manufacture first by Benzedrine, then Amphetamine in 1937 and later Dexedrine in 1946. Not only was this a successful partnership, but it introduced Morsons to the more complex substances and the processes involved.

Since the 1880s Morsons had made sodium glycerophosphate, one of a range of substances included in tonic formulations for which demand increased steadily. When the Works Manager, A. J. Tipping, died suddenly as a young man in 1915, the firm engaged Dr Charles S. Roy as Works Director. He had obtained his Ph.D. in Germany, had studied engineering as well as chemistry and brought with him considerable experience of fine chemical manufacture, especially that of iodides and glycerophosphates, for which Morsons paid him a royalty in the first few years, because he had introduced process improvements which he had developed and patented in 1912; he was then working for Southalls at Birmingham. He and T. D. Morson cooperated in the development of a glass fibre cloth useful for filtration. Its sales produced a small profit which the two men shared in the 1920s; a sample was mounted between glass and used as a fire screen in the days when offices had individual fireplaces.

Production of sodium glycerophosphate had already reached two tons a year in 1914, together with some of the potassium and magnesium salts. Expansion was difficult at this period because the munitions factories nearby were absorbing most of the labour, but some success was achieved by employing women process workers for the first time. The largest demand was for a soluble form of the calcium salt, but Morsons did not develop a process. The experts were E. Merck, of Darmstadt, with whom discussions about a manufacturing and selling arrangement were initiated in 1930. For Merck this was a tariff-avoidance project as much as a transfer of technology. Britain had protected its chemical industry with tariffs as high as 33·33% after their experience before the First World War, it being one of the industries designated under the Key Industry Duty arrangements. In addition, the Imperial Preference scheme allowed duty free-entry for British-made goods to Empire countries, so. Merck could gain entry to a very large market by concluding an agreement with Morson.

After almost two years of negotiation the agreement was signed in July 1933, although letters of intent in February allowed work on the plant to start. A day and a half of final talks in London on 6 and 7 December 1932 had been found to be necessary in order to finalise all the details before the lawyers set to work. Merck agreed to provide their process and a senior production chemist to demonstrate it. Morsons provided all the production facilities. A royalty based on sales would be paid by Morsons and the agreement stipulated that they had an exclusive right to manufacture in Empire countries. Profits were to be shared equally and the agreement was to last for seven years.

Production was soon under way. The first full year was 1935 when over 40,000lb of calcium glycerophosphate was made. A loss of £1,200 was incurred. It was the fourth year before break-even point was reached, after which net profits increased to reach £2,000 by 1939.

The outbreak of war effectively terminated the agreement. By the end of the war, profits had doubled and in 1948 reached

£8,000, without royalties to pay or any sharing of profits. Sales of tonic preparations, in both liquid and sugar-based powder formulations, continued to provide a satisfactory market for a little over ten years. Competition severely trimmed profits in the late 1950s but newer products were replacing tonic proprietary medicines. Output reached a level of 250 tons a year.

From the earliest time of these developments Morsons marketed their own glycerophosphate syrup which they called Vulcan Elixir. It was a very palatable product, popular in the export market. In East Africa, its popularity was said to be due to the label depicting a manly figure wielding a club, leading to the assumption that the tonic had aphrodisiac properties; it was drunk by the Muslim part of the population because of the attraction of having, without breaking their rules, the alcohol it contained.

The strategy represented by all this was an attempt to perpetuate the business on the lines established at the beginning of the century with the addition of the cooperative ventures with Merck and Menley and James. It suffered from an absence of research and from a traditional approach to the management of the business. From a technical point of view there was reliance only upon chemical-processing skills. These were very considerable but insufficient to ensure the introduction of new products, upon which the firm had thrived in the nineteenth century.

May & Baker's solutions to similar problems were to acquire products from other companies but also to invest in research. This produced sulphapyridine (M&B 693) which marked a new departure in medicine – the treatment of the cause of illness, not merely its symptoms.

Few financial figures for pharmaceutical firms in the last quarter of the nineteenth century are available and those that are make comparisons difficult because of the various methods used to keep their books. Morsons did not record all their sales, Howards discounted theirs by 6%. Some expenditure could be paid for directly from receipts which, in Morson's case, was for both personal and business purposes.

The earliest known figure covering Morson's retail and wholesale sales, but excluding some of the sales of chemicals, is £30,113 in 1878. It is likely that turnover had exceeded this ten years previously. The 1900 figures are the first that refer specifically to the inclusion of sales from Homerton. Prior to this, there are references to the accounts operated at three banks, Parr's, London and Counties and the Bank of England, but there are no figures.

The records of financial progress of the Morson firm are far from comprehensive. No attempt at keeping comprehensive annual accounts is discernible from such records as have survived. A firm that grew over a span of fifty years, always in one man's hands and comparatively small, perhaps does not need sophisticated record-keeping and financial controls especially when it was always quite profitable. There was no need to distinguish precisely between business and private expenditure. Using cash from the shop's till must have been the most convenient way of paying for a wide range of business and household expenses. There is no record of difficulty with taxation.

Morson first had an account at the Bank of England in 1841. The ledger records an initial deposit of £115. He was of sufficient reputation and financial standing to be accepted. The fear of bank failure and prestige when doing overseas business were doubtless major considerations in his decision.

The ledgers record virtually no detail of receipts, the great majority being recorded as transfers from other banks. Expenditure is recorded by name of creditor so a knowledge of the business conducted by these names had to be investigated.

While rent for 19 Southampton Row, recorded as a payment to 'Bedford' or 'Duke' is identifiable, some payments of duty, rates and taxes are not. Payments for coal (Charrington's) are recorded but not wages in the early years. The entries appear overwhelmingly to be for raw materials, supplies and building maintenance, but very few for equipment and none for substantial items of equipment. No travel, personal expenditure or school fees have been identified.

The only conclusion possible is that a second bank account was operated and that wages, household expenditure and minor business expenses were paid in cash from the till. This account may have been a joint one for T. N. R. Morson and his wife. Some of Morson's funds may then have been used to supplement Charlotte's income.

Substantial payments to traders in bark, opium, chemicals and to manufacturers of chemicals and solvents, like Bowerbank, appear in all years. There are, however, no figures of payments to indicate the true level of sales.

The total of receipts, year on year, is all that is available to indicate the size of the business. This figure must be treated cautiously, if some payments were credited to the Morsons' joint account. It is revealing that credits for cash deposited in the Bank of England account are few. In the early years the total of receipts varied, from £4,918 in 1841, and rose steadily: only rarely is one year's figure less than the preceding one.

As there is a crude correlation between receipts and the business cycles of the period, the best use of these figures is perhaps to indicate the growth of the business:

1841-45	48%
1845-50	35%
1850-55	24%
1855-60	31%
1860-65	39%
1865-70	12.5%
1870-75	12%

Receipts in this account had increased nearly six times in 35 years.

The smaller rate of growth between 1865 and 1875 is probably a reflection of the trade depression and of German competition. The importation of German chemicals grew rapidly at this time and affected profits on alkaloids particularly. By the turn of the century the small British maker could not compete, some like Joseph Ince deciding that this and other changes justified his decision to retire.

Another reason for the Morson firm's performance was undoubtedly the change of management. Brought up in very comfortable circumstances and entering the business when it was growing and profitable, Morson junior lacked the sharpness in business as well as the technical ability of his father – a not unusual circumstance. A serious blow was dealt when his French wife died in 1878. He lost some interest at this stage. His son took increasing control of the business even though only 26 years old. In any case the size and complexity of the business had grown and was no longer controllable in the old way. The coincidence of this date with the appearance of the earliest balance sheet is an indication of T. P. Morson's efforts to control and improve the business.

When T. N. R. Morson died, his estate was valued at £9,000 for probate purposes. While credit may be due to those who negotiated this figure, it is lower than would be expected of a business operating the pharmacy, warehouse at 31 & 33 Southampton Row and two factories, which were freehold. He owned two houses as well.

While there are some discrepancies in the early figures due perhaps to mistakes in recording and also in the use of cash received at the pharmacy to pay some bills directly, the first balance sheet was drawn up by Saffery (now the accountants Saffery Champness) in 1877 at the time that T. P. Morson became a partner. The sales figure is £29, 361 with a gross profit of 27% at £7,932.

A balance sheet for 1891 reveals sales of £53,000 and a profit of £9,300. The next extant one is for 1894 but for the wholesale business only. This excluded the retail business and some of the trading in chemicals conducted from Homerton. The fact that the sales figure is £52,000 suggests that the 1891 figure is wholesale only. By 1899 the sales were £54,500 with a gross profit of £8,500 and a net, one of £3,500 for the two partners to share.

At the start of the new century sales were increasing with those of 1908 at £57,000. The figures then increased steeply as the war approached and the firm extended its range of technical chemicals. The first balance sheet of the newly incorporated company shows sales of £115,000 and profits at £19,027. The 1915 figure was £221,000, an increase of 92%. The following year provided another 29% increase.

The Bank of England account was closed in 1918. A cash balance of £3,161 15s.5d. was transferred to the new company's account at the London County and Westminster Bank.

T. P. Morson's efforts to expand the business and reorganise its administration bore fruit. The decline in speciality chemical business and a greater reliance on volume products had the effect of reducing profitability. In 1920 a sharp reduction in sales occurred, an experience shared by similar companies operating in Britain.

May & Baker's figures[33] have been reported over a similar period and those for some years are available for Howards.[34] The latter's business was dominated by quinine from the 1840s onwards. It was not until then that their sales grew but they became virtually a one-product company, well over 50% of their sales coming from the salts of quinine. By 1850, yearly sales reached £80,000, probably the largest of the firms operating in London and perhaps in Britain. All the alkaloids apart from quinine appear to have been purchased, but the inorganics (bromides, iodides and citric acid) made up the balance of their turnover. Howards went on to become one of the most important quinine makers in the world and made a scientific contribution to the knowledge of cinchona which was second to none.

May & Baker started business in 1840 when Baker joined May at the beginning of a long spell of success in pharmaceutical trade due to an expanding economy, better products and distribution. In 1878, their turnover had reached £35,000 if we accept the use of the same ratio of turnover to profit that they attained for 1890, even though their profitability at 3% was well below Morson's at 19% on sales of £53,000. In the ten previous years Morson's figures show an average profit of 25% of sales. By 1900, Morson's profit was 14.35%

and M & B's, 10.06%. There was also a big difference in labour productivity: M & B were reported to have 100 employees and Morsons had not more than 55. With the dramatic expansion of sales preceding 1914, Morson's profit fell to 12.5% and M & B's to 4.8%. The turnover, however, rose to £221,000 and £715,000 respectively. Both firms went on expanding until 1921 when Morson's sales fell to £153,000 whereas M & B's fell only to £709,000. However, they incurred a trading loss of £10,000.

After this date, Morson's sales rose only a little and remained steady for many years, rising to £250,000 in 1940 and £376,000 in 1947 with profits at 15-18%. May& Baker were always less profitable but their sales reached £500,000 in the late 1920s.

While combinations and cartels were not unknown before, it was the intense competition of the last quarter of the nineteenth century which led to the formation of cooperative arrangements to maintain prices, share available business and exert pressures on the market. The largest of these was the quinine cartel[35] involving all the European firms, the German and Dutch manufacturers leading the way. The cartel was formally organised in 1893 and succeeded in regulating the production level of its members and to a large extent the price of cinchona bark. These arrangements had a disastrous effect on American producers when their protective tariff was removed. Morsons were not involved though Whiffens and Burbidges were active as well as Howards. In the year the cartel formed, Howards agreed to limit their production to 20,000 kgs and to purchase up to 3,000 kgs from the Germans, who had a production level of 160,000 kgs allocated to them.

Whiffens, Howards and Morsons were the leaders of the Iodine Preparations Combination, which had collapsed in 1880 but was revived in December 1888 and was active until the early 1950s. The original members were German, French and British firms. Böhringer, Schering and Gehe were the German contingent, with all of whom Morson's traded, and Kahlbaum of Berlin. From Paris came Origet and Destreicher. Whiffens, Howards and Morson joined together with the North British Chemical Company of Glasgow.

The Chilean Iodine Corporation was granted a monopoly by its Government and made agreements with other iodine producers in Scotland, Spain, France, Japan and Java. It guaranteed that it would not undersell these smaller producers. The I.P.C. gave its members a 5% discount and all members agreed not to buy iodine from anyone else nor to purchase iodine products that were not made from Chilean iodine. There were thirteen members in 1943, the leading ones being Boots, May & Baker, Morsons, Howards and Whiffens. Others included firms, or their successors, which had been in the van of inorganic chemical production, like Southalls and Burgoyne Burbidges who had absorbed White and Co.

Cost comparisons were made between manufacturers, much time being spent on discussion of yields and refinements to costings so as to make better comparisons. Companies used these sessions to reveal only what they had to and to obtain as much information about costs and customers as they could. Output levels were monitored and on one occasion, even during the 1939-45 war, Morson's plant was closed down for nine months because they had exceeded their quota. The combination was managed by a firm of auditors in Glasgow, who arranged all the meetings and collated figures for the members to consider. Some of the payments by Morson's to the cartel were quite large sums for the time. In 1916, they paid £2,000 – about 2% of the cost of purchases.

There was a similar arrangement about bromine and, in 1903, a Mercurial Preparations Convention was set up. It included Howards, Tyrer, George Atkinson, a subsidiary of Whiffens, Davy Hill & Co., May & Baker but not Morsons. The auditors were Price, Waterhouse who acted as arbitrators. The Bismuth Convention was run on similar lines, with the monopoly supplier, Mining and Chemical Products, joining up with the Bismuth Salt Makers Convention.

Further allocations of business and coordination of prices were made by a Buying Convention which regulated trade, especially for very large buyers, like Boots.

Such cartels certainly had the effect of maintaining prices, protecting the less efficient and making greater profits for the lowest-cost manufacturers. Payments were significant but not large. Morson's 1917 receipts from the Buying Committee were £300, the members being Howards, May & Baker and Hopkin & Williams at that time.

In spite of the efforts to protect business and to promote joint ventures, the performance was disappointing. The reliance on an existing range of well-established products and the expectation that a wide range of personal contacts would produce new business, in fact produced only a marginal increase in turnover. This negative strategy ignored the great technical changes which had started to influence the industry in the 1880s, especially in Germany.

Apart from chemical modifications of substances, like morphine into codeine which Morson had been operating since the late 1830s, and similar operations which were well established, the British fine chemical industry was doing virtually no chemical synthesis. The period before 1914 saw progress in the production of sera and vaccines but the majority of synthetic medicines were imported from Germany. It would have been a disappointment to T. N. R. Morson's generation of pharmacist entrepreneurs that the 1898 *Pharmacopoeia* included monographs for only four synthetic substances; by the 1914 edition this had increased to eighty but almost all were imported.

The fine chemical industry being a small one, the principals and board members, in an age of family firms, all knew one another. Business was conducted on a personal basis with customers, suppliers and employees; for the latter paternalism was the style of the time, because the firms had started from small beginnings. The welfare of the workforce was always an interest of the partners. Morson's in the 1930s did not sack anyone, diverting process labour to maintenance work, with wages reduced generally. The employee preferred this to the dole.

Visits to customers were an important part of a principal's duties. T. P. Morson made at least one visit a year to all important customers, those of long standing being entertained, sometimes with spouses included.

These visits kept everyone in touch with trade and were an opportunity to discuss changes. They dealt with the broader questions of volume, foreign and domestic competition, discounts and payment terms. Order-taking and routine complaints were handled by representatives, who were sometimes on a commission based on turnover. The country was divided into only two or three areas for representatives to cover.

The accent was on product quality and service, some customers relying completely on Morsons for all their chemical and bulk pharmaceutical needs. Thus, they saved the overheads in their purchasing section and Morsons gained sales volume. Even small requests for an isolated need were met. The consequence was a tendency for manufactured items to be made long after their volume had fallen below a profitable level. Another was the importance of ensuring that Morsons purchased many items at price levels which allowed for repackaging costs and profit.

Major purchases were closely supervised and sometimes conducted by a partner. This was always the case for imported supplies, whether in pure form like quinine or crude drugs such as scammony or liquorice. Partners attended the auctions on the exchange which were easily made into opportunities for business and social contact. This tended to become a cosy world somewhat insulated from both business developments and technical progress. Most of the proprietors of such firms were either descendants of founders or had very long associations with their firm. They were also past middle age in the 1930s. It appears from both their performance and the comments made in the 1960s by near-contemporaries still living, that there was an air of complacency.

The reliability of quality and service was paramount and included careful attention to the detail of packaging. The packaging department, staffed exclusively by women, was kept to a high standard of order and cleanliness. Export orders provided a large addition to sales and were frequently of greater total value than sales in the U.K. Orders were sought by local agents and tenders were submitted to the India Office and Crown Agents for the Colonies. Such was the importance of this trade that a shipping manager was employed exclusively for it.

The packaging department might be involved in runs of more than 1,000 bottles or vials, each one filled, labelled and finished (an important operation reflecting house style and using quality paper, or later cellophane, wrap) entirely by hand. In such ways, reputation was jealously guarded.

The financial management was conservative and the methods traditional. Broader questions were discussed with the bank manager and, very occasionally, with a professional accountant. While the partners knew every detail of the business and tended to run it as it had always been run, they were good at reacting to sales opportunities. However, their knowledge of business management was not extensive and longer-term strategies were rarely discussed.

Morson's seem to have been representative of the industry. There was a failure to search for and exploit scientific innovation. It is not surprising, therefore, that there were so many worries about pharmaceutical and fine chemical supplies in the years before 1914, with the reaction after the war that the industry needed protection. These measures, however, produced a patchy response from firms and the inter-war years did not see an improved performance. The cause cannot have been profit margins which remained satisfactory, but volumes were low. It was innovation that was lacking amid generally depressed trade.

In the years following the end of the Second World War, T. D. Morson reached the age of 70 and had suffered several heart attacks. He could no longer direct a new course for the business.

Firms of similar origins, like Howards and Hanburys, had grown faster with a more modern product line. Even so, the upheavals of the 1950s resulted in a widespread reorganisation of the industry and all the firms founded by pharmacist entrepreneurs in the nineteenth century were absorbed into larger ones seeking to diversify or to acquire skills and facilities for the expansion of their trade, often based on the need to exploit their research efforts.

In America, Merck and Co., originally an off-shoot set up in 1891 by the famous firm of E. Merck of Darmstadt, which had been founded in 1827, had had notable successes. After sequestration of the stock in 1917, an auction was held in 1919 at which George Merck bought back control of his firm.

In 1953, Merck joined up with Sharp & Dohme of Philadelphia, for whom Morson's made several products between 1946 and 1956. The formation by Merck of the Merck Sharp and Dohme International Division led to a steady expansion of their overseas operations, exploiting their introduction of new substances. They decided to set up chemical manufacture in support of their pharmaceutical operations in major markets. Thus it was that an approach was made to Morson's resulting in purchase in 1957. This enabled production of the new products derived from their research to start quickly in England.

Morson's facilities and processing expertise were used to supply MSDI subsidiaries in various countries, especially Commonwealth ones.

An initial investment of £500,000 was made to reorganise and re-equip the Ponders End factory, which quickly produced chlorothiazide and hydrochlorothiazide, both of them new diuretics, soon followed by methyl-dopa, an antihypertensive, and Indomethacin, an anti-rheumatic, both original products. Thus the firm was to continue in a new guise the purpose for which it had been created 136 years before.

Notes

1. Private archive; cash book, 1868–71; ledger, 1875–8.
2. Greater London Library; *Minutes of Metropolitan Board of Works, 1869.*
3. Personal archive; John Stevens' Wages Book, Homerton, 1878–1904.
4. Deed of Apprenticeship Thomas Pierre Morson, 1867.
5. *British and Colonial Druggist*, 1910; Supplement: 'Who's Who in the Drug Trade'.

6.   *Chemical News*, 11 October 1867.
7.   Royal College of Surgeons of England; Mss. Add.350 (Lister Cabinet). Copies of these letters were provided by the College librarian, whose help is gratefully acknowledged.
8.   *Proc. Royal Society of Medicine*, Vol. 64, No. 10, October 1971, 1060-3.
9.   *The Chemists and Druggists Year-Book for Scotland*, 1925.
10. *Pharmaceutical Journal*, 10, 2nd series, 1868-9, 390. Morson was in the chair for this meeting held at the time that Martindale went to U. C. H. as Dispenser after several years with T. Morson & Son.
11. Archives of MacFarlan Smith, Edinburgh.
12. *Ibid.*.
13. Martindale, William (1809–1902); F.C.S., F.L.S. President Pharmaceutical Society, 1890; worked for T. N. R. Morson 1864–8; Dispenser, University College Hospital, 1868–73. Took over the retail side of Hopkin & Williams, 1873. Paper on carbolic acid plaster, 1868. Famous for the *Extra Pharmacopoeia* which was published in numerous editions from 1883.
14. Antiseptic Dressing factory, Ladywell, London SW (proprietor: Galen Manufacturing Co. Ltd).
15. *Op.cit.*, note 11 above letters, Alex Macdonald of 66 Southwood Lane, Highgate N6. to Mr A. S. Birnie, J. F. MacFarlan's London Manager, April and May 1927.
16. *Ibid.*
17. Bishop, W. J., *A History of Surgical Dressings*, Robinson & Sons of Chesterfield, 1959.
18. *British Medical Journal*, II (1884), 803.
19. *Pharmaceutical Journal*, 118, 4th series, Vol. 64, 1927, 616.
20. Fisher, Richard B., *Joseph Lister 1827–1912*, London: Macdonald & Jane, 1977.
21. *Chemist & Druggist*, 106, 21 May 1927, 628.
22. Personal archive; Homerton factory memoranda and notes, August 1889.
23. *Pharmaceutical Journal*, 3, 3rd series, 1872-3, 41. The Journal of the Chemical Society reported in 1892 that the doublecyanide was not a combination but a peculiar structure represented by the formula $Zn_4 Hg (CN)_{10}$, "thus it is a tetra-zincic mono mereuric decacyanide."
24. *Op. cit.*, note 7 above; letter, W. H. Perkin to Robert Taubman, dated 20 August 1890.
25. *Op. cit.*, note 11 above; MacFarlan to Galen Manufacturing Co. Ltd, 4 January 1901.

26. *Op. cit.*, note 7 above; Lister letters, 1907. Lister found that sulphate of chromium was more satisfactory than tannic acid for "producing a thread fulfilling all the conditions requisite for the ligature of arteries" except its weak antiseptic property which was obviated by using corrosive sublimate as a germicide. Wellcome Institute MS 6975, item 11/2.

27. *Op. cit.*, note 11 above; Macdonald's notes for Birnie, 1927.

28. *Op. cit.*, note 7 above; catgut treatment method, 1894.

29. *British Medical Journal*, 1 (1908), 125.

30. *The Enfield Gazette and Observer*, 23 November 1928.

31. Porter, Roy, 'Manufacturing Drugs in the Early Consumer Society: The case of Corbyns', *Pharmaceutical Historian*, Vol. 20, No. 2, 5.

32. *Chemist & Druggist*, 85, 5 September 1914, 370.

33. Slinn, Judy, *May & Baker, a history, 1834–1984*, Cambridge: Hobsons Ltd, 1985.

34. Slater, A. W., *Howards, 1797–1837, A Study in Business History*, London University Ph.D. thesis, 1951. (Howard's house publication, 1797–1947.)

35. Royal Pharmaceutical Society – Howard archive (not catalogued).

Appendices

Chapter 6: Attendance at T. N. R. Morson's Reception, June 1848.

1. Fellows of the Royal Society

Rev. J. **BARLOW** 1799–1869.
Secretary, Royal Institution, 1842–1860.

Thomas **BELL** ,1792–1880.
President, Linean Society, 1853–1861;
Dental Surgeon, Guy's Hospital, 1817–1861;
Professor of Zoology, King's College, 1836–1869;
President, Ray Society, 1843–1859; Secretary, Royal Society,
1848–1853. Reporter of Chemical Jury, 1851 Exhibition.

John J. **BENNETT**, 1801–1876.
Keeper, Department of Botany, British Museum, 1858–1870;
Secretary, Linnean Society, 1838–1852

Dr Golding **BIRD**, 1814–1854.
Physician, Guy's Hospital; Professor of Materia Medica,
Guy's Hospital;Paper on Urinary Deposits, 1846;
Guy's Hospital Reports, 1840; Chemical Nature of Mucous and
Purulent Secretions. London Medical Gazette, 1833–1835:
Essays on chemical pathology and clinical medicine.

W. T. **BRANDE**, 1788–1866.
Professor of Chemistry, Society of Apothecaries, 1812;
Professor of Chemistry, Royal Institution, 1813–1834;
Secretary, Royal Society, 1816–1826.

Robert **BROWN**, 1773–1858.
President, Linnean Society, 1849–1853;
Keeper of Banksian Collection, British Museum,
1827–1858; discoverer of Brownian Movement.

Antoine **CLAUDET**, 1797–1867.
Came to London in 1829 to open a glass warehouse;
photographer, Adelaide Gallery 1840–1851; Photographer in
Ordinary to Queen Victoria, 1858; publications:
Royal Society; Society of Arts, 1841–1867.

Dr John **ELLIOTSON**, 1786–1868.
Professor of Medicine, London University, 1832;
first President, Royal Medical & Chirurgical Society of London, 1834.

Thomas **GRAHAM**, 1805– 1869
Professor, Andersonian University, 1830; Professor of Chemistry,
London University, 1837;
Master of the Mint, 1855; reporter, Chemical & Pharmaceutical
Products, 1851 Exhibition.

John E. **GRAY**, 1800–1875.
Keeper, Zoological Department British Museum, 1846–1874;
President, Botanical Society of London, 1844–1851;
married M.E. Gray, conchologist.

Daniel **HANBURY**, 1825–1875.
Son of Daniel Bell Hanbury; *Pharmacographia* with Professor Flückiger,
1874; many contributions to Linnean Society and Pharmaceutical Society.

Luke **HOWARD**, 1772–1854.
Founder of the firm, 1793.

H. **BENCE JONES**, 1813–1873.
Pupil of Graham and Liebig; practised medicine in London,
1846–1862; biography of his friend Faraday, 1870; Honorary Secretary,
R. I., 1860–1872.

Jonathan D. **PEREIRA**, 1804–1853.
A member of many scientific societies; corresponded with the most
famous scientist in all countries.
A major contributor to pharmaceutical reform and lobbyist for the
Pharmaceutical Society with his profession.

Lyon **PLAYFAIR**, 1818–1898.
Studied under Graham, University College, London, 1839–1840;
Professor of Chemistry, School of Mines, London, 1847–1849;
Professor of Chemistry, Edinburgh, 1858–1868; General Postmaster,
1873–1874; M.P. Edinburgh University, 1868–1885;
M.P. for South Leeds, 1885–1892;
Member, Executive Committee, 1851 Exhibition.

Richard H. **SOLLY**, 1778–1858.
Barrister; helped formation of Royal Horticultural Society and
Geological Society;
philanthropist to scientific societies; M.A. 1800; an original promoter
of the Royal Institution; F.L.S. 1826.

Andrew URE, 1778–1857.
M.A. and M.D. Glasgow, 1801; Professor of Chemistry and Natural Philosophy, Andersonian University, 1822; analytical and commercial chemist, London 1830; Analyst to the Board of Customs, 1834.

Nathaniel WALLICH, 1786–1854.
Danish surgeon; Superintendent, Calcutta Botanical Garden; lived in London, contributing his knowledge of East Indian plants; Juror, Vegetable and Animal substances, 1851 Exhibition.

2. Council Members, Pharmaceutical Society, 1848 and later

Messrs Allchin, Bastick, Bell, Davenport, Deane, Dickson, Edwards, Ellis, Garden, Garle,Greenish, Hills, Huxtable, MacFarlan, Meggeson, Palk, Sandford, Savory, Squire, Stone, Waugh, Yarde.

3. Famous Pharmacists/ Chemists

Alfred BIRD, custard powder.

John ROSSITER, founder, British Association of Chemists & Druggists, which folded at its first meeting.

Edward HORNER, original member, drug broker.

Thomas SCOTT,
wholesale druggist, City; witness to Charlotte's wedding,1845.

W. HUSKISSON, manufacture of iodides.

John ELLIS, original committee member.

J. PRESTON, wholesaler

W. JACKSON, auditor, 1848.

W. K. HOPKIN, later founder of Hopkin & Williams.

W. HUDSON, original member.

James BELL, brother of Jacob.

John WILLIAMS, Later President, P. S. G. B., then living at 19 Southampton Row.

B. ORRIDGE, pharmaceutical agent and valuer.

R. STAMPER, original member.

B. HUMPAGE, chemistis agent and valuer.

W. J. BAKER, May & Baker.

C. **MAY**, pharmacist, Plymouth.

W.A.**BAISS**, wholesaler.

4. Medical Men

S. Scott **ALISON**, M.D., M.R.C.S. Edinburgh.

William **HUXTABLE**, M.R.C.S.

J. **PIDDUCK**, F.R.C.P., Bloomsbury dispensary.

John **SNOW**, L.S.A., L.R.C.P., M.R.C.S., 1813–58
    famous for, inter alia, his epidemiological study of cholera in Soho.

Joseph **WILLIAMS**, M.D., M.R.C.S., L.S.A.,
    studied the effects of narcotics in insanity; succeeded Elliotson at
    University College in 1858 as Professor of Medicine.

Robert **WOLLASTON**, F.R.C.S., M.R.C.P., 1801– 65,
    attached to the Scutari hospital in Crimean War; London Hospital and
    Guy's Hospital appointments.

Dr **NORMANDY**, physician;
    author of *A Commercial Handbook of Chemical Analysis*, London:
    George Knight, 1850.

5. Friends in Arts and Sciences

J. **TENNANT**, geologist.

Robert **BENTLEY**, F.L.S., Professor of Botany, King's and P.S.G.B.

Henry J. **JOHNSON**, artist

John **CHURCHILL**, publisher of Pharmaceutical Journal.

Thomas **BAGNOLD**, Captain, Royal Marines;
    inventor and prominent in Society of Arts; died October 1848.

Thomas **LOTT**, F.R.S.A. lawyer.

John Winter **JONES**, Principal Librarian, British Museum, 1866–78.

TOTAL NUMBER OF SIGNATURES: **258**

Chapter 6: T. N. R. Morson's Technical Papers

1. *London Medical Repository*, Vol. XVI, 1821, 447–9; A new Preparation of Bark.
2. *Journal de Pharmacie*, Vol. VII, 1821, 587; Sur les Sophistications de l'extraite de Quinquina.
3. *Poggend. Annal.*, XLII, 1837, 175–6; Darstellung des Aconitin.
4. *Pharmaceutical Journal*, 1 (1841), 14–23; Sketch of the Rise and Progress of Pharmacy.
5. *Pharmaceutical Journal*, 1 (1841–42), 91–2; On a sample of spurious opium.
6. *Pharmaceutical Journal*, 1 (1842), 49–54; On vegetable extracts.
7. *Pharmaceutical Journal*, 2 (1842–43), 355; On the solubility of lead in all water containing free carbonic acid.
8. *Pharmaceutical Journal*, 3 (1844), 424; On Pattinson's process for obtaining magnesia from magnesian limestone.
   See also *P.J.*, 3 (1844), 428 *et seq* (Fownes).
9. *Pharmaceutical Journal*, 3 (1844), 471–8; Observations on certain plants of the genus Piper.
10. *Pharmaceutical Journal*, 4 (1844–5), 503; On a new variety of opium.
11. *Pharmaceutical Journal*, 5 (1845–6); Dragées Minerales.
12. *Pharmaceutical Journal*, 8 (1848–9); On the Decomposition of Chloroform.
13. *Pharmaceutical Journal*, 9 (1848–9), 337, 361, 483, 549; Adulteration of Morphine.
14. *Pharmaceutical Journal*, 13 (1853–4), 331; Substitution of Magnetic Oxide of Iron for Iron in the Metallic State (Quevenne's iron).
15. *Journal de Pharmacie*, Vol. 29, 3rd series, 1856, 216; Sur l'Oxyde de Zinc.
16. *Journal de Pharmacie*, Vol. 35, 3rd series, 1859, 48–9; Observations sur la Nouvelle Résin de Scammonée.
17. *Pharmaceutical Journal*, 2, 3rd series, 1871–2, 921; Substitution of Carbolic or Phenic Acid for Creosote.

Index

293

Printed in the United States
By Bookmasters